# Current Developments in Stroke

## *(Volume 1)*

### *(New Concepts in Stroke Diagnosis and Therapy)*

## Edited by

### Alberto Radaelli

*Division of Cardiac Rehabilitation,*
*San Gerardo Hospital, Monza, Italy*

### Giuseppe Mancia

*University of Milano-Bicocca and IRCCS*
*Istituto Auxologico Italiano, Milan, Italy*

### Carlo Ferrarese

*Department of Neurology, San Gerardo Hospital,*
*University of Milano Bicocca, Monza, Italy*

## &

### Simone Beretta

*Milan Center for Neuroscience (NeuroMi),*
*Milan, Italy*

advertisements or ideas contained in the Work.

## *Limitation of Liability:*

In no event will Bentham Science Publishers, its staff, editors and/or authors, be liable for any damages, including, without limitation, special, incidental and/or consequential damages and/or damages for lost data and/or profits arising out of (whether directly or indirectly) the use or inability to use the Work. The entire liability of Bentham Science Publishers shall be limited to the amount actually paid by you for the Work.

## General:

1. Any dispute or claim arising out of or in connection with this License Agreement or the Work (including non-contractual disputes or claims) will be governed by and construed in accordance with the laws of the U.A.E. as applied in the Emirate of Dubai. Each party agrees that the courts of the Emirate of Dubai shall have exclusive jurisdiction to settle any dispute or claim arising out of or in connection with this License Agreement or the Work (including non-contractual disputes or claims).
2. Your rights under this License Agreement will automatically terminate without notice and without the need for a court order if at any point you breach any terms of this License Agreement. In no event will any delay or failure by Bentham Science Publishers in enforcing your compliance with this License Agreement constitute a waiver of any of its rights.
3. You acknowledge that you have read this License Agreement, and agree to be bound by its terms and conditions. To the extent that any other terms and conditions presented on any website of Bentham Science Publishers conflict with, or are inconsistent with, the terms and conditions set out in this License Agreement, you acknowledge that the terms and conditions set out in this License Agreement shall prevail.

**Bentham Science Publishers Ltd.**
Executive Suite Y - 2
PO Box 7917, Saif Zone
Sharjah, U.A.E.
Email: subscriptions@benthamscience.org

**BENTHAM
SCIENCE**

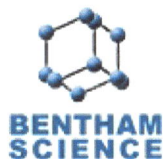

# CONTENTS

# Foreword

Stroke is likely the neurological disease with the most relevant developments in all the research fields, from knowledge of the mechanisms leading to brain tissue death to codification of rehabilitation mainstays, through better definition of risk factors and consequent improvement of primary and secondary prevention, diagnosis with advanced imaging or by identification of genetic mechanisms in rare cases, treatments of the acute phase of ischemic events, with the well-established role of i.v. thrombolysis now backed up by combined endovascular treatments and with the potentialities of neuroprotection and neuroregeneration, or of iatrogenic hemorrhagic stroke, with the advent of antidotes for the new generation of direct oral anticoagulants.

As a consequence, a terribly huge literature on stroke has been produced: by typing the word "stroke" one may find approximately 140000 papers indexed in PubMed in the last 20 years. Hence, a book summarizing all the "new concepts in stroke diagnosis and therapy" is highly appreciated. The Authors report the present knowledge on all the above mentioned issue, with updated and well selected reference literature. The book can be a good "traveling companion" for neurologists working daily on stroke patient management and having little time to look for scientific literature, but also a guide for stroke basic and clinical researchers to pick up the most recent information and to get suggestions for further research.

My compliments to the Authors and "enjoy the reading" to all the readers.

**Prof. Danilo Toni, MD**
Associate Professor of Neurology
Director Emergency Department Stroke Unit
Hospital Policlinico Umberto I
Dept. of Neurology and Psychiatry, Sapienza Univerisity
00185 Roma, Italy

# Preface 1

Stroke prevention, diagnosis and therapy are all evolving fields that give us the idea of how in progress is the clinical job and the scientific work. Stroke in particular deserves a special mention as it is perceived both by patients and by physicians and it is one of the most feared and invalidating condition.

In this regard, every single step able to improve prevention, accelerate diagnosis and therapy is welcome and need to be rapidly shared with all the scientific community.

On the one hand, despite the stabilization of stroke events in civilized countries other emerging countries contribute to new events so keeping a high prevalence of stroke worldwide. In this regard, stroke prevention still represents one of the missing opportunities and the recognition and treatment of old and new risk factors are mandatory. On the other hand, imaging and therefore diagnosis and therapeutic opportunities are now available to treat faster than ever ischemic events in order to reduce overall cerebral damage and therefore disability. These new possibilities nevertheless should not remain restricted to few golden clinical and scientific realities but be rapidly shared and diffused to the emerging countries where the prevalence of stroke is growing.

This book aims to be an aid to the diffusion and discussion of what is new in the field and what are some of the new directions of prevention, diagnosis and therapy. At least, eighty five per cent of strokes are of ischemic origin and are therefore the results of a missed prevention in vascular atherosclerosis and thrombosis. This has always been a "cardiology" field. It is evident that a tighter cooperation between cardiologists and neurologists is needed in order to share expertise and to create more powerful tools to improve prevention, diagnosis and therapy of vascular events that involve in a similar dramatic way both the heart and the brain.

***Dr. Alberto Radaelli***
Director of the Division of Cardiac Rehabilitation,
San Gerardo Hospital,
Monza,
Italy

# Preface 2

Only few decades ago stroke was considered a devastating condition with high mortality, high disability, without adequate prevention strategies, any tool to perform accurate diagnosis and consequently without any effective treatment available.

Scientific and technological advances in the last few years have dramatically changed the scenario: epidemiologic, genetic, imaging, biological and therapeutic advances have made it possible to effectively prevent strokes, to perform accurate differential diagnosis of stroke type and of location of vessel occlusion and new treatments for acute phase have recently demonstrated dramatic results.

In the context of this new scenario, new concepts for stroke diagnosis and therapy emerged, and this book specifically addresses this point.

Major experts and opinion leaders in respective fields extensively review and discuss new advances in the knowledge of the role of stroke risk factor for their prevention; new technological tools to perform *in vivo* imaging of cerebral collateral circulation and ischemic penumbra are widely described and their relevance for more accurate diagnosis and prognosis is discussed.

Diagnostic challenges in rare aethiologies of stroke are described in detail and new studies on recanalization and neuroprotection strategies are reported, with analysis of their impact on stroke health organization.

Finally, the hemorrhagic risk associated to older and new anticoagulants is discussed and new studies on stroke recovery are presented.

The reader of this new book may obtain a state-of-the-art knowledge of stroke diagnosis and treatment options to address the challenges of this severe, but now treatable disease.

*Dr. Carlo Ferrarese,*
Professor of Neurology. Director of the Department of Neurology,
San Gerardo Hospital,
University of Milano Bicocca,
Monza,
Italy

# List of Contributors

| | |
|---|---|
| **Antonio Coca** | Hypertension and Vascular Risk Unit. Department of Internal Medicine, Institute of Medicine and Dermatology, Hospital Clinic (IDIBAPS), University of Barcelona, Barcelona, Spain |
| **Alberto Radaelli** | Division of Cardiac Rehabilitation, San Gerardo Hospital, Monza, Italy |
| **Alessandro Versace** | Laboratory of Experimental Stroke Research, School of Medicine, University of Milano Bicocca, Monza, Italy |
| **Anna Bersano** | Cerebrovascular Unit, IRCCS Foundation Neurological Institute "C. Besta", Via Celoria 11, Milan 20133, Italy |
| **Antonio Vincenti** | Electrophysiology Unit, Multimedica IRCCS Sesto San Giovanni, Milan, Italy |
| **Barbara Casolla** | NESMOS (Neuroscience Mental Healt and Sensory Organs) Department, School of Medicine and Psychology, Sapienza University, Rome, Italy |
| **Carlo Ferrarese** | Department of Neurology, Director of the Department of Neurology, San Gerardo Hospital, University of Milano Bicocca, Monza, Italy |
| **Carole Frindel** | Université de Lyon, CREATIS, CNRS UMR5220, Inserm U1206, INSA-Lyon, Université Claude Bernard Lyon 1, France |
| **Cristina Sierra** | Hypertension and Vascular Risk Unit. Department of Internal Medicine, Institute of Medicine and Dermatology, Hospital Clinic (IDIBAPS), University of Barcelona, Barcelona, Spain, |
| **David Carone** | Laboratory of Experimental Stroke Researc, School of Medicine, University of Milano-Bicocca, Monza, Italy<br>Milan Center for Neuroscience (NeuroMi), Milan, Italy |
| **David Rousseau** | Université de Lyon, CREATIS, CNRS UMR5220, Inserm U1206, INSA-Lyon, Université Claude Bernard Lyon 1, France |
| **Elio Clemente Agostoni** | Department of Neuroscience, Neurology and Stroke Unit of the ASST: "Grande Ospedale Metropolitano Niguarda", Milan, Italy |
| **Elisa Cuccione** | Laboratory of Experimental Stroke Research, School of Medicine, University of Milano Bicocca, Monza, Italy |
| **Fausto De Angeli** | Laboratory of Experimental Stroke Research, School of Medicine, University of Milano Bicocca, Monza, Italy |
| **Francesco Orzi** | NESMOS (Neuroscience Mental Health and Sensory Organs) Department, School of Medicine and Psichology, Sapienza University, Rome, Italy |
| **Francesca Maria Salmeri** | Department of Biomedical, Dental Sciences and Morphological and Functional Images, University of Messina, Messina, Italy |

| | |
|---|---|
| **Giuseppe Mancia** | University of Milano-Bicocca and IRCCS Istituto Auxologico Italiano, Milan, Italy |
| **Gianvito Martino** | Institute of Experimental Neurology, Division of Neuroscience, San Raffaele Scientific Institute, *Via* Olgettina 58, 20132 Milan, Italy |
| **Giada Padovano** | Laboratory of Experimental Stroke Research, School of Medicine, University of Milano Bicocca, Monza, Italy |
| **Gianluca Luigi Russo** | Institute of Experimental Neurology, Division of Neuroscience, San Raffaele Scientific Institute, Via Olgettina 58, 20132 Milan, Italy |
| **Giuliano Sette** | NESMOS (Neuroscience Mental Healt and Sensory Organs) Department, School of Medicine and Psichology, Sapienza University, Rome, Italy |
| **Giulia Soraci** | University of "La Cattolica Sacro Cuore", Rome, Italy |
| **Leandro Provinciali** | Department of Experimental and Clinical Medicine, Neurological Section, Marche Polytechnic University, Ancona, Italy |
| **Leslie Wenning** | Department of Physiology, Pharmacology and Neuroscience, The City University of New York School of Medicine, The Sophie Davis School of Biomedical Education, The City College of New York, New York, NY USA; Department of Anesthesiology, NYU Langone Medical Center, New York, NY, USA |
| **Luca Soraci** | Department of Biomedical, Dental Sciences and Morphological and Functional Images, University of Messina, Messina, Italy |
| **Marco Longoni** | Department of Neuroscience, Neurology and Stroke Unit of the ASST: "Grande Ospedale Metropolitano Niguarda", Milan, Italy |
| **Maria Elas Gambuzza** | Ministry of Health, Messina, Italy |
| **Marco Bacigaluppi** | Neuroimmunology Unit, Institute of Experimental Neurology, Division of Neuroscience, San Raffaele Scientific Institute, Via Olgettina 58, 20132 Milan, Italy |
| **Mathilde Giacalone** | Université de Lyon, CREATIS, CNRS UMR5220, Inserm U1206, INSA-Lyon, Université Claude Bernard Lyon 1, France |
| **Michela Coccia** | Department of Experimental and Clinical Medicine, Neurological Section, Marche Polytechnic University, Ancona, Italy |
| **Michela Ranieri** | Cerebrovascular Unit, IRCCS Foundation Neurological Institute "C. Besta", Via Celoria 11, Milan 20133, Italy |
| **Monica Carpenedo** | Hematology and Transplant Unit, San Gerardo Hospital, Monza, Italy |
| **Norbert Nighoghossian** | Université de Lyon, CREATIS, CNRS UMR5220, Inserm U1206, INSA-Lyon;Université Claude Bernard Lyon 1, France |

| Patricia Ann Broderick | Department of Physiology, Pharmacology and Neuroscienc, The City University of New York School of Medicine, The Sophie Davis Program in Biomedical Education, The City College of New York, New York, NY, USA<br>Department of Biology, CUNY Grad. Ctr., New York, NY, USA<br>Department of Neurology, NYU Langone Medical Center and Comprehensive Epilepsy Center, New York, NY, USA |
|---|---|
| Paolo Castiglioni | IRCCS Fondazione Don Carlo Gnocchi, Milan, Italy |
| Paolo La Spina | Department of Clinical and Experimental Medicine, University of Messina, Messina, Italy |
| Robin Zagala | Université de Lyon, CREATIS, CNRS UMR5220, Inserm U1206, INSA-Lyon, Université Claude Bernard Lyon 1, France |
| Simone Beretta | Laboratory of Experimental Stroke Research, School of Medicine, University of Milano Bicocca, Monza, Italy |
| Serena Candela | NESMOS (Neuroscience Mental Health and Sensory Organs) Department, School of Medicine and Psichology, Sapienza University, Rome, Italy |
| Tae-Hee Cho | Université de Lyon, CREATIS, CNRS UMR5220, Inserm U1206, INSA-Lyon, Université Claude Bernard Lyon 1, France |
| Vincenza Sofo | Department of Biomedical, Dental Sciences and Morphological and Functional Images, University of Messina, Messina, Italy |
| Yves Berthezène | Université de Lyon, CREATIS, CNRS UMR5220, Inserm U1206, INSA-Lyon, Université Claude Bernard Lyon 1, France |
| Yong-Sheng Li | Department of Physiology, Pharmacology and Neuroscienc, The City University of New York School of Medicine, The Sophie Davis Program in Biomedical Education, The City College of New York, New York, NY, USA<br>Department of Anesthesiology, NYU Langone Medical Center, New York, NY, USA |

# Current Developments in Stroke

2

# Current Developments in Stroke

*Volume # 1*

**New Concepts in Stroke Diagnosis and Therapy**

Editors: Alberto Radaelli, Giuseppe Mancia, Carlo Ferrarese & Simone Beretta

eISSN (Online): 2542-5129

ISSN (Print): 2542-5110

eISBN (Online): 978-1-68108-421-3

ISBN (Print): 978-1-68108-422-0

# Stroke and Hypertension

**Cristina Sierra** and **Antonio Coca**\*

*Hypertension and Vascular Risk Unit. Department of Internal Medicine, Hospital Clinic (IDIBAPS), University of Barcelona, Barcelona, Spain*

**Abstract:** Stroke, the third most-common cause of mortality after cancer and heart disease in developed countries, is one of the most common causes of cognitive impairment and vascular dementia. Stroke pathogenesis and its consequences are not completely elucidated, with various factors and biological mechanisms probably having a role. After age, hypertension is the leading modifiable cardiovascular risk factor for ischaemic/haemorrhagic stroke, small vessel disease predisposing to lacunar infarction, cerebral white matter lesions (cWML), and cerebral microbleeds. Primary stroke prevention, involving hypertension therapy and blood pressure (BP) control is now standard. At the same time, elevated post-stroke BP levels increase the risk of recurrent stroke, with recent trials suggesting that BP reduction with combinations of hypertension therapy reduces stroke recurrence. This chapter reviews the evidence on hypertension as a stroke risk factor and the part played by hypertension therapy in first/recurrent stroke prevention.

**Keywords:** Cerebral microbleeds, Cerebral small vessel disease, Cognitive impairment, Hemorrhagic stroke, Hypertension, Hypertension therapy, Ischemic stroke, Lacunar infarction, Recurrent stroke, Vascular dementia, White matter lesions.

## INTRODUCTION

Stroke, the third most-frequent cause of death after cancer and heart disease in developed countries, is one of the most common causes of cognitive impairment and vascular dementia [1]. Stroke entails high economic and public health

---

\* **Corresponding author Antonio Coca:** Hypertension and Vascular Risk Unit, Hospital Clinic., Villarroel 170, Barcelona 08036, Spain, Tel: + 34 932275759, E-mail: acoca@clinic.ub.es

**Alberto Radaelli, Giuseppe Mancia, Carlo Ferrarese & Simone Beretta (Eds.)**

impacts. Age is the first all-stroke risk factor [1]. The stroke rate doubles each 10 years in both males and females > 55 years of age, with > 80% of strokes occurring in persons aged ≥ 65 years. Due to the aging population, the burden of stroke will rise substantially in forthcoming years. Elderly people's increased vulnerability to stroke is related to changes in the aging brain and with a higher prevalence of established stroke risk factors, including hypertension (HT), atrial fibrillation, carotid stenosis and cardiovascular (CV) disease.

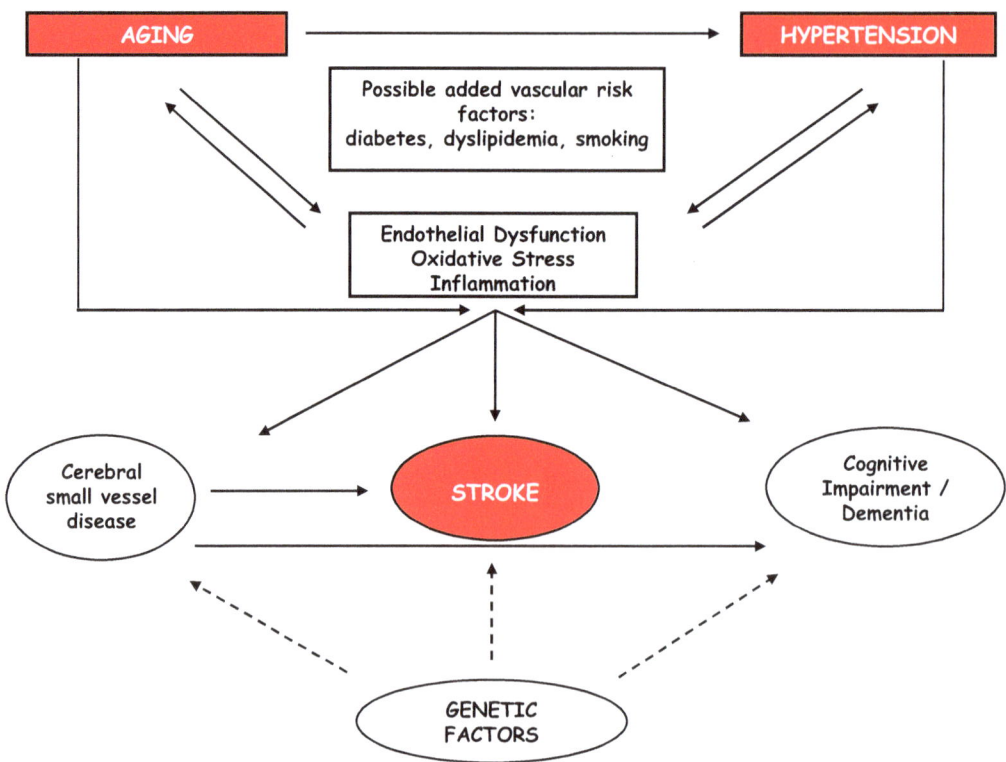

**Fig. (1).** Multiple connected biological mechanisms that participate in the pathogenesis of stroke (Adapted from Sierra C *et al.* [2]).

Stroke pathogenesis and its consequences are not completely elucidated, with various factors and biological mechanisms possibly playing a role (Fig. **1**) [2]. Elevated blood pressure (BP) is a major stroke risk factor, with an established, continuous relationship between stroke and BP [1, 3]. However, trials of hypertension therapy demonstrate that relatively-small BP reductions (5-6 mmHg in diastolic BP (DBP), 10-12 mmHg in systolic BP (SBP) for 3-5 years) cut the stroke risk by > 33% [3]. Primary stroke prevention through BP control and hypertension treatment is now standard [1, 3]. In the same way, elevated post-stroke BP increases the recurrent stroke risk [3, 4], with some trials demonstrating that BP lowering plus combination hypertension therapy has benefits in lowering stroke recurrence [3, 4].

HT, known to be the leading factor for macrovascular cerebral complications, such as stroke and, therefore, vascular dementia [1, 3, 5], may also predispose to more-subtle cerebral changes due to narrowing of the arterioles or pathological microvascular changes. Cerebral microvascular disease has been suggested as a factor in vascular cognitive impairment [6, 7]. The complex underlying mechanisms of HT-related cognitive changes are not completely elucidated. Associations between cerebral white matter lesions (cWML) and BP elevation indirect suggest that long-term structural/functional brain changes may result in worse cognitive functioning when BP control is poor or absent. At the same time, some evidence suggests hypertension therapy may aid the prevention of cognitive impairment/vascular dementia by controlling BP [5].

Older age and HT are consistently reported as the leading risk factors for cWML, which, in turn is a leading factor in the prognosis of stroke and cognitive impairment/dementia [1, 3, 5, 6, 8]. Hypertensives present more and a greater area of cWML than normotensives [6, 8]. At the same time, treated and controlled hypertensives have been shown to have a lower prevalence of cWML than untreated/treated uncontrolled hypertensives [9]. A randomized BP-lowering trial of perindopril *vs.* placebo in normotensives and hypertensives with cerebrovascular disease (CeVD) found average total new WML volume was significantly lower in actively treated patients than in the placebo group [10].

The idea that, in hypertensives, cWML may be an early, silent marker of brain damage is strongly supported by recent evidence.

## STROKE EPIDEMIOLOGY

HT increases the stroke risk six-fold [11], with stroke being most common complication in hypertensives (Fig. **2**) [12]. As stated, stroke, one of the leading causes of death worldwide and of disability in developed countries, entails a substantial economic burden and has a large public health impact. In developed countries, ischaemic stroke represent approximately 80% of all strokes and haemorrhagic stroke 20%. Incidence rates, often stated as 2 per 1000 persons, rise steeply from < 1 per 1000 in people aged <45 years, to > 15 per 1000 in subjects aged ≥ 85 years, but vary widely [13]. In developed countries, around 75% of all strokes take place in subjects aged > 65 years. Around 80% of people survive the first four weeks post-stroke and 70% survive for ≥ 1 year. Prevalence rates are > 8 per 1000 adults with an accentuated age gradient [13], suggesting future pressure on health services. Disability is common and, sometimes, severe, in stroke survivors, requiring increased formal/informal care.

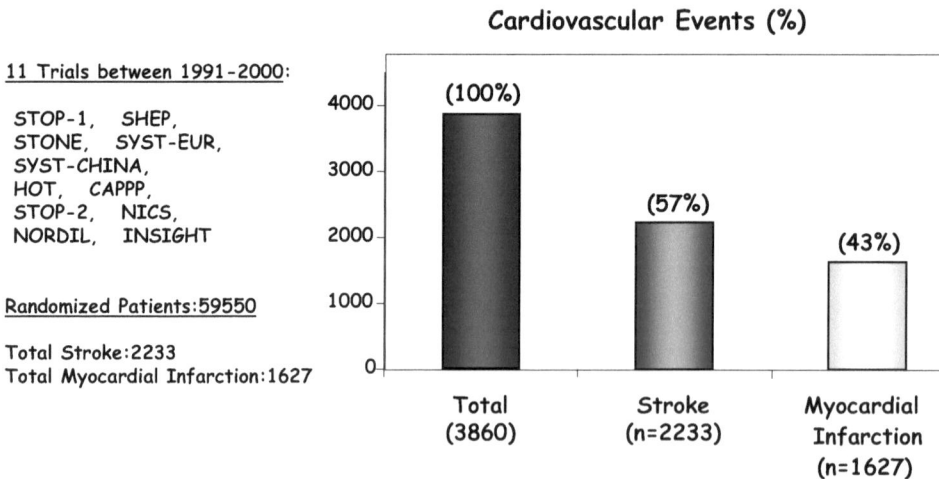

**Cardiovascular Events (%)**

11 Trials between 1991-2000:

STOP-1, SHEP,
STONE, SYST-EUR,
SYST-CHINA,
HOT, CAPPP,
STOP-2, NICS,
NORDIL, INSIGHT

Randomized Patients:59550

Total Stroke:2233
Total Myocardial Infarction:1627

Total (3860) (100%)
Stroke (n=2233) (57%)
Myocardial Infarction (n=1627) (43%)

**Fig. (2).** Number of fatal and non-fatal cerebral strokes and fatal and non-fatal myocardial infarctions reported in large prospective hypertension trials published after 1990 (Adapted from Kjieldsen *et al.* [13]).

## PATHOPHISIOLOGY OF BRAIN VASCULAR DAMAGE INDUCED BY HIGH BLOOD PRESSURE

The brain is highly susceptible to the damaging effects of BP elevation. Systolic and diastolic HT in both males and females are known risk factors for ischaemic/ haemorrhagic stroke. HT is a leading risk factor for two types of vascular complications: those of atherosclerosis (including cerebral infarction), and those of hypertensive small vessel disease (including intra-cerebral haemorrhage, lacunar infarcts, and cWML). Some silent lesions (lacunar infarcts and cWML) can only be detected by radiology.

Stroke can be classified by clinical factors, clinical-radiologic correlates or radiologic findings alone. Topographically, infarcts are classified as cortical (anterior cerebral artery, middle cerebral artery branches, posterior cerebral artery territory, external watershed infarcts) or subcortical (lacunar, striatocapsular, anterior choroidal artery territory, white matter medullary, internal watershed infarcts). Broadly, HT is more likely to be involved in subcortical infarcts (lacunar infarcts, WML).

The course of chronic elevated BP involves hypertensive cerebral angiopathy, secondary reparative changes and adaptive processes at all cerebrovascular structural/functional levels (Table **1**). HT results in marked adaptive changes in the cerebral circulation (including greater cerebral vessel resistance and loss of physiological autoregulation). Hypertensive encephalopathy is due to sudden, maintained BP elevation that surpasses the upper limit of cerebral blood flow autoregulation. The cerebral circulation adapts to less-severe chronic HT through changes predisposing to stroke due to arterial occlusion/rupture.

**Table 1. Main physiopathological cerebrovascular changes associated with high blood pressure.**

| |
|---|
| Mechanical stress (endothelial lesion) |
| Endothelial dysfunction (loss of vasodilatory capacity) |
| Increased vascular permeability |
| Opened ionic channels |
| Hypertrophy of smooth muscle vascular vessels (reduced lumen) |
| Contraction of smooth muscle vascular vessels (increased vascular resistance) |
| Synthesis of collagen fibre (vascular stiffness) |
| Transudation of plasmatic products to the arterial wall |

Stroke is a generic term that encompasses focal infarction, cerebral haemorrhage, and subarachnoid haemorrhage. Atherothromboembolism and thrombotic occlusion of the lipohyalinotic small-diameter end arteries are the leading causes of cerebral infarcts. Microaneurysm rupture is the first cause of HT-associated intra-cerebral haemorrhage, while rupture of aneurysms in the circle of Willis is the leading cause of non-traumatic subarachnoid haemorrhage.

Due to their high prevalence in clinical lacunar syndromes and the hypertensive lipohyalinotic changes seen at autopsy in small penetrating vessels, lacunar infarcts are the infarct subtype most closely and directly associated with HT [14]. The influence of HT is less direct in other infarct types and is mediated by its effects on atherogenesis in large extracranial or intracranial vessels. Lacunae are small infarcts or, occasionally, Charcot-Bouchard microaneurysm-related haemorrhages.

## RELATIONSHIP BETWEEN HIGH BLOOD PRESSURE AND RISK OF STROKE

Taken together, large observational studies demonstrate that usual BP levels show a log-linear, positive and continuous correlation with the stroke risk [15], a correlation that holds true over a wide BP range, from SBP levels down to 115 mmHg and DBP levels down to 70 mmHg [15]. Findings from prospective observational studies demonstrate a direct, continuous correlation between usual BP levels and initial stroke risk, with an extended difference in usual BP of only 9/5 mmHg correlating with a rise of about one third in the stroke risk: the effects are similar in hyper- and normotensives [16, 17]. Thus, each 5-6 mmHg reduction in usual DBP entails a 38% lower stroke risk [17]. Elevated BP correlates with ischaemic and haemorrhagic strokes, although the association may be closer for haemorrhagic events. The BP/stroke risk relationship remains almost the same after adjusting for serum cholesterol, smoking, alcohol and previous CV disease [15]. There seem to be similar correlations between BP and the recurrent stroke risk, although much of the evidence is contained in smaller cohort/observational studies [15]. The United Kingdom Transient Ischaemic Attack (UK TIA) Collaborative Group data revealed a 10 mmHg reduction in usual SBP was associated with a 28% recurrent stroke risk reduction [18].

While the continuous relationship between SBP/DBP and stroke is established, epidemiological evidence from the MRFIT study suggests SBP may have strong deleterious effects on CeVD [19]. Increased arterial stiffness is known to result in increases in characteristic aortic impedance and pulse wave velocity, thereby raising SBP and pulse pressures, of which large-artery stiffness is the main determinant. SHEP study data show rises of 11% in the stroke risk and 16% in the all-cause mortality risk for each 10-mm Hg rise in pulse pressure [20]. A longitudinal study by Laurent and colleagues [21] demonstrated that aortic stiffness, assessed by carotid-femoral pulse wave velocity, independently predicted fatal stroke in essential hypertensives.

## HYPERTENSION THERAPY AND CEREBROVASCULAR DAMAGE PREVENTION

Epidemiological studies demonstrate that each 5-6 mmHg reduction in usual DBP is associated with a 38% lower stroke risk [17], while clinical trials demonstrate that a 10 mmHg lowering in usual SBP is associated with a 28% lowering in the recurrent stroke risk [18]. Some evidence suggests that hypertension therapy may play a role in preventing cognitive impairment/vascular dementia by BP control [3, 5].

### Primary Stroke Prevention

Around 50% of strokes are thought to be preventable through changes in modifiable risk factors, of which HT is the most important, contributing to 60% of all strokes, and life-styles. A 1996 review of seventeen RCT of hypertension therapy by MacMahon [22] demonstrated a net BP lowering (10-12 mmHg SBP and 5-6 mmHg DBP) and 38% (SD 4) lowering in the incidence of stroke, with corresponding reductions in fatal/non-fatal events. Due to the similarity of the proportional treatment effects in patients at higher or lower risk, the absolute effects of therapy on stroke directly varied according to the background stroke risk, with the largest potential benefits seen in subjects with previous CeVD. Overviews of RCT by the *Blood Pressure Lowering Treatment Trialists* Collaboration [23] in 2000 showed that placebo-controlled trials of calcium antagonists reduced the stroke risk by 39% (95% confidence intervals (CI) 15-56) and that placebo-controlled trials of angiotensin-converting-enzyme inhibitors (ACEi) reduced the stroke risk by 30% (95% CI 15-43), with no significant differences between groups of regimens. More-intense therapy was associated with a 20% stroke risk reduction (95% CI 2-35) compared with normal BP lowering, although differences between the normal and intensive BP lowering strategies were only 3 mmHg. Later meta-analyses of RCT confirmed an approximately 30% to 40% stroke risk reduction with BP lowering [24].

A subsequent meta-analysis of 147 RCT found that beta-blockers reduced strokes by 17% compared with the 29% attributed to other agents, but had similar effects to other agents in preventing coronary events and heart failure, and a higher efficacy than other agents in patients with a recent coronary event [25].

The International Society of Hypertension statement on BP lowering and stroke prevention [15] recommended any of the 5 classes of hypertension drugs (diuretics, betablockers, calcium channel blockers, ACEi, angiotensin receptor blockers (ARBs)) due to the priority in BP reduction "per se". At the same time, trials in hypertensives have suggested a protective effect of ARBs on primary stroke prevention. The LIFE [26] study compared losartan and atenolol in hypertensives aged > 55 years with electrocardiographically-detected LVH. Losartan significantly reduced CV endpoints (13%) with minimal differences in BP changes between therapies. The benefit of losartan was principally due to a 25% decrease in the stroke rate (p=0.001), with no differences in myocardial infarction or total mortality. The SCOPE [27] study included hypertensives aged 70-89 years randomly assigned to candesartan or placebo with open-label active hypertension therapy added as required. The primary composite endpoint (combination of CV death, stroke and myocardial infarction) was reduced by a non-significant 10.9%. Of the primary endpoint components, only the reduction in non-fatal stroke (27.8%; 95% CI: 1.3-47.2; p=0.04) was significant, although there were marked differences in BP lowering (3.2/1.6 mmHg) between patients receiving and esartan and placebo.

The Aliskiren Trial in Type 2 Diabetes Using Cardio-Renal Endpoints (ALTITUDE) study was terminated early due to lack of benefits and a raised risk of stroke using dual inhibition of the renin-angiotensin system, even though a BP reduction of 1.3/0.6mmHg was found in patients with diabetes and renal disease [28]. After re-analysis, ONTARGET Trial data failed to confirm that dual renin-angiotensin system inhibition is associated with an elevated stroke risk in diabetics with/without nephropathy [29]. Due to the absence of clinical benefits and the higher incidence of renal adverse events, dual renin-angiotensin system blockade cannot be recommended in this type of patient.

The 2013 European Guidelines stated, in summary, that there is no indisputable evidence that the capacity of major drug classes to provide protection against overall CV risk or cause-specific CV events (stroke and myocardial infarction), varies [3].

BP reduction is, overall, of greater importance that the specific drugs used, but meta-analyses shown some antihypertensive classes can provide direct neuroprotection: renin-angiotensin system and calcium-channel blockers and thiazide diuretics are the drug classes that have the greatest effect on primary prevention of stroke.

## A Special Situation: Primary Stroke Prevention in the Very Elderly

Age and HT are recognized as the leading risk factors for stroke, which is often seen as a disease of the elderly. Until the results of the HYVET study [30] in 3845 patients aged $\geq$ 80 years with sustained SBP $\geq$ 160 mmHg were recently reported, the benefits of therapy in subjects with HT aged $\geq$ 80 years had not been established. Subjects included were randomized to the diuretic, indapamide (sustained release 1.5 mg) or matching placebo. Fatal/nonfatal stroke was the primary end point. The intention to-treat-analysis showed active treatment was associated with a 30% reduction of the primary end point (P=0.06). Analysis of secondary end points showed statistically-significant reductions of 39% in stroke mortality (P=0.05), 21% in all-cause mortality (P<0.02), and 64% in heart failure (P<0.001).

## Secondary Stroke Prevention

Hypertension therapy may be the most important intervention for secondary ischaemic stroke prevention. The Chinese Post-Stroke Antihypertensive Treatment Study (PATS) [31] which randomized 5665 patients with a recent TIA or minor stroke (hemorrhagic or ischemic) to indapamide or placebo was the first large study that demonstrated the effectiveness of HT treatment in secondary stroke prevention. Subjects were included regardless of baseline BP, and the average period from qualifying event to randomization was 30 months. Average SBP was 153 mm Hg in the placebo arm and 154 mm Hg in the indapamide arm at baseline. Over the average 24-month follow-up, average SBP was reduced by 6.7 in the placebo arm and 12.4 mm Hg in the indapamide arm. The main outcome (recurrent stroke) occurred in 44.1% of subjects in the placebo arm and 30.9% of subjects in the indapamide arm (reduction in RR, 30%; 95% CI, 14-43).

A 2003 systematic review of the link between BP reduction and secondary stroke prevention and other vascular events encompassed seven RCT with a combined total of 15,527 participants with ischemic/haemorrhagic stroke who were studied from three weeks to fourteen months after the event and followed for two to five years [32]. Hypertension drug therapy correlated with statistically-significant all-recurrent stroke reductions, with the overall reductions in stroke and all vascular events being associated with the degree of BP lowering achieved, while the results on the relative benefits of specific hypertension regimens in secondary prevention of stroke were unclear.

The HOPE trial [33] studied the effects of ramipril in subjects with an elevated risk of CV events: 11% of subjects had suffered a previous stroke, enabling analysis of the efficacy of secondary prevention of stroke. However, the results demonstrated a 17% reduction in the RR of stroke recurrence, which was not statistically significant.

The PROGRESS trial [34], specifically designed to test a BP-lowering regimen that included an ACEi in 6,105 patients with stroke/transient ischemic attack (TIA) in the previous five years stratified randomization by intention-to-use single (perindopril) or combination (perindopril plus indapamide) therapy in both hypertensives and normotensives. Perindopril+indapamide lowered BP by an average of 12/5 mmHg and the recurrent stroke risk by 43% (95% CI: 30-54) (Fig. **3**) in both hypertensive and normotensive groups. No benefit was observed when perindopril was given alone (average BP reduction: 5/3 mmHg). The subsequent MOSES study of the ARB, eprosartan for secondary prevention of stroke showed that when eprosartan was compared with nitrendipine in subjects with a prior stroke, although there was a comparable reduction in BP, there were fewer cerebrovascular and CV events in subjects receiving eprosartan [35]. The included 1,405 high-risk hypertensives with cerebral events during the previous two years, who were randomized to eprosartan or nitrendipine (average follow-up 2.5 years). The primary end point was a composite (total mortality and all CV and cerebrovascular events, including all recurrent events. The combined primary end point was significantly lower in subjects receiving eprosartan, principally due to fewer cerebrovascular events.

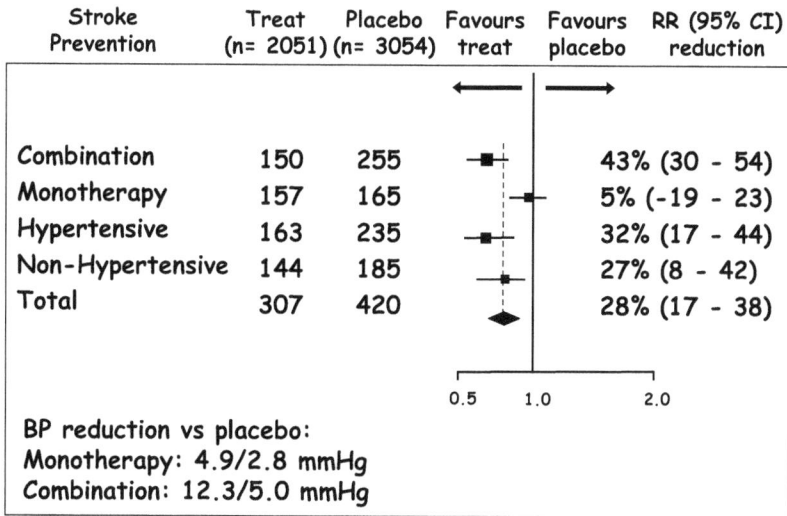

| Stroke Prevention | Treat (n= 2051) | Placebo (n= 3054) | Favours treat | Favours placebo | RR (95% CI) reduction |
|---|---|---|---|---|---|
| Combination | 150 | 255 | | | 43% (30 - 54) |
| Monotherapy | 157 | 165 | | | 5% (-19 - 23) |
| Hypertensive | 163 | 235 | | | 32% (17 - 44) |
| Non-Hypertensive | 144 | 185 | | | 27% (8 - 42) |
| Total | 307 | 420 | | | 28% (17 - 38) |

0.5          1.0          2.0

BP reduction vs placebo:
Monotherapy: 4.9/2.8 mmHg
Combination: 12.3/5.0 mmHg

**Fig. (3).** Long-term blood pressure lowering and secondary prevention of stroke in the the PROGRESS trial. Adapted from reference [34].

The large Prevention Regimen for Effectively Avoiding Second Strokes (PROFESS) trial [36], a large-scale study of post-stroke hypertension therapy analysed the efficacy of telmisartan compared with placebo in preventing the recurrence of ischaemic stroke. The study randomized 2,0332 subjects with previous ischaemic stroke to telmisartan or placebo ≤ 90 days after an ischaemic event. No association was found between telmisartan and reductions in recurrent stroke (HR 0.95; 95% CI 0.86-1.04) or major CV events (HR, 0.94; 95% CI, 0.87-1.01) throughout the average 2.5-year follow-up. Factors that may have biased the results included the facts that the BP-lowering group was underpowered statistically and that there were small differences in BP between arms (difference in SBP: 5.4 mm Hg at one month and 4.0 mm Hg at one year) caused by lack of adherence to telmisartan and more-aggressive treatment with other hypertensive therapies in the placebo arm which could have reduced the impact of therapy on stroke recurrence.

Combined analysis of the PROFESS and TRASCEND [37] trials to analyse whether telmisartan was effective in ACEi-intolerant subjects with CV disease or T2DM and end-organ damage showed the incidence of the composite end point (stroke, myocardial infarction or vascular death) was 12.8% for telmisartan compared with 13.8% for placebo (HR 0.91; 95% CI 0.85-0.98, p = 0.013) [38].

The question of whether the recurrent stroke risk is related to higher or lower SBP remains unanswered. A *post hoc* observational evaluation of the PROFESS study assessed possible associations between maintaining low-normal or high-normal SBP levels with the recurrent stroke risk [39]. The primary outcome was the first recurrence of any type of stroke and the secondary outcome was a composite (stroke, myocardial infarction, death from vascular causes). During the follow up, SBP levels in the very low–normal (<120 mm Hg), high (140-150 mmHg) and very high (>150 mmHg) range were associated with a higher recurrent stroke risk, supporting the suggestion that there is a J curve in BP levels in secondary stroke prevention. However, there remain limited data that specifically evaluate the optimal BP target in secondary stroke prevention.

The recent Secondary Prevention of Small Subcortical Strokes (SPS3) trial [40] randomized (open label) 3,020 patients with lacunar stroke to two target SBP control levels (<150 *vs.* <130 mmHg). Mean baseline SBP was 145 mmHg in the <150 mmHg arm and 144 mmHg in the <130 mmHg arm. At twelve months, average SBP was 138 mmHg in the <150 mmHg arm compared with 127 mmHg in the <130mmHg arm. The primary outcome (recurrent stroke) occurred in 152 subjects in the <150 mmHg arm compared with 125 in the <130mmHg arm, although the difference was not statistically-significant (HR, 0.81; 95% CI, 0.64-1.03). Fifteen subjects in the <150mmHg and twenty-three subjects in the <130mmHg arm presented serious hypotensive complications (0.40%/year; HR, 1.53; 95% CI, 0.80-2.93). A very-recent *post-hoc* evaluation of the SPS3 data [41] assessed the correlation between average BP achieved six months post-randomization and recurrent stroke, major vascular events, and all-cause mortality and found that after an average follow up of 3.7 years, a J-shaped association between BP achieved and the outcomes measured was apparent, with the lowest risk being for SBP circa 124 mmHg and DBP circa 67 mmHg. The all-event risk nadir was between 120-128 mmHg SBP and between 65-70 mmHg DBP. Future studies should evaluate the impact of excessive BP reduction, especially in elderly subjects with pre-existing vascular disease. At present the only specifically-designed trial examining this issue is the ongoing European Society of Hypertension-Chinese Hypertension League Stroke in Hypertension Optimal Treatment trial (SHOT) [42], a prospective, multinational, RCT with a 3x2 factorial design that compared a) three SBP targets (<145-135; <135-125; <125 mmHg) and b) two LDL-C targets (2.8-1.8; <1.8mmol/l), which will include 7500 patients aged ≥ 65 years (2500 European, 5000 Chinese) with HT and a stroke/ TIA in the six months pre-randomization. Hypertension and statin treatments are initiated or modified using suitable registered agents chosen by the researchers in order to maintain patients within the randomized SBP and LDL-C windows. BP is measured each three months and LDL-C each six months. Ambulatory BP will be measured yearly. The primary outcome is time to fatal/non-fatal stroke, while secondary outcomes include the time to first major CV event; cognitive decline (assessed using the Montreal Cognitive test); and dementia. All major outcomes will be adjudicated by committees blinded to randomized allocation.

In summary, according to the American Heart Association [4] and the 2013 European Hypertension Guidelines [43], hypertension treatment is recommended for recurrent stroke prevention:

• Initiation of BP therapy is indicated for previously-untreated patients with ischaemic stroke or TIA who, after the first few days, have established SBP ≥140 mm Hg or DBP ≥90 mm Hg *(Class I; Level of Evidence B)*.
• Initiation of therapy for patients with SBP <140 mm Hg and DBP <90 mm Hg is of unclear benefit *(Class IIb; Level of Evidence C)*.
• Goals for target BP level or reduction from pre-treatment baseline are unclear and should be individualized, but SBP <140 mm Hg and DBP <90 mm Hg are reasonable *(Class IIa; Level of Evidence B)*. For patients with recent lacunar stroke, a target SBP of <130 mm Hg may be reasonable *(Class IIb; Level of Evidence B)*.

**Hypertension Therapy and Early Cerebral Damage**

Cross-sectional, population-based MRI studies have demonstrated that treated, controlled hypertensives have a lower prevalence of cWML than untreated and treated uncontrolled controlled hypertensives [9]. Van Dijk and colleagues [44], studied 1,805 subjects aged 65-75 years from ten European cohorts in whom BP measurements were initiated 5-20 years before brain-MRI, and found that subjects with poorly-controlled HT had a greater risk of severe cWML than those without cWML or those with controlled or untreated HT. Increased SBP and DBP correlated with more severe cWML and reduced DBP with more severe periventricular cWML. The authors suggest that successful HT treatment could lower the cWML risk but that reducing DBP could have a potential negative effect on severe periventricular cWML. However, the lack of differences between controlled and untreated hypertensives might be because untreated hypertensives had less-severe or shorter-lasting HT. Another study in 845 subjects found that baseline HT was significantly associated with an increased risk of severe cWML on brain-MRI at four years of follow-up. When BP levels and hypertension drug intake were taken into account, the risk of severe cWML was significantly reduced in subjects with normal BP taking hypertension medication compared with those with high BP also taking medication [45].

A longitudinal study by Schmidt and colleagues [46] evaluated volunteers aged 50-75 years without neuropsychiatric disease had MRI at baseline, three years (204 subjects) and six years (191 subjects). At three years, only baseline DBP and cWML significantly predicted the progression of white matter hyperintensities. At six years, the baseline cWML grade predicted cWML progression better than age and HT [46].

A MRI substudy of the PROGRESS study recently found that the average total new cWML volume was significantly reduced in the active treatment arm compared with the placebo arm [10]. A *post hoc* analysis also showed that the greatest beneficial effect of hypertension therapy on cWML progression was seen in patients with severe cWML at study entry.

# EVIDENCE OF THE RELATIONSHIP BETWEEN TREATMENT OF OTHER ASSOCIATED RISK FACTORS AND STROKE PREVENTION

## Type 2 Diabetes Mellitus

Type 2 diabetes mellitus (T2DM) is a leading risk factor for vascular events, but there are no specific guidelines for T2DM therapy in stroke patients. Correct glycaemic control of T2DM may lower the impact and burden of microvascular complications and the small-artery atherosclerosis risk. Thus, current secondary CV disease-prevention guidelines endorse glucose and HbA1c objectives of near-normoglycaemic levels (*i.e.*, glycated haemoglobin <7%) in patients with T2DM and recent stroke [4, 47].

Subgroup analyses of clinical trials suggest therapy could effectively reduce the stroke risk. Although the PROactive trial reported a lowered stroke incidence in selected patients receiving pioglitazone [48], the other risks of thiazolidinedione treatment must be considered.

Three large RCT comparing aggressive glycaemic control with standard control in T2DM patients with antecedents of CV disease, stroke, or additional vascular risk factors evidenced no reductions in CV events or mortality in patients on intensive glucose therapy. While not designed to measure stroke outcomes, the trials showed no lowering of stroke incidence due to tight glycaemic control.

The ACCORD trial randomly assigned 10,251 patients to intensive therapy targeting HbA1c ≤6% *vs.* a standard HbA1c of 7-7.9%. After an average of 3.5 years of follow-up the trial was halted due to an increased mortality risk in patients randomized to intensive therapy. No significant differences in nonfatal stroke rates or the primary end point (composite of nonfatal heart attack, nonfatal stroke, and death due to a CV cause) were demonstrated [49].

The ADVANCE trial, in which 11,140 patients with T2DM and a history of macrovascular disease or other risk factors were randomly assigned to intensive glucose control (target HbA1c ≤6.5%) or standard glucose control (target >7%), with 9% of subjects having a previous stroke, also found no benefits in secondary CV event prevention. There were no significant reductions in macrovascular events alone, although there were no significant between-group differences in mortality [50]. Lastly, the Veterans Affairs Diabetes Trial assigned 1,791 patients with T2DM to intensive blood glucose therapy or standard therapy and found no significant between-group differences. The results of these trials suggest glycaemic targets should not be lowered to HbA1c <6.5% in subjects with a high added CV risk or with a previous stroke or TIA [51].

## Dyslipidemia

While there are established correlations between dyslipidaemia and coronary heart disease and between LDL-cholesterol reductions and mortality due to coronary heart disease, the relationship between dyslipidaemia and stroke is less clear. However, results from trials and meta-analyses show an association between serum cholesterol and ischaemic, rather than haemorrhagic, stroke [52 - 54].

The Heart Protection Study [52] randomized 17,265 subjects to simvastatin or placebo to study the effect of statins on stroke incidence of stroke in subjects without CeVD but with a high risk of vascular disease. Simvastatin reduced stroke, coronary death, nonfatal myocardial infarction and revascularization by 24%, and stroke alone by 1.6%. In a Heart Protection Study substudy, 3,280 patients with a history of stroke or TIA in the 4.3 years after randomization were followed for 4.8 years. Simvastatin significantly reduced the incidence of the composite of major events by 20%, but not the stroke risk.

In the Jupiter trial [54] 17, 802 healthy males and females with low-density lipoprotein cholesterol levels and high-sensitivity C-reactive protein levels were randomly treated with rosuvastatin 20 mg or placebo. After 1.9 years, rosuvastatin reduced the risk of fatal/ nonfatal stroke by 48% compared with placebo.

The SPARCL study [55], a specific trial of statins in secondary stroke prevention, evaluated the efficacy of high-dose atorvastatin after stroke or TIA in 4,731 subjects with a history of ischaemic stroke or TIA who were randomized to atorvastatin 80 mg/day or placebo. After a median follow-up of 4.9 years, atorvastatin significantly reduced fatal/nonfatal stroke by 16% and major CV events by 21%.

# IS THERE A NEUROPROTECTIVE EFFECT OF RENIN-ANGIOTENSIN SYSTEM BLOCKADE?

As stated, two large primary prevention RCT in hypertensives demonstrated that losartan [26] and candesartan [27] were superior to atenolol or conventional therapy in stroke prevention. A smaller secondary prevention study in hypertensives with a previous stroke found that another ARB, eprosartan, provided greater cerebrovascular protection than nitrendipine [35]. While definitive conclusions are different to establish when comparing trials involving divergent patient types and therapeutic comparisons, the above-mentioned studies may suggest that ARB proportion greater cerebrovascular protection. Varying, and almost certainly complementary, mechanisms, are suggested as explanations for this seeming trend: these include regression of left ventricular hypertrophy, protection against atrial enlargement and supraventricular arrhythmias, effects on endothelial function, risk biomarkers and vascular remodelling, and angiotensin II/ AT-2 receptor- mediated specific neuroprotective effects [56]. Evidence for the purported improved outcomes comes from specific mechanisms involving the renin-angiotensin blockade, the specific AT-1 receptor antagonism, increased angiotensin II and AT-2 receptor stimulation, effects that have not been shown for ACEi: this provides an explanation as to why ACEi do not show significantly improved stroke protection compared with other conventional hypertension therapy, unlike ARB therapy. Even so, these supposed benefits require confirmation in further trials.

## CONCLUSION

Stroke is the third most-frequent cause of death after cancer and heart disease in developed countries and one of the most common reasons for developing cognitive impairment and vascular dementia. The pathogenesis of stroke and its consequences are not fully understood. In addition to age, hypertension is the most important modifiable cardiovascular risk factor for cerebral small vessel disease including lacunar infarction, white matter lesions, and cerebral microbleeds, all them predictors of future ischemic or hemorrhagic stroke. Primary stroke prevention by antihypertensive therapy and blood pressure control is well established. Likewise, higher blood pressure levels after stroke increase the risk of recurrent stroke and recent trials indicate that BP reduction with combined antihypertensive therapy is beneficial in reducing stroke recurrence.

## TAKE HOME MESSAGES

- Stroke, the third most-frequent cause of death after cancer and heart disease in developed countries, is one of the most common reasons for cognitive impairment and vascular dementia.
- Hypertension is the most important modifiable CV risk factor for developing CeVD including stroke, small vessel disease, and cognitive impairment.
- Older age and hypertension are constantly reported to be the main risk factors for cerebral small vessel disease that includes lacunar infarcts, cWML, and microbleeds.
- The primary prevention of stroke through hypertension therapy and BP control has been established by RCT.
- Any of the five classes of hypertension drugs and their combinations (diuretics, betablockers, calcium channel blockers, ACEi, angiotensin receptor blockers) may be used for stroke prevention in hypertensive patients. The priority is the BP reduction "per se".
- Treatment of hypertension and BP control is the most important action for secondary prevention of ischemic stroke.

## CONFLICT OF INTEREST

The authors confirm that they have no conflict of interest to declare for this publication.

## ACKNOWLEDGEMENTS

Declared none.

## REFERENCES

[1]   Goldstein LB, Bushnell CD, Adams RJ, *et al.* Guidelines for the primary prevention of stroke: a guideline for healthcare professionals from the American Heart Association/American Stroke Association. Stroke 2011; 42: 517-84. https://www.ncbi.nlm.nih.gov/pubmed?term=Creager%20MA% 5BAuthor%5D&cauthor=true&cauthor_uid=21127304.

[2]   Sierra C, Coca A, Schiffrin EL. Vascular mechanisms in the pathogenesis of stroke. Curr Hypertens Rep 2011; 13(3): 200-7.
[http://dx.doi.org/10.1007/s11906-011-0195-x] [PMID: 21331606]

[3]     ESH/ESC Guidelines for the management of arterial hypertension. TheTask Force for the management of arterial hypertension of the European Society of Hypertension (ESH) and of the European Society of Cardiology (ESC). J Hypertens 2013; 2013: 1281-357.

[4]     Kernan WN, Ovbiagele B, Black HR, *et al.* Guidelines for the prevention of stroke in patients with stroke and transient ischemic attack: a guideline for healthcare professionals from the American Heart Association/American Stroke Association. Stroke 2014; 45(7): 2160-236.
        [http://dx.doi.org/10.1161/STR.0000000000000024] [PMID: 24788967]

[5]     Gorelick PB, Scuteri A, Black SE, *et al.* Vascular contributions to cognitive impairment and dementia: a statement for healthcare professionals from the American heart association/american stroke association. Stroke 2011; 42(9): 2672-713.
        [http://dx.doi.org/10.1161/STR.0b013e3182299496] [PMID: 21778438]

[6]     Pantoni L. Cerebral small vessel disease: from pathogenesis and clinical characteristics to therapeutic challenges. Lancet Neurol 2010; 9(7): 689-701.
        [http://dx.doi.org/10.1016/S1474-4422(10)70104-6] [PMID: 20610345]

[7]     Sierra C, Doménech M, Camafort M, Coca A. Hypertension and mild cognitive impairment. Curr Hypertens Rep 2012; 14(6): 548-55.
        [http://dx.doi.org/10.1007/s11906-012-0315-2] [PMID: 23073614]

[8]     Sierra C. Essential hypertension, cerebral white matter pathology and ischemic stroke. Curr Med Chem 2014; 21(19): 2156-64.
        [http://dx.doi.org/10.2174/0929867321666131227155140] [PMID: 24372222]

[9]     Liao D, Cooper L, Cai J, *et al.* Presence and severity of cerebral white matter lesions and hypertension, its treatment, and its control. The ARIC Study. Atherosclerosis Risk in Communities Study. Stroke 1996; 27(12): 2262-70.
        [http://dx.doi.org/10.1161/01.STR.27.12.2262] [PMID: 8969791]

[10]    Dufouil C, Chalmers J, Coskun O, *et al.* Effects of blood pressure lowering on cerebral white matter hyperintensities in patients with stroke. The PROGRESS Magnetic resonance imaging substudy. Circulation 2005; 112: 1644-50.
        [http://dx.doi.org/10.1161/CIRCULATIONAHA.104.501163] [PMID: 16145004]

[11]    National Stroke Association. Stroke prevention: the importance of risk factors. Stroke 1991; 1: 17-20.

[12]    Kjeldsen SE, Julius S, Hedner T, Hansson L. Stroke is more common than myocardial infarction in hypertension: analysis based on 11 major randomized intervention trials. Blood Press 2001; 10(4): 190-2.
        [http://dx.doi.org/10.1080/08037050152669684] [PMID: 11800055]

[13]    Kavanagh S, Knapp M, Patel A. Costs and disability among stroke patients. J Public Health Med 1999; 21(4): 385-94.
        [http://dx.doi.org/10.1093/pubmed/21.4.385] [PMID: 11469359]

[14]    Fisher CM. Lacunes: small, deep cerebral infarcts. Neurology 1965; 15: 774-84.
        [http://dx.doi.org/10.1212/WNL.15.8.774] [PMID: 14315302]

[15]    Chalmers J, Todd A, Chapman N, *et al.* International Society of Hypertension (ISH): statement on

blood pressure lowering and stroke prevention. J Hypertens 2003; 21(4): 651-63.
[http://dx.doi.org/10.1097/00004872-200304000-00001] [PMID: 12658005]

[16]  MacMahon S, Peto R, Cutler J, *et al.* Blood pressure, stroke, and coronary heart disease. Part 1, Prolonged differences in blood pressure: prospective observational studies corrected for the regression dilution bias. Lancet 1990; 335(8692): 765-74.
[http://dx.doi.org/10.1016/0140-6736(90)90878-9] [PMID: 1969518]

[17]  Collins R, Peto R, MacMahon S, *et al.* Blood pressure, stroke, and coronary heart disease. Part 2, Short-term reductions in blood pressure: overview of randomised drug trials in their epidemiological context. Lancet 1990; 335(8693): 827-38.
[http://dx.doi.org/10.1016/0140-6736(90)90944-Z] [PMID: 1969567]

[18]  Rodgers A, MacMahon S, Gamble G, Slattery J, Sandercock P, Warlow C. Blood pressure and risk of stroke in patients with cerebrovascular disease. BMJ 1996; 313(7050): 147.
[http://dx.doi.org/10.1136/bmj.313.7050.147] [PMID: 8688776]

[19]  Stamler J, Stamler R, Neaton JD. Blood pressure, systolic and diastolic, and cardiovascular risks. US population data. Arch Intern Med 1993; 153(5): 598-615.
[http://dx.doi.org/10.1001/archinte.1993.00410050036006] [PMID: 8439223]

[20]  Domanski MJ, Davis BR, Pfeffer MA, Kastantin M, Mitchell GF. Isolated systolic hypertension: prognostic information provided by pulse pressure. Hypertension 1999; 34(3): 375-80.
[http://dx.doi.org/10.1161/01.HYP.34.3.375] [PMID: 10489379]

[21]  Laurent S, Katsahian S, Fassot C, *et al.* Aortic stiffness is an independent predictor of fatal stroke in essential hypertension. Stroke 2003; 34(5): 1203-6.
[http://dx.doi.org/10.1161/01.STR.0000065428.03209.64] [PMID: 12677025]

[22]  MacMahon S. Blood pressure and the prevention of stroke. J Hypertens Suppl 1996; 14(6): S39-46.
[PMID: 9023715]

[23]  Blood Pressure Lowering Treatment Trialists Collaboration. Effects of ACE inhibitors, calcium antagonists, and other blood-pressure-lowering drugs: results of prospectively designed overviews of randomised trials. Lancet 2000; 355: 1955-64.
[PMID: 10859041]

[24]  Lawes CM, Bennett DA, Feigin VL, Rodgers A. Blood pressure and stroke: an overview of published reviews. Stroke 2004; 35(3): 776-85.
[http://dx.doi.org/10.1161/01.STR.0000116869.64771.5A] [PMID: 14976329]

[25]  Law MR, Morris JK, Wald NJ. Use of blood pressure lowering drugs in the prevention of cardiovascular disease: meta-analysis of 147 randomised trials in the context of expectations from prospective epidemiological studies. BMJ 2009; 338: b1665.
[http://dx.doi.org/10.1136/bmj.b1665] [PMID: 19454737]

[26]  Dahlöf B, Devereux RB, Kjeldsen SE, *et al.* Cardiovascular morbidity and mortality in the Losartan Intervention For Endpoint reduction in hypertension study (LIFE): a randomised trial against atenolol. Lancet 2002; 359(9311): 995-1003.
[http://dx.doi.org/10.1016/S0140-6736(02)08089-3] [PMID: 11937178]

[27]  Lithell H, Hansson L, Skoog I, *et al.* The Study on Cognition and Prognosis in the Elderly (SCOPE):

principal results of a randomized double-blind intervention trial. J Hypertens 2003; 21(5): 875-86.
[http://dx.doi.org/10.1097/00004872-200305000-00011] [PMID: 12714861]

[28]  Parving H-H, Brenner BM, McMurray JJ, *et al.* Cardiorenal end points in a trial of aliskiren for type 2 diabetes. N Engl J Med 2012; 367(23): 2204-13.
[http://dx.doi.org/10.1056/NEJMoa1208799] [PMID: 23121378]

[29]  Mann JF, Anderson C, Gao P, *et al.* Dual inhibition of the renin-angiotensin system in high-risk diabetes and risk for stroke and other outcomes: results of the ONTARGET trial. J Hypertens 2013; 31(2): 414-21.
[http://dx.doi.org/10.1097/HJH.0b013e32835bf7b0] [PMID: 23249829]

[30]  Beckett NS, Peters R, Fletcher AE, *et al.* Treatment of hypertension in patients 80 years of age or older. N Engl J Med 2008; 358(18): 1887-98.
[http://dx.doi.org/10.1056/NEJMoa0801369] [PMID: 18378519]

[31]  PATS Collaborating Group. Post-stroke antihypertensive treatment study. A preliminary result. Chin Med J (Engl) 1995; 108(9): 710-7.
[PMID: 8575241]

[32]  Rashid P, Leonardi-Bee J, Bath P. Blood pressure reduction and secondary prevention of stroke and other vascular events: a systematic review. Stroke 2003; 34(11): 2741-8.
[http://dx.doi.org/10.1161/01.STR.0000092488.40085.15] [PMID: 14576382]

[33]  Heart Outcomes Prevention Evaluation Study Investigators. Effects of ramipril on cardiovascular and microvascular outcomes in people with diabetes mellitus: results of the HOPE study and MICRO-HOPE substudy. Lancet 2000; 355(9200): 253-9.
[http://dx.doi.org/10.1016/S0140-6736(99)12323-7] [PMID: 10675071]

[34]  Randomised trial of a perindopril-based blood-pressure-lowering regimen among 6,105 individuals with previous stroke or transient ischaemic attack. Lancet 2001; 358(9287): 1033-41.
[http://dx.doi.org/10.1016/S0140-6736(01)06178-5] [PMID: 11589932]

[35]  Schrader J, Lüders S, Kulschewski A, *et al.* Morbidity and mortality after stroke, eprosartan compared with nitrendipine for secondary prevention: principal results of a prospective randomized controlled study (MOSES). Stroke 2005; 36(6): 1218-26.
[http://dx.doi.org/10.1161/01.STR.0000166048.35740.a9] [PMID: 15879332]

[36]  Yusuf S, Diener HC, Sacco RL, *et al.* Telmisartan to prevent recurrent stroke and cardiovascular events. N Engl J Med 2008; 359(12): 1225-37.
[http://dx.doi.org/10.1056/NEJMoa0804593] [PMID: 18753639]

[37]  Yusuf S, Teo K, Anderson C, *et al.* Effects of the angiotensin-receptor blocker telmisartan on cardiovascular events in high-risk patients intolerant to angiotensin-converting enzyme inhibitors: a randomised controlled trial. Lancet 2008; 372(9644): 1174-83.
[http://dx.doi.org/10.1016/S0140-6736(08)61242-8] [PMID: 18757085]

[38]  Diener HC. Preventing stroke: the PRoFESS, ONTARGET, and TRANSCEND trial programs. J Hypertens Suppl 2009; 27(5): S31-6.
[http://dx.doi.org/10.1097/01.hjh.0000357906.60778.7f] [PMID: 19587553]

[39]  Ovbiagele B, Diener HC, Yusuf S, *et al.* Level of systolic blood pressure within the normal range and

risk of recurrent stroke. JAMA 2011; 306(19): 2137-44.
[http://dx.doi.org/10.1001/jama.2011.1650] [PMID: 22089721]

[40]   White CL, Szychowski JM, Pergola PE, *et al.* Can blood pressure be lowered safely in older adults with lacunar stroke? The Secondary Prevention of Small Subcortical Strokes study experience. J Am Geriatr Soc 2015; 63(4): 722-9.
[http://dx.doi.org/10.1111/jgs.13349] [PMID: 25850462]

[41]   Odden MC, McClure LA, Sawaya BP, *et al.* Achieved Blood Pressure and Outcomes in the Secondary Prevention of Small Subcortical Strokes Trial. Hypertension 2016; 67(1): 63-9.
[http://dx.doi.org/10.1161/HYPERTENSIONAHA.115.06480] [PMID: 26553236]

[42]   Zanchetti A, Liu L, Mancia G, *et al.* Blood pressure and LDL-cholesterol targets for prevention of recurrent strokes and cognitive decline in the hypertensive patient: design of the European Society of Hypertension-Chinese Hypertension League Stroke in Hypertension Optimal Treatment randomized trial. J Hypertens 2014; 32(9): 1888-97.
[http://dx.doi.org/10.1097/HJH.0000000000000254] [PMID: 24979303]

[43]   Mancia G, Fagard R, Narkiewicz K, *et al.* 2013 ESH/ESC Guidelines for the management of arterial hypertension: the Task Force for the management of arterial hypertension of the European Society of Hypertension (ESH) and of the European Society of Cardiology (ESC). J Hypertens 2013; 31(7): 1281-357.
[http://dx.doi.org/10.1097/01.hjh.0000431740.32696.cc] [PMID: 23817082]

[44]   van Dijk EJ, Breteler MM, Schmidt R, *et al.* The association between blood pressure, hypertension, and cerebral white matter lesions: cardiovascular determinants of dementia study. Hypertension 2004; 44(5): 625-30.
[http://dx.doi.org/10.1161/01.HYP.0000145857.98904.20] [PMID: 15466662]

[45]   Dufouil C, de Kersaint-Gilly A, Besançon V, *et al.* Longitudinal study of blood pressure and white matter hyperintensities: the EVA MRI Cohort. Neurology 2001; 56(7): 921-6.
[http://dx.doi.org/10.1212/WNL.56.7.921] [PMID: 11294930]

[46]   Schmidt R, Enzinger C, Ropele S, Schmidt H, Fazekas F. Progression of cerebral white matter lesions: 6-year results of the Austrian Stroke Prevention Study. Lancet 2003; 361(9374): 2046-8.
[http://dx.doi.org/10.1016/S0140-6736(03)13616-1] [PMID: 12814718]

[47]   Saposnik G, Goodman SG, Leiter LA, *et al.* Applying the evidence: do patients with stroke, coronary artery disease, or both achieve similar treatment goals? Stroke 2009; 40(4): 1417-24.
[http://dx.doi.org/10.1161/STROKEAHA.108.533018] [PMID: 19213947]

[48]   Dormandy JA, Charbonnel B, Eckland DJ, *et al.* Secondary prevention of macrovascular events in patients with type 2 diabetes in the PROactive Study (PROspective pioglitAzone Clinical Trial In macroVascular Events): a randomised controlled trial. Lancet 2005; 366(9493): 1279-89.
[http://dx.doi.org/10.1016/S0140-6736(05)67528-9] [PMID: 16214598]

[49]   Gerstein HC, Miller ME, Genuth S, *et al.* Long-term effects of intensive glucose lowering on cardiovascular outcomes. N Engl J Med 2011; 364(9): 818-28.
[http://dx.doi.org/10.1056/NEJMoa1006524] [PMID: 21366473]

[50]   Patel A, MacMahon S, Chalmers J, *et al.* Intensive blood glucose control and vascular outcomes in patients with type 2 diabetes. N Engl J Med 2008; 358(24): 2560-72.
[http://dx.doi.org/10.1056/NEJMoa0802987] [PMID: 18539916]

[51]    Duckworth W, Abraira C, Moritz T, *et al.* Glucose control and vascular complications in veterans with type 2 diabetes. N Engl J Med 2009; 360(2): 129-39.
[http://dx.doi.org/10.1056/NEJMoa0808431] [PMID: 19092145]

[52]    Collins R, Armitage J, Parish S, Sleight P, Peto R. Effects of cholesterol-lowering with simvastatin on stroke and other major vascular events in 20536 people with cerebrovascular disease or other high-risk conditions. Lancet 2004; 363(9411): 757-67.
[http://dx.doi.org/10.1016/S0140-6736(04)15690-0] [PMID: 15016485]

[53]    Randomised trial of cholesterol lowering in 4444 patients with coronary heart disease: the Scandinavian Simvastatin Survival Study (4S). Lancet 1994; 344(8934): 1383-9.
[PMID: 7968073]

[54]    Everett BM, Glynn RJ, MacFadyen JG, Ridker PM. Rosuvastatin in the prevention of stroke among men and women with elevated levels of C-reactive protein: justification for the Use of Statins in Prevention: an Intervention Trial Evaluating Rosuvastatin (JUPITER). Circulation 2010; 121(1): 143-50.
[http://dx.doi.org/10.1161/CIRCULATIONAHA.109.874834] [PMID: 20026779]

[55]    Amarenco P, Bogousslavsky J, Callahan A III, *et al.* High-dose atorvastatin after stroke or transient ischemic attack. N Engl J Med 2006; 355(6): 549-59.
[http://dx.doi.org/10.1056/NEJMoa061894] [PMID: 16899775]

[56]    De la Sierra A, Sierra C. Cerebral white matter lesions, risk of stroke and cerebrovascular protection with angiotensin receptor blockers. Curr Drug Ther 2006; 1: 9-16.
[http://dx.doi.org/10.2174/157488506775268452]

# CHAPTER 2

# Autonomic Nervous System Dysfunction and Risk of Stroke

**Alberto Radaelli**[a,*]**, Paolo Castiglioni**[b] **and Giuseppe Mancia**[c]

[a] *Division of Cardiac Rehabilitation, Ospedale San Gerardo, Monza, Italy*

[b] *IRCCS Fondazione Don C. Gnocchi, Milan, Italy*

[c] *University of Milano-Bicocca and IRCCS Istituto Auxologico Italiano, Milan, Italy*

**Abstract:** Cerebrovascular disease is predicted to remain the second leading cause of mortality reaching almost eight million annual deaths by 2030. Cerebral arteries are innervated and are therefore potential targets for autonomic nervous system dysfunction. In particular, a dynamic baroreflex mediated sympathetic modulation of cerebral blood flow has been demonstrated, confirming the role that the autonomic nervous system exerts on cerebral flow regulation. Moreover, it has been shown that the vagus nerve may influence neuro-inflammation therefore producing an inflammatory mediated vascular damage in case of dysfunction. Dynamic interactions between cerebral blood flow and the autonomic nervous system activity are therefore important and can be analyzed by studying the rhythms that characterize both cerebral blood flow, blood pressure and heart rate. With this regard, variability analysis performed together with techniques that investigate cerebral blood flow distribution and together with functional evaluation of the brain could provide new insight on the role played by the autonomic nervous system in the progression of cerebral vascular disease.

**Keywords:** Autonomic nervous system activity, Baroreflex function, Blood pressure variability, Heart rate variability, Neuro inflammation, Parasympathetic activity, Stroke, Sympathetic activity.

---

* **Corresponding author Alberto Radaelli:** Divisione di Riabilitazione Cardiologica – Ospedale San Gerardo, Via Pergolesi, 33, 20052 Monza (MI), Italy; Tel: +39 039 2332631; Fax: +39 039 2333086; E-mail: albertorada13@gmail.com

# INTRODUCTION

Since the last three decades, stroke remains the second most common cause of mortality [1] and recently, it has become the third leading cause of global disease burden if we consider disability-adjusted life years [2]. Cerebrovascular disease is predicted to remain the second leading cause of mortality reaching almost eight million annual deaths by 2030 [3]. Hypertension and aging are the most important risk factors for stroke. Both of them share the presence of important alterations of the activity of the autonomic nervous system. In particular, there is a clear evidence now that an increase in the activity of the sympathetic nervous system plays an important role not only in the development of hypertension but also of the related organ damage [4]. In addition to this, it is becoming more and more evident that autonomic nervous system dysfunction does not play an ancillary role in cardiovascular disease but is able to promote atherosclerosis and vascular remodeling [5 - 7]. So far emphasis has been placed on the effect of stroke on autonomic nervous system and not on the role that an alteration of autonomic nervous system activity could play in the genesis of strokes. The issue is important as autonomic nervous system dysfunction is a common condition shared by many diseases. Moreover, evidence is accumulating indicating that the autonomic nervous system plays an important role in the dynamic regulation of cerebral blood flow that has to adapt continuously to changes in blood pressure. The aim of this review is therefore to discuss the actual evidence on the influence that the autonomic nervous system activity has on cerebral blood flow and on the possible effect of an alteration of the autonomic nervous system activity on the cerebral circulation.

## Stroke Subtypes

Strokes can be subdivided into three subtypes [8]: 1) ischemic strokes, caused by an occluded vessel, (80% of strokes), 2) intracerebral hemorrhages (15% of all strokes), and 3) subarachnoid hemorrhages (5%). In humans ischemic strokes occur most often in the brain region supplied by the middle cerebral arteries which are relatively large vessels arising from the circle of Willis. Occlusion of one of these arteries produces a large area of ischemic injury and neuronal death. Ischemic strokes can be further subdivided into: large artery atherothrombotic strokes, (40% of strokes), lacunar strokes (20% of stroke) that occur when small intracranial arteries are occluded (Fig. **1**). In 20% of the patients, strokes are caused by a cardiac emboli lodging in a cerebral artery and originating from the heart and much more rarely from the aorta, other large arteries or the venous side of the circulation [9]. Additionally, hemodynamic strokes are the result of cerebral hypoperfusion in the absence of a clot nor emboli.

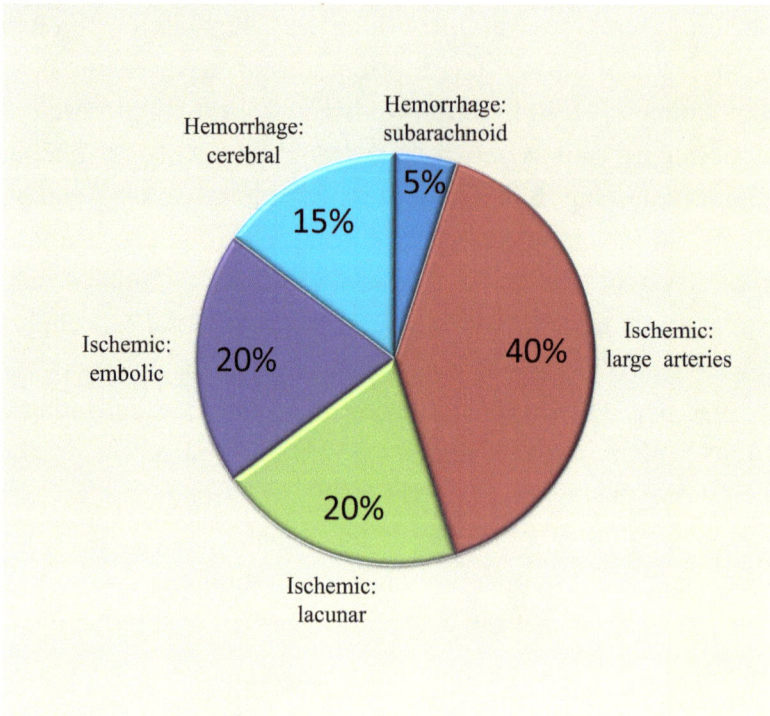

**Fig. (1).** Percent distribution of different types of stroke.

## Cerebral Blood Vessels Innervation

Cerebral arteries are innervated and therefore they are potential targets for autonomic nervous system (ANS) dysfunction. Two types of cerebral vessels innervation are distinguished [10]. Extrinsic innervation: the pial arteries on the surface of the brain receive innervation from the peripheral nervous system. The majority of these nerves arise from the superior cervical ganglion, although a small percentage of nerves also arise from the sphenopalatine, otic and trigeminal ganglia [11]. Intrinsic innervation: the parenchymal arterioles supplying the cerebral cortex receive innervation from within the cerebral parenchyma [12] *i.e.*

noradrenergic, serotoninergic, cholinergic or GABAergic afferents from subcortical neurons located in various nuclei within the brain including the locus coeruleus and raphe nucleus [11]. The postjunctional neurotransmitter as well as their receptor expression varies across the cerebrovascular tree. Norepinephrine (NE) acting on alpha 1 adrenoreceptors characterizes the middle cerebral artery [13, 14] but the parenchymal arterioles express mostly beta adrenergic receptors, the effect of NE being respectively vasoconstriction and vasodilatation [15].

## *Sympathetic Innervation*

The sympathetic innervation of the cerebral circulation arises in the hypothalamus, first order neurons projecting to the intermediolateral cell column of the spinal cord. Second order neurons arise from the sympathetic chain and proceed to synapse with third order neurons in the superior cervical ganglion [16]. The innervation has a unilateral distribution with respect to the midline, its projection to the cerebral vessels being provided by sympathetic nerves that run along the carotid arteries. Nerves (particularly dense in the more proximal large artery portions), follow the vessels out to the pia and along the brain surface to join the penetrating vessels for a short distance into the cerebral parenchyma. The largest part of the adrenergic supply of the intraparenchymal vessels is supplied by the locus coeruleus [17]. The sympathetic nerve terminals are predominantly located close to smooth muscle cells in the outer media. In the cerebral vessels sympathetic innervation accounts for about half the nerves observed in the vessel walls. The innervation is most dense anteriorly with a sparser supply in the vertebro-basilar territory in which it arises largely from the stellate ganglion.

The main transmitter of the cerebral sympathetic nerves is NE. In addition, however, sympathetic nerves release the vasoconstrictor neuropeptide Y, which is widely distributed not only in the brain but also in the peripheral nervous system. Fibers that contain neuropeptide Y form a dense network around cerebral arteries.

## *Parasympathetic Innervation*

The parasympathetic system arises from the superior salivatory nucleus, emerging from the brain in the facial (VII Th cranial) nerve, with a subsequent fiber distribution to the pterygopalatine (sphenopalatine) and optic ganglia and carotid miniganglia. Pharmacologically, the system is characterized by the presence of acetylcholine, vasoactive intestinal peptides and peptide histidine methionine and perhaps other substances [16]. Their effect is a vasodilator one, *via* one or more of its peptidergic neurotransmitters.

## Cerebral Blood Flow Auto-regulation

The human brain is exquisitely sensitive to even brief reductions of oxygen supply by the perfusing blood. Elaborate mechanisms have evolved to maintain optimal cerebral blood flow (CBF) and to ensure a favourable balance between oxygen supply and demand [18]. Niels A. Lassen was one of the first to demonstrate the complexity of cerebral autoregulation, *i.e.* the process by which CBF is kept at a constant level when mean systemic arterial pressure changes between 50-150 mmHg [19]. It is now well established that this phenomenon is mediated and modulated by several mechanism such as intrinsic changes of vascular muscle tone in response to the distending intravascular pressure [20], the vasomotor effects of arterial carbon dioxide and oxygen tension, the vasodilatation caused by cerebral metabolic by-products [17] and the relaxing influence of neuronal nitric oxide production [21 - 24]. It has also been shown that the lower and upper BP limits of the autoregulation plateau, *i.e.*, the blood pressure range over which CBF is maintained constant, is different under different circumstances [25], both showing, for example, an increase in hypertensive patients and a reset towards lower values when BP is reduced by treatment. Autoregulation is impaired or lost in the ischemic or otherwise damaged brain areas [20], with ominous consequences for the survival of cerebral tissue [25].

A question under discussion since a long time is whether innervation of the cerebral arteries participates in the brain autoregulation and has a substantial influence on CBF in health and disease. This is because most of the evidence has by necessity been obtained in animals or animal models of stroke and other diseases [26 - 33], the few usually insufficiently controlled and technically limited studies in humans being unable to fully understand the physiological and pathophysiological role of cerebrovascular innervation [34, 35], which thus still remains the subject of considerable controversy [34, 35]. Over time, however, data on an important role played by the autonomic nervous system on CBF regulation in humans and on the participation of neural factors to the brain perfusion, at least during cerebral ischaemia or after subarachnoid hemorrhage, have grown, as reported by a recent review [18].

## *Sympathetic Regulation of CBF*

Surgical excision of the stellate ganglion appears to provide a modest (maximum +20%) increase in CBF, moreover minor CBF reductions (5-10%) have been shown to accompany electrical stimulation of sympathetic nerves to the brain [26, 27, 36 - 39]. These observations suggest that in physiological conditions the sympathetic nervous system has a limited potential influence on the brain circulation, with no significant tonic contribution to its basic vasomotor tone. However, sympathetic stimulation does produce a profound fall in CBF if cerebral vessels have been previously dilated by hypercapnia, an observation that generated the "dual control" hypothesis, *i.e.*, that the cerebral circulation is comprised of two resistances in series. Extra-parenchymal vessels are thought to be regulated largely by the autonomic nervous system, while intra-parenchymal vessels (responsible for half the resistance under physiological conditions) are governed primarily by intrinsic metabolic and myogenic factors [29].

Other findings on the importance of sympathetic vascular influences for the brain circulation are the following. First, although in presence of normal blood pressure values cerebral vessels escape from the vasoconstrictor response to sympathetic stimulation, this does not occur during acute hypertension, in which an increase of sympathetic influences can attenuate the resulting CBF increase and exert a protective effect on the brain [40 - 42]. Second, in stroke prone spontaneously hypertensive (spSH) rats (a model of hypertension with a strikingly high incidence of stroke) sympathetic influences can enhance the ability of the cerebral arteries to autoregulate blood flow [27] in intact vessels but perhaps also in vessels within the ischemic area [18], and to reduce the incidence of hemorrhagic strokes by putting the parenchymal brain arterioles and microvasculature at a reduced risk of damage when blood pressure fluctuates. Third, under these circumstances, a sympathetic activation may oppose a CBF increase, thereby preventing or attenuating the fluid accumulation and plasma protein extravasation into the cerebral tissue that follows a breakdown of the blood-brain barrier, and limiting cerebral oedema. Fourth, although in physiological conditions cerebral autoregulation is not affected by sympathetic influences, these influences may have a non- marginal role in disease. That is, there are elements to suggest that direct innervation of cerebral arteries from cervical ganglia (as well as stimulation of adrenergic receptors by circulating catecholamines) may have a protective effect against stroke and its consequences.

Sympathetic nerves are also thought to exert trophic influences upon the vessels that they innervate, as shown by the observation that sympathectomy reduces the hypertrophy of the arterial wall that develops in response to chronic hypertension [7]. This has been shown to occur also in spSH rats in which sympathetic denervation of the cerebral arteries by superior cervical ganglionectomy prevents the development of wall hypertrophy [32] and reduces the wall thickness and distensibility of the pial arteries [33]. It is also possible that sympathetic nerve activation plays a protective role on the smaller parenchymal arterioles where NE causes vasodilatation [15].

Little is known on the role, if any, of the dense adrenergic innervation of the choroid plexus, and thus of the capacitance vessel component of the brain circulation. Alterations of the constrictor tone and diameter of large cerebral vein, however, can mechanically affect blood pressure gradient and perfusion across the brain, with a possible non negligible influence upon intracranial pressure [43, 44].

### *Parasympathetic Regulation of Cerebral Blood Flow*

Although stimulation of parasympathetic nerves elicits a rise of cortical blood flow, there is no convincing evidence that under physiological conditions cholinergic mechanisms contribute significantly to CBF regulation. Furthermore, parasympathetic nerves have not been shown to be involved in the vasodilator response to hypercapnia [29], thereby failing to become a determinant of brain perfusion under $CO_2$, as it is the case for sympathetic influences. However, in young Long Evans rats, sectioning of the parasympathetic nerve fibers innervating the circle of Willis increased the damage induced by focal cerebral ischemia [31], similar results being obtained in spontaneously hypertensive rats [30]. Thus, it appears that parasympathetic nerve fiber activation may play a protective role in cerebral ischemia, possibly because its ability to induce dilatation of small arteries located in an ischemic territory [45] limits the damage caused by a focal reduction of brain perfusion. This has also been observed in a recent study on a canine model of cerebral ischemia, in which a post-stroke non-invasive parasympathetic nerve stimulation limited the ischemic–dependent brain damage [46]. It should be added that this protective parasympathetic effect may not be identical in all areas of the brain. The effect of vasoactive intestinal peptides has been shown to be much less in the posterior circulation than in the anterior one. Moreover the activity of the parasympathetic nervous system has shown effects other than the vasomotor ones, such as modulation of neuro-inflammation (see below).

## Vagal Modulation of Neuro-inflammation

Certain neurotransmitters may exert an anti-inflammatory effect on the brain *via* receptors located in microglia and astrocytes [47]. It is well known that this is the case for amines and more specifically NE which can act as a powerful endogenous neuroimmunomodulator, its anti-inflammatory properties possibly helping to maintain an immunosuppressive environment within the brain [48]. Interestingly, such anti-inflammatory role may be shared by the central parasympathetic neural innervation because the solitary nucleus, the major viscero sensory station receiving the information carried by afferent vagal pathways, provides input to the locus coeruleus, which is the major source of NE in the brain [49]. Indeed, electrophysiological and biochemical studies in the rat have shown that vagus nerve stimulation increases the firing rate of noradrenergic neurons [50] as well as the extracellular concentration of NE in the hippocampus and cortex [51]. Therefore, the anti-inflammatory role of sympathetic fibers in the brain may be shared by vagal nerve influences *via* modulation of central adrenergic transmission, vagal stimulation thus possibly reducing brain inflammation.

Animal studies have shown that electrical, chemical or mechanical stimulation of peripheral efferent vagal fibers is accompanied by a reduced production of pro inflammatory cytokines in various animal models of inflammation [52]. Furthermore, an inverse relationship between indices of vagal activity and inflammatory markers has been observed in man, in whom an increase of heart rate variability has been associated with a reduction of inflammatory markers [53]. The vagus, and more in general the cholinergic system, thus appear to have not only a central but also a peripheral antiinflammatory effect, which may have an implication for neuroinflammation because systemic inflammation favours the one developing in the brain [52]. Recent findings have indicated that the spleen may play an important role in the peripheral vagal anti-inflammatory effects [54]. There is still a considerable uncertainty, however, on the relative importance of the central *vs* the peripheral cholinergic anti-inflammatory mechanisms. On one hand, activation of central vagal or cholinergic influences [55] have been reported to offer protection against acute ischemic brain injury and counteracts the inflammatory response that follows hemorrhagic stroke. However, in another study central administration of muscarine was ineffective at reducing cerebral oedema in splenectomised rats, suggesting that the spleen, and thus the peripheral mechanism, is key in these processes [56, 57].

### *Baroreflex Modulation of Cerebral Blood Flow*

As CBF is autoregulated across a wide range of blood pressure values (from 50 to 150 mmHg), it seems that the arterial baroreflex may be relatively unimportant for CBF control. Consistent with this notion animal studies using carotid baroreceptor stimulation or baroreceptor denervation protocols have failed to demonstrate any consistent baroreflex modulation of steady state measures of CBF [58]. Nevertheless, Liu *et al.* observed that a high baroreflex sensitivity could delay stroke events and provided evidence in rats that BRS is an independent predictor of stroke in hypertension [59]. Interestingly, impaired baroreflex gain and BRS were reported also in patients who suffered from cardiovascular events (Fig. **2**) [60].

Moreover, at difference with previous studies that analyzed the static component of cerebral autoregulation (CA), there is evidence now that baroreflex modulates the dynamic component of CA, that is, the ability to regulate blood flow against rapidly changing blood pressure values [61]. Baroreflex sensitivity and dynamic CA are in fact inversely related. Therefore subjects with lower baroreflex sensitivity and greater blood pressure variability (BPV) have better dynamic CA (and *vice versa*). This suggests moreover that, in absence of stroke, dynamic CA may adjust over time to optimize CBF control depending on the prevailing level of baroreflex sensitivity or BPV. Such neuroplasticity could explain why spontaneously hypertensive persons with baroreflex impairment and elevated BPV have augmented dynamic CA compared to normotensive controls [62]. However, if such compensatory interactions were not able to take place, as might occur after a stroke, the brain would be rendered more vulnerable to excess variations in blood pressure.

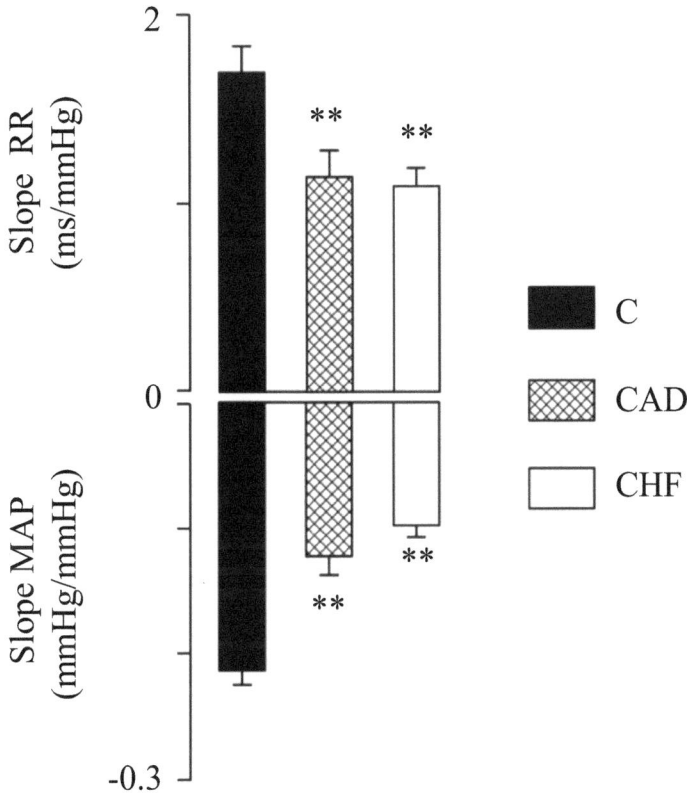

**Fig. (2).** Upper panel: baroreflex sensitivity on heart rate as slope of RR interval increases *versus* the degree of neck suction stimulation (slope RR): lower panel: baroreflex gain as slope of mean arterial pressure decreases *versus* the degree of neck suction stimulation (slope MAP). Average values in 31 congestive heart failure patients (CHF) with reduced left-ventricle ejection fraction, in 29 coronary artery disease patients (CAD) without previous myocardial infarction and with preserved left ventricle ejection fraction, and in 29 matched controls (C); the ** indicates significant differences *versus* controls at $p<0.01$ (from [60] with permission).

A dynamic baroreflex mediated sympathetic modulation of CBF at frequencies greater than 0.05 Hz (or faster than 20 seconds) was also demonstrated [42], confirming the role that the autonomic nervous system exerts on the dynamic component of cerebral blood flow regulation. A CBF modulation by baroreflex was also demonstrated in humans by showing the presence in mean CBF velocity of low frequency oscillations, a marker of sympathetic efferent activity to the vessel dependent on intact baroreflex control, these oscillations in CBF being moreover consistently associated with oscillations in other cardiovascular signals [63]. Two other studies that used repetitive lower-body negative pressure to generate and compare arterial pressure oscillations and CBF velocity oscillations, confirmed the increased transfer function gain and decreased phase shifts suggestive of a deterioration of dynamic blood flow regulation by phentolamine and during ganglion block by trimetaphan [41, 42].

## Autonomic Nervous System and the Risk of Stroke

In the description of autonomic effects on cerebral vessels we have to take into account also the systemic effects (*i.e.* on blood pressure) that an alteration of the activity of the autonomic nervous system produces.

### *Blood Pressure Level, Blood Pressure Variability and Risk of Stroke*

#### *Autonomic Nervous System Dysfunction and the Development of Hypertension*

Hypertension is a well-recognized major risk factor for stroke [64], an increase of BP above the values regarded as epidemiologically optimal (115 mmHg systolic) accounting for no less than two thirds of all cerebrovascular events [65]. It is also well known that the risk of stroke increases progressively with the severity of hypertension and that this is the case for both sexes, in all ethnicities and at all ages [65]. To confirm these observations the National High Blood Pressure Education Program has shown a 70-80% reduction in the morbidity attributable to hypertension, mainly heart attack and stroke [64], the control of hypertension producing a one third decrease in stroke risk for each 10 mmHg decrease in systolic blood pressure [65]. In addition to strokes hypertension contributes to dementia [66]. It is known in fact that hypertension promotes alterations in small arteries and arterioles supplying the deep hemispheric white matter and basal ganglia, resulting in a condition known as small vessel disease whose pathological substrates is arteriolosclerosis [67]. Small vessel disease in turn has been recognized as a major cause of vascular cognitive impairment contributing up to 45% of dementia cases [66].

Crucial to the argument of the present chapter, however, is the evidence that a dysfunction of the autonomic nervous system, *i.e.*, increased sympathetic and decreased parasympathetic activity, is involved in the generation and maintenance of hypertension [4]. In animal models of hypertension both a sympathetic activation and a reduced vagal cardiac and extracardiac tone have been repeatedly found in association with high blood pressure levels [68 - 70]. In humans, similar relationships have been documented with different techniques of quantification of sympathetic (urinary and plasma NE, NE spillover from sympathetic nerve terminals, microneurographic recordings of efferent post ganglionic sympathetic nerve firing, cardiovascular variability) or parasympathetic (overall or restricted heart rate variabilities) nerve activity in virtually all hypertension phenotypes [71 - 76]. For example, an increased sympathetic activity has been observed in individuals with a family history of hypertension [76], in subjects with borderline hypertension [71] and in established hypertension [73]. Sympathetic activity has been shown to increase with the increasing BP levels as well as with the progression of the magnitude and extension of the BP-related damage to target organs [77] with a peak level in patients exhibiting resistance to treatment even when consisting of three or more antihypertensive drugs [78]. A sympathetic activation has been found in young, middle age and elderly patients, including those with a selective increase of systolic BP or isolated systolic hypertension. A parallel reduction of the parasympathetic influences have also been frequently observed [72, 74]. These observations strongly support the conclusion that *via* its role in the determination of BP levels an autonomic nervous dysfunction plays a major role in the determination of the risk of stroke as well.

## *Autonomic Nervous System Dysfunction Alters BP Variability*

In the last three decades the ability to measure BP over the 24 hours has documented that BP undergoes striking variations over the day and night [79]. Evidence has also been obtained that the extent of variations may be markedly different between subjects with an overall increase in hypertension and in aged individuals [80, 81]. Most importantly, studies in spSHRs have shown that an increase of BP variability may cause stroke [82] and that in humans under prolonged invasive or non-invasive BP monitoring BP variability bears a direct relationship with the prevalence and severity of target organ damage, which is higher in subjects in whom the 24-hour BP variability is higher even after adjusting for differences in mean BP [80, 81]. Finally, clinical studies on large number of hypertensive individuals or populations undergoing intermittent ambulatory blood pressure recording have shown increasing values of 24-hour BP variability to be associated with an increased progression of death and cardiovascular events including stroke [83 - 88]. Interestingly this has been found to occur also for more specific BP variability phenomena within the 24 hours, the BP fluctuations occurring from day to night have been shown to predict cardiovascular risk, non-dipping subjects or subjects with rising BP pattern at night being at increased risk of CV events [89] and mortality [90]. An increased morning BP surge on waking from sleep has also been associated with higher incidence of cardiovascular outcomes [89, 91 - 93]. In elderly hypertensive patients the association was particularly clear for silent cerebral infarcts defined by brain magnetic resonance imaging [91, 94]. A higher prevalence of peak BP values during the day has been found to carry a greater cardiovascular risk [95]. In most instances the increased risk persisted after adjusting for the mean BP level and other confounding variables [96] indicating the independent nature of the relationship.

BP variability is importantly modulated by the activity of the autonomic nervous system [79], which mediates both pro and antioscillatory reflex influences. In experimental animals reflex influences from the arterial baroreceptors exert an important buffering action on spontaneous BP variations [97], with baroreflex impairment producing a marked increase (threefold or more) of BP oscillations [98]. The same phenomenon has been observed in man [99] in which the relationship between baroreflex sensitivity and BP variability is so close that an inverse relationship between the two can be documented throughout the 24 hours [100]. However, 24 hour BP variations are known to be determined to a substantial degree by behavioural influences on the cardiovascular system (reduction of BP during sleep, increase during exercise and emotional stimuli, increase by environmental challenges *etc.*), which are largely transmitted *via* sympathetic nerves to the heart and the vasculature. It has been shown in fact that in man 1) sympathetic nerve activity bears a direct relationship with the extent of the BP variations, particularly during the day time period [101] and 2) a decrease of BP variability occurs in patients with an impairment of the autonomic nervous system produced by familial amyloid polyneuropathy [102]. This makes the sympathetic nervous system indirectly responsible also for the adverse role of BP variability on stroke.

## *Autonomic Nervous System Activity and Dynamic Regulation of Cerebral Blood Flow*

It has been shown that both the sympathetic and the parasympathetic nervous system exert a patterned stimulation both at the blood vessels and at the heart giving rise to periodic fluctuations of blood pressure and heart rate. These fluctuations have been observed also in the cerebral blood flow [63]. This is an interesting observation, it seems in fact that a dynamic, rhythmical modulation augments the efficiency of the cardiovascular system. A patterned stimulation is able in fact to increase the acetylcholine and norepinephrine release more than constant frequency stimulation and to evoke at different frequencies different neurotransmitters release [103]. Moreover while oscillations slower than 1 Hz result in cycle of vasoconstriction and vasodilation the amplitude of the oscillations decreases with the increase of the frequency of stimulation. Therefore the vasculature respond to faster frequencies of sympathetic nervous activity with steady tone and to lower frequencies with oscillations. The reduction of these fluctuations or an alteration in the pattern of stimulation could represent therefore a risk factor for future cardiovascular events (for more detailed information see the excellent review by SC Malpas [103]) and could be revealed by simultaneously recording cerebral blood flow, blood pressure, heart rate and respiration.

## Summary

Autonomic nervous system dysfunction is a widespread condition that characterizes both people with hypertension [4, 104], the most important risk factor for stroke, and people with other metabolic (diabetes mellitus overall) or cardiovascular diseases. It has been shown that even mild autonomic nervous system dysfunction is able to increase cardiovascular risk [105 - 107]. As far as the cerebral circulation is concerned, contrary to what previously thought, it is now known that the autonomic nervous system exerts a protective role in pathological conditions such as cerebral ischemia or sudden changes in blood pressure with autonomic dysfunction leading to an increased risk of stroke and to a worse evolution of the stroke itself. Autonomic dysfunction can lead in fact to an increase of the level of blood pressure and to an increase of BPV, to an impaired response of CBF to different challenges with a consequent increase of the wall related stress and vascular damage (Fig. **3**). In this situation it has been observed that cerebral autoregulation of the smaller intraparenchymal arteries becomes more efficient in order to protect the cerebral parenchyma. Later on nevertheless, with the persistence of autonomic nervous system dysfunction, neuro inflammation, endothelial dysfunction and vascular atherosclerosis will affect the arterial wall and this together with the increased vascular stress will produce alterations of the autoregulatory mechanisms and occlusions even of the smaller intraparenchymal arteries (Fig. **3**). It is now clear in fact that the autonomic nervous system plays a crucial and independent role in the genesis of cardiovascular diseases and in their progression. In animal models, beta blockers in fact decreased both stress induced and diet induced atherosclerosis [108]. Therefore autonomic imbalance is much more than a surrogate marker of increased CHD risk [103].

## Methodological Aspects and Future Perspectives

Dynamic changes of CBF and dynamic interactions among CBF, the autonomic nervous system and blood pressure and heart rate changes should be investigated in the future. At this regard variability analysis that has been widely used in cardiology, provided encouraging results in recent studies even in the neurological field. The more studied components of cardiovascular variability are those related to the heart rate. Countless studies demonstrated the influence of autonomic regulation on heart rate variability (HRV), quantified in terms of beat-by-beat changes of the time interval between consecutive R peaks of the electrocardiogram, R-R intervals. The more popular indices of HRV for assessing the autonomic regulation are based on time-domain analysis (like the standard deviation of the beat-to-beat time series) and on frequency-domain analysis. In this latter case, HRV is expressed as spectral powers of specific frequency bands, *i.e.*, a low-frequency (LF, from 0.05 to 0.15 Hz) and a high-frequency (HF, from 0.15 to 0.40 Hz) band [109, 110]. The HF power is considered index of vagal modulations of heart rate, and the ratio between LF and HF powers is considered a reliable measure of the cardiac sympatho/vagal balance [109, 110]. Spectral analysis is also performed on beat-to-beat values of systolic and diastolic blood pressure, being the LF powers of BPV considered to reflect sympathetic modulations of vascular resistances generated by a resonance in the baroreflex loop [111, 112].

Nevertheless, conventional time-domain and frequency-domain measures of cardiovascular variability have some limits when applied to the clinical field and cannot reveal more delicate and subtle changes in cardiovascular dynamics. This picture is changing with the introduction of new measures for assessing aspects not related to the amplitude of the HRV fluctuations, but to their complex dynamics. One of these aspects is related to the "self-similarity" of cardiovascular time series. This means that the original beat-to-beat series can be split into small segments, and these smaller pieces of data may appear similar to the original series, at least in a statistical sense, if plotted at higher time resolution after having properly rescaled their amplitude by means of a scale exponent, $\alpha$. This makes cardiovascular series, like the heart rate, analogous to fractal objects (a geometric fractal can be split into smaller parts and still each fragment looks like the original when enlarged). The scale exponent $\alpha$ characterizes the fractal dynamics and is usually calculated with the "detrended fluctuation analysis" algorithm [113]. This algorithm originally suggested that the heart rate actually has a "bi-fractal" nature, with a short-term exponent $\alpha_1$ (for scales shorter than 12 beats) and a long-term exponent $\alpha_2$ (for scales longer than 12 beats). The cardiac autonomic outflows strongly influence $\alpha_1$, that increases when the sympatho/vagal balance increases [114, 115]. An altered $\alpha_1$ coefficient was associated with dysfunctions of the autonomic cardiovascular control, being predictor of mortality in patients with congestive heart failure or in individuals after acute myocardial infarction [116 - 118].

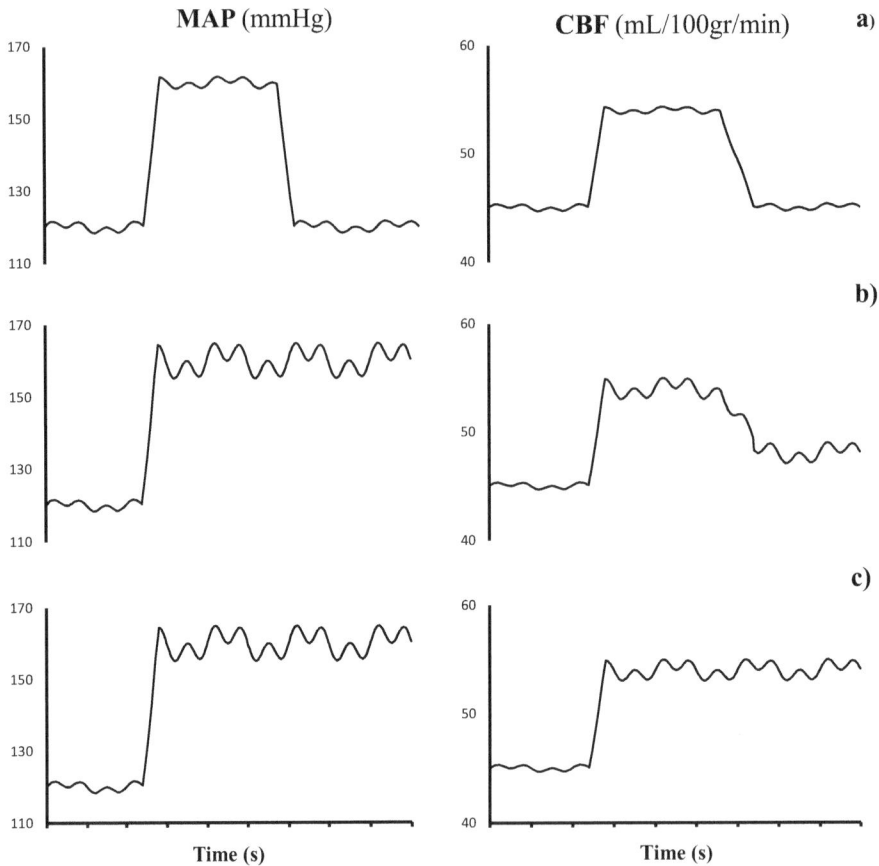

**Fig. (3).** Schematic description of Mean Arterial Pressure (MAP) and Cerebral Blood Flow (CBF) dynamics in different conditions of cardiovascular and cerebrovascular autoregulation. Panels **a)**: increased sympathetic activity with preserved baroreflex function and cerebral flow autoregulation; panels **b)**: increased sympathetic activity with impairment of baroreflex and short lasting impairment of cerebral flow autoregulation; panels **c)**: increased sympathetic activity with long lasting impairment of baroreflex and cerebral flow autoregulation.

Another feature of HRV that can be associated to the autonomic control is the level of "irregularity", quantified by measures of entropy. Actually, the autonomic control acts continuously on the heart rate in response to external stimuli, making the heart rate irregular and unpredictable, thus increasing its entropy. Autonomic dysfunctions are expected to decrease the effects of external stimuli, making the heart rate more regular and predictable, and therefore decreasing its entropy [118]. Measures of HRV entropy obtained with different algorithms confirmed that the autonomic cardiovascular control is a major determinant of entropy [119, 120].

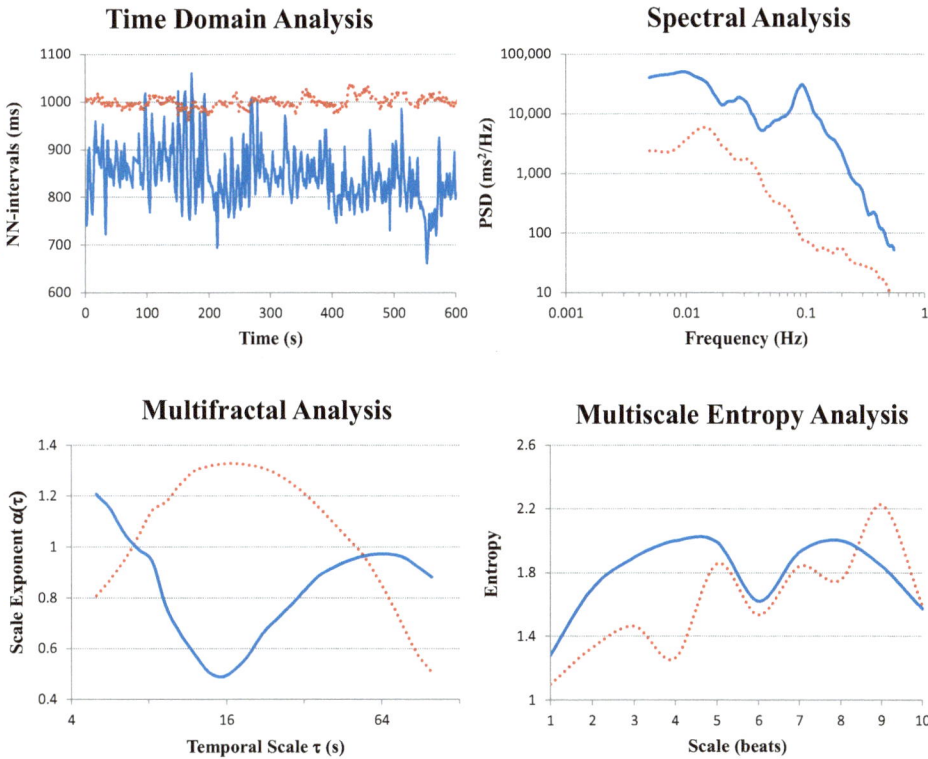

**Fig. (4).** Example of time-domain and frequency-domain analysis (upper panels) and of more advanced complexity-based analysis (lower panels) in a coronary artery disease patient, (CAD, red dotted line), with preserved left ventricular ejection fraction and in a control subject (C, continuous blue line) matched by age and gender. Time domain analysis reveals a dramatic decrease of the overall HRV, as quantified by a lower standard deviation in CAD patient (11.9 ms) than in C (58.8 ms). Spectral analysis shows that the decreased variability in CAD regards a wide band of frequencies and is associated to the disappearance of the 0.1 Hz spectral peak. In addition, multifractal analysis shows that the reduction in variability quantified by the traditional time-domain and spectral methods is accompanied by a complete alteration of the self-similarity profile, being the minimum occurring in C at the scale $\tau$ of 16 s, and equal to $\alpha=0.5$, replaced in CAD by a maximum that reaches the level of $\alpha=1.3$. Furthermore, multiscale entropy points out a decrease of irregularity (low entropy) in CAD compared to C scales shorter than 4 beats.

The more advanced research in these fields are aimed at focusing complexity measures over separate scales or fractal components with the purpose to identify more sensitive indices of autonomic alterations (Fig. **4**). For instance, multiscale entropy [121] can help predict outcomes [122] and appears potential predictor of stroke in evolution [123] in non-atrial fibrillation ischemic stroke patients. Multifractal approaches [115, 124] have been also introduced to describe the superimposition of sympathetic and parasympathetic fractal controls on heart rate [125, 126].

Some complexity measures of HRV have advantages over conventional measures considering risk stratification purposes. These advantages include: less dependency on heart rate, less inter individual and intra individual variation [127, 128], smaller relative changes of individual values over time after myocardial infarction and relatively good comparability of individual values between long-term and short-term electrocardiographic recordings [128].

Variability analysis of cardiovascular signals and dynamic autonomic tasks on the other hand should be performed together with technique that investigate cerebral blood flow distribution like positron emission tomography (PET) with radiolabelled water ($^{15}$O-H$_2$O) or with functional magnetic resonance imaging (fMRI) that maps changes in local blood in response to local neuronal activity (see the excellent review by H.D. Critchley and C.J. Mathias [129]).

## CONCLUSION

New evidences show the importance of the activity of the autonomic nervous system in the dynamic regulation of CBF. This with other observations highlights the role played by the autonomic nervous system in the protection of cerebral parenchyma and the potential damage that could derive from autonomic nervous system dysfunction.

Interventions aimed at improving autonomic function could therefore help to reduce risk of stroke. Different interventions have been shown to improve autonomic function: 1) physical exercise, that has been shown to improve autonomic function, to reduce blood pressure, to reduce the risk of developing heart failure and to improve autonomic function after stroke [130 - 133]; 2) vagal stimulation, that has been shown in a canine model can limit the damage caused by cerebral ischemia [46] and in humans to be able to decrease sympathetic nerve activity and blood pressure levels [134]; 3) Omega 3 dietary supplements, that have been shown to improve autonomic function in coronary and heart failure patients and to reduce arrhythmic risk in post myocardial infarction patients [135 - 138]; 4) body weight reduction [139]; 5) behaviours aimed at reducing psychological stress [140, 141]; 6) pharmacological interventions (beta blockers, Ace inhibitors).

We hope that future studies investigating the dynamic regulation of cerebral blood flow will demonstrate the importance of restoring autonomic function in the prevention of cerebral strokes.

## TAKE HOME MESSAGES

Autonomic nervous system is actively involved in dynamic regulation of cerebral blood flow and exerts a protective role in pathological conditions such as cerebral ischemia or sudden changes in blood pressure. An impairment of the activity of autonomic nervous system therefore can lead to an increased risk of stroke and to a worse evolution of the stroke itself.

## CONFLICT OF INTEREST

The authors confirm that they have no conflict of interest to declare for this publication.

## ACKNOWLEDGEMENTS

Declared none.

## REFERENCE

[1]     Lozano R, Naghavi M, Foreman K, *et al*. Global and regional mortality from 235 causes of death for 20 age groups in 1990 and 2010: a systematic analysis for the Global Burden of Disease Study 2010. Lancet 2012; 380(9859): 2095-128.
[http://dx.doi.org/10.1016/S0140-6736(12)61728-0] [PMID: 23245604]

[2]     Murray CJ, Vos T, Lozano R, *et al*. Disability-adjusted life years (DALYs) for 291 diseases and injuries in 21 regions, 19902010: a systematic analysis for the Global Burden of Disease Study 2010. Lancet 2012; 380(9859): 2197-223.
[http://dx.doi.org/10.1016/S0140-6736(12)61689-4] [PMID: 23245608]

[3]     Johnston SC, Mendis S, Mathers CD. Global variation in stroke burden and mortality: estimates from monitoring, surveillance, and modelling. Lancet Neurol 2009; 8(4): 345-54.
[http://dx.doi.org/10.1016/S1474-4422(09)70023-7] [PMID: 19233730]

[4]     Mancia G, Grassi G. The autonomic nervous system and hypertension. Circ Res 2014; 114(11): 1804-14.
[http://dx.doi.org/10.1161/CIRCRESAHA.114.302524] [PMID: 24855203]

[5]    Hansson GK. How to chew up cells: lessons for the atherosclerotic plaque. Circ Res 2012; 111(6): 669-71.
       [http://dx.doi.org/10.1161/CIRCRESAHA.112.268151] [PMID: 22935531]

[6]    Bevan RD, Tsuru H. Functional and structural changes in the rabbit ear artery after sympathetic denervation. Circ Res 1981; 49(2): 478-85.
       [http://dx.doi.org/10.1161/01.RES.49.2.478] [PMID: 7249283]

[7]    Mangoni AA, Mircoli L, Giannattasio C, Mancia G, Ferrari AU. Effect of sympathectomy on mechanical properties of common carotid and femoral arteries. Hypertension 1997; 30(5): 1085-8.
       [http://dx.doi.org/10.1161/01.HYP.30.5.1085] [PMID: 9369260]

[8]    Dorrance AM, Fink G. Effects of stroke on the autonomic nervous system. Compr Physiol 2015; 5(3): 1241-63.
       [http://dx.doi.org/10.1002/cphy.c140016] [PMID: 26140717]

[9]    Warlow C, Sudlow C, Dennis M, Wardlaw J, Sandercock P. Stroke. Lancet 2003; 362(9391): 1211-24.
       [http://dx.doi.org/10.1016/S0140-6736(03)14544-8] [PMID: 14568745]

[10]   Owman C. Neurogenic control of the vascular system: Focus on cerebral circulation. Handbook of physiology, the nervous system, intrinsic regulatory systems of the brain. Paulson OB: Strandgaard 2011; pp. 225-80.

[11]   Hamel E. Perivascular nerves and the regulation of cerebrovascular tone. J Appl Physiol (1985) 2006 Mar; 100(3): 1059-64.

[12]   Cipolla MJ. The cerebral circulation. San Rafael, CA: Morgan & Claypool Life Sciences 2009.

[13]   Duckworth JW, Wellman GC, Walters CL, Bevan JA. Aminergic histofluorescence and contractile responses to transmural electrical field stimulation and norepinephrine of human middle cerebral arteries obtained promptly after death. Circ Res 1989; 65(2): 316-24.
       [http://dx.doi.org/10.1161/01.RES.65.2.316] [PMID: 2752543]

[14]   Högestätt ED, Andersson KE. On the postjunctional alpha-adrenoreceptors in rat cerebral and mesenteric arteries. J Auton Pharmacol 1984; 4(3): 161-73.
       [http://dx.doi.org/10.1111/j.1474-8673.1984.tb00093.x] [PMID: 6149225]

[15]   Lincoln J. Innervation of cerebral arteries by nerves containing 5-hydroxytryptamine and noradrenaline. Pharmacol Ther 1995; 68(3): 473-501.
       [http://dx.doi.org/10.1016/0163-7258(95)02017-9] [PMID: 8788567]

[16]   Goadsby PJ. Autoregulation and autonomic control of the cerebral circulation: implications and pathophysiology. In: Mathias CJ, Bannister R, Eds. Autonomic failure: A textbook of clinical disorders of the autonomic nervous system. Oxford: OUP Oxford 2015; pp. 169-74.

[17]   Raichle ME, Hartman BK, Eichling JO, Sharpe LG. Central noradrenergic regulation of cerebral blood flow and vascular permeability. Proc Natl Acad Sci USA 1975; 72(9): 3726-30.
       [http://dx.doi.org/10.1073/pnas.72.9.3726] [PMID: 810805]

[18]   ter Laan M, van Dijk JM, Elting JW, Staal MJ, Absalom AR. Sympathetic regulation of cerebral blood flow in humans: a review. Br J Anaesth 2013; 111(3): 361-7.
       [http://dx.doi.org/10.1093/bja/aet122] [PMID: 23616589]

[19]   Lassen NA. Cerebral blood flow and oxygen consumption in man. Physiol Rev 1959; 39(2): 183-238.
       [PMID: 13645234]

[20]   Davis MJ, Hill MA. Signaling mechanisms underlying the vascular myogenic response. Physiol Rev
       1999; 79(2): 387-423.
       [PMID: 10221985]

[21]   Duchemin S, Boily M, Sadekova N, Girouard H. The complex contribution of NOS interneurons in the
       physiology of cerebrovascular regulation. Front Neural Circuits 2012; 6: 51.
       [http://dx.doi.org/10.3389/fncir.2012.00051] [PMID: 22907993]

[22]   Jones SC, Radinsky CR, Furlan AJ, Chyatte D, Perez-Trepichio AD. Cortical NOS inhibition raises
       the lower limit of cerebral blood flow-arterial pressure autoregulation. Am J Physiol 1999; 276(4 Pt 2):
       H1253-62.
       [PMID: 10199850]

[23]   Paulson OB, Strandgaard S, Edvinsson L. Cerebral autoregulation. Cerebrovasc Brain Metab Rev
       1990; 2(2): 161-92.
       [PMID: 2201348]

[24]   Talman WT, Nitschke Dragon D. Neuronal nitric oxide mediates cerebral vasodilatation during acute
       hypertension. Brain Res 2007; 1139: 126-32.
       [http://dx.doi.org/10.1016/j.brainres.2007.01.008] [PMID: 17291465]

[25]   Drummond JC. The lower limit of autoregulation: time to revise our thinking? Anesthesiology 1997;
       86(6): 1431-3.
       [http://dx.doi.org/10.1097/00000542-199706000-00034] [PMID: 9197320]

[26]   Sadoshima S, Busija D, Brody M, Heistad D. Sympathetic nerves protect against stroke in stroke-
       prone hypertensive rats. A preliminary report. Hypertension 1981; 3(3 Pt 2): I124-7.
       [http://dx.doi.org/10.1161/01.HYP.3.3_Pt_2.I124] [PMID: 7262975]

[27]   Sadoshima S, Busija DW, Heistad DD. Mechanisms of protection against stroke in stroke-prone
       spontaneously hypertensive rats. Am J Physiol 1983; 244(3): H406-12.
       [PMID: 6829782]

[28]   Pires PW, Rogers CT, McClain JL, Garver HS, Fink GD, Dorrance AM. Doxycycline, a matrix
       metalloprotease inhibitor, reduces vascular remodeling and damage after cerebral ischemia in stroke-
       prone spontaneously hypertensive rats. Am J Physiol Heart Circ Physiol 2011; 301(1): H87-97.
       [http://dx.doi.org/10.1152/ajpheart.01206.2010] [PMID: 21551278]

[29]   Moskowitz MA, Sharp MC, MacFarlane R. Autonomic and neurohumoral control of cerebral
       circulation. In: Mathias CJ, Bannister R, Eds. Autonomic failure: A textbook of clinical disorders of
       the autonomic nervous system. Oxford: OUP Oxford 2015; pp. 90-6.

[30]   Koketsu N, Moskowitz MA, Kontos HA, Yokota M, Shimizu T. Chronic parasympathetic sectioning
       decreases regional cerebral blood flow during hemorrhagic hypotension and increases infarct size after
       middle cerebral artery occlusion in spontaneously hypertensive rats. J Cereb Blood Flow Metab 1992;
       12(4): 613-20.
       [http://dx.doi.org/10.1038/jcbfm.1992.85] [PMID: 1618940]

[31]   Kano M, Moskowitz MA, Yokota M. Parasympathetic denervation of rat pial vessels significantly increases infarction volume following middle cerebral artery occlusion. J Cereb Blood Flow Metab 1991; 11(4): 628-37.
[http://dx.doi.org/10.1038/jcbfm.1991.114] [PMID: 2050751]

[32]   Hart MN, Heistad DD, Brody MJ. Effect of chronic hypertension and sympathetic denervation on wall/lumen ratio of cerebral vessels. Hypertension 1980; 2(4): 419-23.
[http://dx.doi.org/10.1161/01.HYP.2.4.419] [PMID: 7399625]

[33]   Baumbach GL, Heistad DD, Siems JE. Effect of sympathetic nerves on composition and distensibility of cerebral arterioles in rats. J Physiol 1989; 416: 123-40.
[http://dx.doi.org/10.1113/jphysiol.1989.sp017753] [PMID: 2607446]

[34]   van Lieshout JJ, Secher NH. Point: Counterpoint: Sympathetic activity does/does not influence cerebral blood flow. Point: Sympathetic activity does influence cerebral blood flow. J Appl Physiol (1985) 2008 Oct; 105(4): 1364-6.

[35]   Strandgaard S, Sigurdsson ST. Point:Counterpoint: Sympathetic activity does/does not influence cerebral blood flow. Counterpoint: Sympathetic nerve activity does not influence cerebral blood flow. J Appl Physiol (1985) 2008 Oct; 105(4): 1366-7.

[36]   Jeng JS, Yip PK, Huang SJ, Kao MC. Changes in hemodynamics of the carotid and middle cerebral arteries before and after endoscopic sympathectomy in patients with palmar hyperhidrosis: preliminary results. J Neurosurg 1999; 90(3): 463-7.
[http://dx.doi.org/10.3171/jns.1999.90.3.0463] [PMID: 10067914]

[37]   Shenkin HA, Cabieses F, Van Den Noordt G. The effect of bilateral stellectomy upon the cerebral circulation of man. J Clin Invest 1951; 30(1): 90-3.
[http://dx.doi.org/10.1172/JCI102421] [PMID: 14803562]

[38]   Shenkin HA. Cervical sympathectomy on patients with occlusive cerebrovascular disease. Arch Surg 1969; 98(3): 317-20.
[http://dx.doi.org/10.1001/archsurg.1969.01340090093015] [PMID: 5766278]

[39]   Suzuki J, Iwabuchi T, Hori S. Cervical sympathectomy for cerebral vasospasm after aneurysm rupture. Neurol Med Chir (Tokyo) 1975; 15(pt 1): 41-50.
[http://dx.doi.org/10.2176/nmc.15pt1.41] [PMID: 60719]

[40]   Zhang R, Zuckerman JH, Iwasaki K, Wilson TE, Crandall CG, Levine BD. Autonomic neural control of dynamic cerebral autoregulation in humans. Circulation 2002; 106(14): 1814-20.
[http://dx.doi.org/10.1161/01.CIR.0000031798.07790.FE] [PMID: 12356635]

[41]   Mitsis GD, Zhang R, Levine BD, Tzanalaridou E, Katritsis DG, Marmarelis VZ. Autonomic neural control of cerebral hemodynamics. IEEE Eng Med Biol Mag 2009; 28(6): 54-62.
[http://dx.doi.org/10.1109/MEMB.2009.934908] [PMID: 19914889]

[42]   Hamner JW, Tan CO, Lee K, Cohen MA, Taylor JA. Sympathetic control of the cerebral vasculature in humans. Stroke 2010; 41(1): 102-9.
[http://dx.doi.org/10.1161/STROKEAHA.109.557132] [PMID: 20007920]

[43]   Jordan J, Shannon JR, Diedrich A, *et al.* Interaction of carbon dioxide and sympathetic nervous system activity in the regulation of cerebral perfusion in humans. Hypertension 2000; 36(3): 383-8.

[http://dx.doi.org/10.1161/01.HYP.36.3.383] [PMID: 10988269]

[44]    Zhang R, Crandall CG, Levine BD. Cerebral hemodynamics during the Valsalva maneuver: insights from ganglionic blockade. Stroke 2004; 35(4): 843-7.
[http://dx.doi.org/10.1161/01.STR.0000120309.84666.AE] [PMID: 14976327]

[45]    Suzuki N, Hardebo JE, Kåhrström J, Owman C. Selective electrical stimulation of postganglionic cerebrovascular parasympathetic nerve fibers originating from the sphenopalatine ganglion enhances cortical blood flow in the rat. J Cereb Blood Flow Metab 1990; 10(3): 383-91.
[http://dx.doi.org/10.1038/jcbfm.1990.68] [PMID: 2329125]

[46]    Borsody MK, Yamada C, Bielawski D, *et al.* Effects of noninvasive facial nerve stimulation in the dog middle cerebral artery occlusion model of ischemic stroke. Stroke 2014; 45(4): 1102-7.
[http://dx.doi.org/10.1161/STROKEAHA.113.003243] [PMID: 24549865]

[47]    Heneka MT, OBanion MK. Inflammatory processes in Alzheimers disease. J Neuroimmunol 2007; 184(1-2): 69-91.
[http://dx.doi.org/10.1016/j.jneuroim.2006.11.017] [PMID: 17222916]

[48]    OSullivan JB, Ryan KM, Curtin NM, Harkin A, Connor TJ. Noradrenaline reuptake inhibitors limit neuroinflammation in rat cortex following a systemic inflammatory challenge: implications for depression and neurodegeneration. Int J Neuropsychopharmacol 2009; 12(5): 687-99.
[http://dx.doi.org/10.1017/S146114570800967X] [PMID: 19046481]

[49]    Zec N, Kinney HC. Anatomic relationships of the human nucleus of the solitary tract in the medulla oblongata: a DiI labeling study. Auton Neurosci 2003; 105(2): 131-44.
[http://dx.doi.org/10.1016/S1566-0702(03)00027-4] [PMID: 12798209]

[50]    Manta S, Dong J, Debonnel G, Blier P. Enhancement of the function of rat serotonin and norepinephrine neurons by sustained vagus nerve stimulation. J Psychiatry Neurosci 2009; 34(4): 272-80.
[PMID: 19568478]

[51]    Roosevelt RW, Smith DC, Clough RW, Jensen RA, Browning RA. Increased extracellular concentrations of norepinephrine in cortex and hippocampus following vagus nerve stimulation in the rat. Brain Res 2006; 1119(1): 124-32.
[http://dx.doi.org/10.1016/j.brainres.2006.08.048] [PMID: 16962076]

[52]    Rosas-Ballina M, Tracey KJ. Cholinergic control of inflammation. J Intern Med 2009; 265(6): 663-79.
[http://dx.doi.org/10.1111/j.1365-2796.2009.02098.x] [PMID: 19493060]

[53]    Sloan RP, McCreath H, Tracey KJ, Sidney S, Liu K, Seeman T. RR interval variability is inversely related to inflammatory markers: the CARDIA study. Mol Med 2007; 13(3-4): 178-84.
[PMID: 17592552]

[54]    Huston JM, Ochani M, Rosas-Ballina M, *et al.* Splenectomy inactivates the cholinergic antiinflammatory pathway during lethal endotoxemia and polymicrobial sepsis. J Exp Med 2006; 203(7): 1623-8.
[http://dx.doi.org/10.1084/jem.20052362] [PMID: 16785311]

[55]    Ottani A, Giuliani D, Mioni C, *et al.* Vagus nerve mediates the protective effects of melanocortins against cerebral and systemic damage after ischemic stroke. J Cereb Blood Flow Metab 2009; 29(3):

512-23.
[http://dx.doi.org/10.1038/jcbfm.2008.140] [PMID: 19018269]

[56]    Ay I, Lu J, Ay H, Gregory Sorensen A. Vagus nerve stimulation reduces infarct size in rat focal cerebral ischemia. Neurosci Lett 2009; 459(3): 147-51.
[http://dx.doi.org/10.1016/j.neulet.2009.05.018] [PMID: 19446004]

[57]    Lee ST, Chu K, Jung KH, *et al.* Cholinergic anti-inflammatory pathway in intracerebral hemorrhage. Brain Res 2010; 1309: 164-71.
[http://dx.doi.org/10.1016/j.brainres.2009.10.076] [PMID: 19900419]

[58]    Heistad DD, Marcus ML. Total and regional cerebral blood flow during stimulation of carotid baroreceptors. Stroke 1976; 7(3): 239-43.
[http://dx.doi.org/10.1161/01.STR.7.3.239] [PMID: 942613]

[59]    Liu AJ, Ma XJ, Shen FM, Liu JG, Chen H, Su DF. Arterial baroreflex: a novel target for preventing stroke in rat hypertension. Stroke 2007; 38(6): 1916-23.
[http://dx.doi.org/10.1161/STROKEAHA.106.480061] [PMID: 17446420]

[60]    Radaelli A, Castiglioni P, Balestri G, *et al.* Increased pulse wave velocity and not reduced ejection fraction is associated with impaired baroreflex control of heart rate in congestive heart failure. J Hypertens 2010; 28(9): 1908-12.
[http://dx.doi.org/10.1097/HJH.0b013e32833c2088] [PMID: 20577129]

[61]    Tzeng YC, Lucas SJ, Atkinson G, Willie CK, Ainslie PN. Fundamental relationships between arterial baroreflex sensitivity and dynamic cerebral autoregulation in humans. J Appl Physiol (1985) 2010 May; 108(5): 1162-8.

[62]    Serrador JM, Sorond FA, Vyas M, Gagnon M, Iloputaife ID, Lipsitz LA. Cerebral pressure-flow relations in hypertensive elderly humans: transfer gain in different frequency domains. J Appl Physiol (1985) 2005 Jan; 98(1): 151-9.

[63]    Cencetti S, Lagi A, Cipriani M, Fattorini L, Bandinelli G, Bernardi L. Autonomic control of the cerebral circulation during normal and impaired peripheral circulatory control. Heart 1999; 82(3): 365-72.
[http://dx.doi.org/10.1136/hrt.82.3.365] [PMID: 10455091]

[64]    Moser M, Roccella EJ. The treatment of hypertension: a remarkable success story. J Clin Hypertens (Greenwich) 2013; 15(2): 88-91.
[http://dx.doi.org/10.1111/jch.12033] [PMID: 23339725]

[65]    Lawes CM, Bennett DA, Feigin VL, Rodgers A. Blood pressure and stroke: an overview of published reviews. Stroke 2004; 35(4): 1024.
[PMID: 15053002]

[66]    Gorelick PB, Scuteri A, Black SE, *et al.* Vascular contributions to cognitive impairment and dementia: a statement for healthcare professionals from the American heart association/american stroke association. Stroke 2011; 42(9): 2672-713.
[http://dx.doi.org/10.1161/STR.0b013e3182299496] [PMID: 21778438]

[67]    Faraco G, Iadecola C. Hypertension: a harbinger of stroke and dementia. Hypertension 2013; 62(5): 810-7.

[http://dx.doi.org/10.1161/HYPERTENSIONAHA.113.01063] [PMID: 23980072]

[68]    Folkow B. Physiological aspects of primary hypertension. Physiol Rev 1982; 62(2): 347-504.
        [PMID: 6461865]

[69]    Oparil S. The sympathetic nervous system in clinical and experimental hypertension. Kidney Int 1986;
        30(3): 437-52.
        [http://dx.doi.org/10.1038/ki.1986.204] [PMID: 3537449]

[70]    Mark AL. The sympathetic nervous system in hypertension: a potential long-term regulator of arterial
        pressure. J Hypertens Suppl 1996; 14(5): S159-65.
        [PMID: 9120673]

[71]    Anderson EA, Sinkey CA, Lawton WJ, Mark AL. Elevated sympathetic nerve activity in borderline
        hypertensive humans. Evidence from direct intraneural recordings. Hypertension 1989; 14(2): 177-83.
        [http://dx.doi.org/10.1161/01.HYP.14.2.177] [PMID: 2759678]

[72]    Grassi G, Cattaneo BM, Seravalle G, Lanfranchi A, Mancia G. Baroreflex control of sympathetic
        nerve activity in essential and secondary hypertension. Hypertension 1998; 31(1): 68-72.
        [http://dx.doi.org/10.1161/01.HYP.31.1.68] [PMID: 9449393]

[73]    Grassi G, Seravalle G, Bertinieri G, *et al.* Sympathetic and reflex alterations in systo-diastolic and
        systolic hypertension of the elderly. J Hypertens 2000; 18(5): 587-93.
        [http://dx.doi.org/10.1097/00004872-200018050-00012] [PMID: 10826562]

[74]    Julius S, Randall OS, Esler MD, Kashima T, Ellis C, Bennett J. Altered cardiac responsiveness and
        regulation in the normal cardiac output type of borderline hypertension. Circ Res 1975; 36(6) (Suppl.
        1): 199-207.
        [http://dx.doi.org/10.1161/01.RES.36.6.199] [PMID: 1132080]

[75]    Mancia G, Grassi G, Giannattasio C, Seravalle G. Sympathetic activation in the pathogenesis of
        hypertension and progression of organ damage. Hypertension 1999; 34(4 Pt 2): 724-8.
        [http://dx.doi.org/10.1161/01.HYP.34.4.724] [PMID: 10523349]

[76]    Yamada Y, Miyajima E, Tochikubo O, *et al.* Impaired baroreflex changes in muscle sympathetic nerve
        activity in adolescents who have a family history of essential hypertension. J Hypertens Suppl 1988;
        6(4): S525-8.
        [http://dx.doi.org/10.1097/00004872-198812040-00165] [PMID: 3241250]

[77]    Grassi G, Seravalle G, Quarti-Trevano F, *et al.* Sympathetic and baroreflex cardiovascular control in
        hypertension-related left ventricular dysfunction. Hypertension 2009; 53(2): 205-9.
        [http://dx.doi.org/10.1161/HYPERTENSIONAHA.108.121467] [PMID: 19124679]

[78]    Seravalle GL, Volpe M, Ganz F, *et al.* Neuroadrenergic profile in patients with resistant hypertension:
        9C.03. J Hypertens 2011; 29: e141. [Ref Type].
        [http://dx.doi.org/10.1097/00004872-201106001-00348]

[79]    Parati G, Ochoa JE, Lombardi C, Bilo G. Blood pressure variability: assessment, predictive value, and
        potential as a therapeutic target. Curr Hypertens Rep 2015; 17(4): 537.
        [http://dx.doi.org/10.1007/s11906-015-0537-1] [PMID: 25790801]

[80]    Parati G, Pomidossi G, Albini F, Malaspina D, Mancia G. Relationship of 24-hour blood pressure
        mean and variability to severity of target-organ damage in hypertension. J Hypertens 1987; 5(1): 93-8.

[http://dx.doi.org/10.1097/00004872-198702000-00013] [PMID: 3584967]

[81]    Frattola A, Parati G, Cuspidi C, Albini F, Mancia G. Prognostic value of 24-hour blood pressure variability. J Hypertens 1993; 11(10): 1133-7.
        [http://dx.doi.org/10.1097/00004872-199310000-00019] [PMID: 8258679]

[82]    Miao CY, Xie HH, Zhan LS, Su DF. Blood pressure variability is more important than blood pressure level in determination of end-organ damage in rats. J Hypertens 2006; 24(6): 1125-35.
        [http://dx.doi.org/10.1097/01.hjh.0000226203.57818.88] [PMID: 16685213]

[83]    Mancia G, Parati G, Hennig M, *et al.* Relation between blood pressure variability and carotid artery damage in hypertension: baseline data from the European Lacidipine Study on Atherosclerosis (ELSA). J Hypertens 2001; 19(11): 1981-9.
        [http://dx.doi.org/10.1097/00004872-200111000-00008] [PMID: 11677363]

[84]    Mancia G, Parati G. The role of blood pressure variability in end-organ damage. J Hypertens Suppl 2003; 21(6): S17-23.
        [http://dx.doi.org/10.1097/00004872-200307006-00004] [PMID: 14513947]

[85]    Sega R, Corrao G, Bombelli M, *et al.* Blood pressure variability and organ damage in a general population: results from the PAMELA study (Pressioni Arteriose Monitorate E Loro Associazioni). Hypertension 2002; 39(2 Pt 2): 710-4.
        [http://dx.doi.org/10.1161/hy0202.104376] [PMID: 11882636]

[86]    Tatasciore A, Renda G, Zimarino M, *et al.* Awake systolic blood pressure variability correlates with target-organ damage in hypertensive subjects. Hypertension 2007; 50(2): 325-32.
        [http://dx.doi.org/10.1161/HYPERTENSIONAHA.107.090084] [PMID: 17562971]

[87]    Manios E, Tsagalis G, Tsivgoulis G, *et al.* Time rate of blood pressure variation is associated with impaired renal function in hypertensive patients. J Hypertens 2009; 27(11): 2244-8.
        [http://dx.doi.org/10.1097/HJH.0b013e328330a94f] [PMID: 19644388]

[88]    Sander D, Kukla C, Klingelhöfer J, Winbeck K, Conrad B. Relationship between circadian blood pressure patterns and progression of early carotid atherosclerosis: A 3-year follow-up study. Circulation 2000; 102(13): 1536-41.
        [http://dx.doi.org/10.1161/01.CIR.102.13.1536] [PMID: 11004145]

[89]    Metoki H, Ohkubo T, Kikuya M, *et al.* Prognostic significance for stroke of a morning pressor surge and a nocturnal blood pressure decline: the Ohasama study. Hypertension 2006; 47(2): 149-54.
        [http://dx.doi.org/10.1161/01.HYP.0000198541.12640.0f] [PMID: 16380533]

[90]    Hansen TW, Li Y, Boggia J, Thijs L, Richart T, Staessen JA. Predictive role of the nighttime blood pressure. Hypertension 2011; 57(1): 3-10.
        [http://dx.doi.org/10.1161/HYPERTENSIONAHA.109.133900] [PMID: 21079049]

[91]    Kario K, Pickering TG, Umeda Y, *et al.* Morning surge in blood pressure as a predictor of silent and clinical cerebrovascular disease in elderly hypertensives: a prospective study. Circulation 2003; 107(10): 1401-6.
        [http://dx.doi.org/10.1161/01.CIR.0000056521.67546.AA] [PMID: 12642361]

[92]    Kario K, Ishikawa J, Pickering TG, *et al.* Morning hypertension: the strongest independent risk factor for stroke in elderly hypertensive patients. Hypertens Res 2006; 29(8): 581-7.
        [http://dx.doi.org/10.1291/hypres.29.581] [PMID: 17137213]

[93]    Amici A, Cicconetti P, Sagrafoli C, *et al.* Exaggerated morning blood pressure surge and cardiovascular events. A 5-year longitudinal study in normotensive and well-controlled hypertensive elderly. Arch Gerontol Geriatr 2009; 49(2): e105-9.
[http://dx.doi.org/10.1016/j.archger.2008.10.003] [PMID: 19070375]

[94]    Kario K. Prognosis in relation to blood pressure variability: pro side of the argument. Hypertension 2015; 65(6): 1163-9.
[http://dx.doi.org/10.1161/HYPERTENSIONAHA.115.04800] [PMID: 25916727]

[95]    Rothwell PM, Howard SC, Dolan E, *et al.* Prognostic significance of visit-to-visit variability, maximum systolic blood pressure, and episodic hypertension. Lancet 2010; 375(9718): 895-905.
[http://dx.doi.org/10.1016/S0140-6736(10)60308-X] [PMID: 20226988]

[96]    Pringle E, Phillips C, Thijs L, *et al.* Systolic blood pressure variability as a risk factor for stroke and cardiovascular mortality in the elderly hypertensive population. J Hypertens 2003; 21(12): 2251-7.
[http://dx.doi.org/10.1097/00004872-200312000-00012] [PMID: 14654744]

[97]    Cowley AW Jr, Liard JF, Guyton AC. Role of baroreceptor reflex in daily control of arterial blood pressure and other variables in dogs. Circ Res 1973; 32(5): 564-76.
[http://dx.doi.org/10.1161/01.RES.32.5.564] [PMID: 4713198]

[98]    Ramirez AJ, Bertinieri G, Belli L, *et al.* Reflex control of blood pressure and heart rate by arterial baroreceptors and by cardiopulmonary receptors in the unanaesthetized cat. J Hypertens 1985; 3(4): 327-35.
[http://dx.doi.org/10.1097/00004872-198508000-00004] [PMID: 4045185]

[99]    Ripley RC, Hollifield JW, Nies AS. Sustained hypertension after section of the glossopharyngeal nerve. Am J Med 1977; 62(2): 297-302.
[http://dx.doi.org/10.1016/0002-9343(77)90326-6] [PMID: 835607]

[100]   Mancia G, Parati G, Pomidossi G, Casadei R, Di Rienzo M, Zanchetti A. Arterial baroreflexes and blood pressure and heart rate variabilities in humans. Hypertension 1986; 8(2): 147-53.
[http://dx.doi.org/10.1161/01.HYP.8.2.147] [PMID: 3080371]

[101]   Narkiewicz K, Winnicki M, Schroeder K, *et al.* Relationship between muscle sympathetic nerve activity and diurnal blood pressure profile. Hypertension 2002; 39(1): 168-72.
[http://dx.doi.org/10.1161/hy1201.097302] [PMID: 11799097]

[102]   Carvalho MJ, van Den Meiracker AH, Boomsma F, *et al.* Diurnal blood pressure variation in progressive autonomic failure. Hypertension 2000; 35(4): 892-7.
[http://dx.doi.org/10.1161/01.HYP.35.4.892] [PMID: 10775557]

[103]   Malpas SC. Sympathetic nervous system overactivity and its role in the development of cardiovascular disease. Physiol Rev 2010; 90(2): 513-57.
[http://dx.doi.org/10.1152/physrev.00007.2009] [PMID: 20393193]

[104]   Grassi G, Mark A, Esler M. The sympathetic nervous system alterations in human hypertension. Circ Res 2015; 116(6): 976-90.
[http://dx.doi.org/10.1161/CIRCRESAHA.116.303604] [PMID: 25767284]

[105]   Lahiri MK, Kannankeril PJ, Goldberger JJ. Assessment of autonomic function in cardiovascular

disease: physiological basis and prognostic implications. J Am Coll Cardiol 2008; 51(18): 1725-33.
[http://dx.doi.org/10.1016/j.jacc.2008.01.038] [PMID: 18452777]

[106] Katz A, Liberty IF, Porath A, Ovsyshcher I, Prystowsky EN. A simple bedside test of 1-minute heart rate variability during deep breathing as a prognostic index after myocardial infarction. Am Heart J 1999; 138(1 Pt 1): 32-8.
[http://dx.doi.org/10.1016/S0002-8703(99)70242-5] [PMID: 10385760]

[107] Curtis BM, OKeefe JH Jr. Autonomic tone as a cardiovascular risk factor: the dangers of chronic fight or flight. Mayo Clin Proc 2002; 77(1): 45-54.
[http://dx.doi.org/10.4065/77.1.45] [PMID: 11794458]

[108] Hedblad B, Wikstrand J, Janzon L, Wedel H, Berglund G. Low-dose metoprolol CR/XL and fluvastatin slow progression of carotid intima-media thickness: Main results from the Beta-Blocker Cholesterol-Lowering Asymptomatic Plaque Study (BCAPS). Circulation 2001; 103(13): 1721-6.
[http://dx.doi.org/10.1161/01.CIR.103.13.1721] [PMID: 11282901]

[109] Task Force of the European Society of Cardiology and the North American Society of Pacing and Electrophysiology. Heart rate variability: standards of measurement, physiological interpretation and clinical use Circulation 1996; 93(5): 1043-65.
[http://dx.doi.org/10.1161/01.CIR.93.5.1043] [PMID: 8598068]

[110] Kamath MV, Fallen EL. Power spectral analysis of heart rate variability: a noninvasive signature of cardiac autonomic function. Crit Rev Biomed Eng 1993; 21(3): 245-311.
[PMID: 8243093]

[111] Castiglioni P, Di Rienzo M, Veicsteinas A, Parati G, Merati G. Mechanisms of blood pressure and heart rate variability: an insight from low-level paraplegia. Am J Physiol Regul Integr Comp Physiol 2007; 292(4): R1502-9.
[http://dx.doi.org/10.1152/ajpregu.00273.2006] [PMID: 17122332]

[112] Julien C. The enigma of Mayer waves: Facts and models. Cardiovasc Res 2006; 70(1): 12-21.
[http://dx.doi.org/10.1016/j.cardiores.2005.11.008] [PMID: 16360130]

[113] Peng CK, Havlin S, Stanley HE, Goldberger AL. Quantification of scaling exponents and crossover phenomena in nonstationary heartbeat time series. Chaos 1995; 5(1): 82-7.
[http://dx.doi.org/10.1063/1.166141] [PMID: 11538314]

[114] Tulppo MP, Kiviniemi AM, Hautala AJ, *et al.* Physiological background of the loss of fractal heart rate dynamics. Circulation 2005; 112(3): 314-9.
[http://dx.doi.org/10.1161/CIRCULATIONAHA.104.523712] [PMID: 16009791]

[115] Castiglioni P, Parati G, Di Rienzo M, Carabalona R, Cividjian A, Quintin L. Scale exponents of blood pressure and heart rate during autonomic blockade as assessed by detrended fluctuation analysis. J Physiol 2011; 589(Pt 2): 355-69.
[http://dx.doi.org/10.1113/jphysiol.2010.196428] [PMID: 21115648]

[116] Mäkikallio TH, Huikuri HV, Hintze U, *et al.* Fractal analysis and time- and frequency-domain measures of heart rate variability as predictors of mortality in patients with heart failure. Am J Cardiol 2001; 87(2): 178-82.
[http://dx.doi.org/10.1016/S0002-9149(00)01312-6] [PMID: 11152835]

[117]  Tapanainen JM, Thomsen PE, Køber L, *et al.* Fractal analysis of heart rate variability and mortality after an acute myocardial infarction. Am J Cardiol 2002; 90(4): 347-52.
[http://dx.doi.org/10.1016/S0002-9149(02)02488-8] [PMID: 12161220]

[118]  Sassi R, Cerutti S, Lombardi F, *et al.* Advances in heart rate variability signal analysis: joint position statement by the e-Cardiology ESC Working Group and the European Heart Rhythm Association co-endorsed by the Asia Pacific Heart Rhythm Society. Europace 2015; 17(9): 1341-53.
[http://dx.doi.org/10.1093/europace/euv015] [PMID: 26177817]

[119]  Porta A, Gnecchi-Ruscone T, Tobaldini E, Guzzetti S, Furlan R, Montano N. Progressive decrease of heart period variability entropy-based complexity during graded head-up tilt. J Appl Physiol (1985 ) 2007 Oct; 103(4): 1143-9.

[120]  Porta A, Castiglioni P, Bari V, *et al.* K-nearest-neighbor conditional entropy approach for the assessment of the short-term complexity of cardiovascular control. Physiol Meas 2013; 34(1): 17-33.
[http://dx.doi.org/10.1088/0967-3334/34/1/17] [PMID: 23242201]

[121]  Costa M, Goldberger AL, Peng CK. Multiscale entropy analysis of biological signals. Phys Rev E Stat Nonlin Soft Matter Phys 2005; 71(2 Pt 1): 021906.
[http://dx.doi.org/10.1103/PhysRevE.71.021906] [PMID: 15783351]

[122]  Tang SC, Jen HI, Lin YH, *et al.* Complexity of heart rate variability predicts outcome in intensive care unit admitted patients with acute stroke. J Neurol Neurosurg Psychiatry 2015; 86(1): 95-100.
[http://dx.doi.org/10.1136/jnnp-2014-308389] [PMID: 25053768]

[123]  Chen CH, Huang PW, Tang SC, *et al.* Complexity of heart rate variability can predict stroke-i--evolution in acute ischemic stroke patients. Sci Rep 2015; 5: 17552.
[http://dx.doi.org/10.1038/srep17552] [PMID: 26619945]

[124]  Kantelhardt JW, Zschiegner SA, Koscielny-Bunde E, Bunde A, Havlin S, Stanley HE. Multifractal detrended fluctuation analysis of nonstationary time series. Physica A 2002; 316: 87-114.
[http://dx.doi.org/10.1016/S0378-4371(02)01383-3]

[125]  Gierałtowski J, Hoyer D, Schneider U, Żebrowski JJ. Formation of functional associations across time scales in the fetal autonomic control systema multifractal analysis. Auton Neurosci 2015; 190: 33-9.
[http://dx.doi.org/10.1016/j.autneu.2015.03.007] [PMID: 25892613]

[126]  Makowiec D, Rynkiewicz A, Wdowczyk-Szulc J, Zarczyńska-Buchowiecka M, Gałaska R, Kryszewski S. Aging in autonomic control by multifractal studies of cardiac interbeat intervals in the VLF band. Physiol Meas 2011; 32(10): 1681-99.
[http://dx.doi.org/10.1088/0967-3334/32/10/014] [PMID: 21926460]

[127]  Maestri R, Pinna GD, Porta A, *et al.* Assessing nonlinear properties of heart rate variability from short-term recordings: are these measurements reliable? Physiol Meas 2007; 28(9): 1067-77.
[http://dx.doi.org/10.1088/0967-3334/28/9/008] [PMID: 17827654]

[128]  Perkiömäki JS, Zareba W, Ruta J, *et al.* Fractal and complexity measures of heart rate dynamics after acute myocardial infarction. Am J Cardiol 2001; 88(7): 777-81.
[http://dx.doi.org/10.1016/S0002-9149(01)01851-3] [PMID: 11589848]

[129]  Critchley HD, Mathias CJ. Functional neuroimaging of autonomic control. In: Mathias CJ, Bannister R, Eds. Autonomic failure: A textbook of clinical disorders of the autonomic nervous system. Oxford:

OUP Oxford 2015; pp. 143-68.

[130] Francica JV, Bigongiari A, Mochizuki L, *et al.* Cardiac autonomic dysfunction in chronic stroke women is attenuated after submaximal exercise test, as evaluated by linear and nonlinear analysis. BMC Cardiovasc Disord 2015; 15: 105.
[http://dx.doi.org/10.1186/s12872-015-0099-9] [PMID: 26420632]

[131] Andersen K, Mariosa D, Adami HO, *et al.* Dose-response relationship of total and leisure time physical activity to risk of heart failure: a prospective cohort study. Circ Heart Fail 2014; 7(5): 701-8.
[http://dx.doi.org/10.1161/CIRCHEARTFAILURE.113.001010] [PMID: 25185250]

[132] Coats AJ, Adamopoulos S, Radaelli A, *et al.* Controlled trial of physical training in chronic heart failure. Exercise performance, hemodynamics, ventilation, and autonomic function. Circulation 1992; 85(6): 2119-31.
[http://dx.doi.org/10.1161/01.CIR.85.6.2119] [PMID: 1591831]

[133] Iwane M, Arita M, Tomimoto S, *et al.* Walking 10,000 steps/day or more reduces blood pressure and sympathetic nerve activity in mild essential hypertension. Hypertens Res 2000; 23(6): 573-80.
[http://dx.doi.org/10.1291/hypres.23.573] [PMID: 11131268]

[134] Heusser K, Tank J, Engeli S, *et al.* Carotid baroreceptor stimulation, sympathetic activity, baroreflex function, and blood pressure in hypertensive patients. Hypertension 2010; 55(3): 619-26.
[http://dx.doi.org/10.1161/HYPERTENSIONAHA.109.140665] [PMID: 20101001]

[135] Gruppo Italiano per lo Studio della Sopravvivenza nellInfarto miocardico. Dietary supplementation with n-3 polyunsaturated fatty acids and vitamin E after myocardial infarction: results of the GISSI-Prevenzione trial. Lancet 1999; 354(9177): 447-55.
[http://dx.doi.org/10.1016/S0140-6736(99)07072-5] [PMID: 10465168]

[136] Christensen JH, Gustenhoff P, Korup E, *et al.* Effect of fish oil on heart rate variability in survivors of myocardial infarction: a double blind randomised controlled trial. BMJ 1996; 312(7032): 677-8.
[http://dx.doi.org/10.1136/bmj.312.7032.677] [PMID: 8597736]

[137] Christensen JH, Skou HA, Fog L, *et al.* Marine n-3 fatty acids, wine intake, and heart rate variability in patients referred for coronary angiography. Circulation 2001; 103(5): 651-7.
[http://dx.doi.org/10.1161/01.CIR.103.5.651] [PMID: 11156875]

[138] Radaelli A, Cazzaniga M, Viola A, *et al.* Enhanced baroreceptor control of the cardiovascular system by polyunsaturated Fatty acids in heart failure patients. J Am Coll Cardiol 2006; 48(8): 1600-6.
[http://dx.doi.org/10.1016/j.jacc.2006.05.073] [PMID: 17045894]

[139] Grassi G, Seravalle G, Cattaneo BM, *et al.* Sympathetic activation in obese normotensive subjects. Hypertension 1995; 25(4 Pt 1): 560-3.
[http://dx.doi.org/10.1161/01.HYP.25.4.560] [PMID: 7721398]

[140] Kawachi I, Sparrow D, Vokonas PS, Weiss ST. Decreased heart rate variability in men with phobic anxiety (data from the Normative Aging Study). Am J Cardiol 1995; 75(14): 882-5.
[http://dx.doi.org/10.1016/S0002-9149(99)80680-8] [PMID: 7732994]

[141] Watkins LL, Grossman P, Krishnan R, Sherwood A. Anxiety and vagal control of heart rate. Psychosom Med 1998; 60(4): 498-502.
[http://dx.doi.org/10.1097/00006842-199807000-00018] [PMID: 9710297]

CHAPTER 3

# Stroke and the Immune System: Therapeutic Targeting of Toll-Like Receptors

**Vincenza Sofo[1], Luca Soraci[1], Francesca Maria Salmeri[1], Giulia Soraci[2], Paolo La Spina[3] and Maria Elsa Gambuzza[4,*]**

[1] *Department of Biomedical and Dental Sciences, University of Messina, Messina, Italy*

[2] *University of "La Cattolica Sacro Cuore" Rome, Italy,*

[3] *Department of Clinical and Experimental Medicine, University of Messina, Messina, Italy*

[4] *Ministry of Health, Messina, Italy*

**Abstract:** Local and systemic inflammatory responses have been shown to play an important role in post-stroke damage. Recent studies suggest that the innate immune cells contribute to stroke-induced brain injury by activating an inflammatory response that further increases local ischemic damage. Innate immune signaling, *via* Toll-like receptors (TLRs), has been shown to be involved in several neuropathological processes. This chapter summarizes the current knowledge concerning the involvement of TLRs in acute ischemic brain injury. In particular, the therapeutic role of TLR2 and TLR4 antagonists will be discussed. Moreover, since TLR3 stimulation could play a beneficial role through the production of anti-inflammatory molecules, including I type interferons (IFNs), the potential benefits of TLR3 agonist administration to counteract stroke-related inflammation will be also focused.

**Keywords:** DAMPs, IFNα/β, Immunomodulators TLR-targeting, Inflammatory Responses, Innate Immunity, Ischemia/Reperfusion, Pro-inflammatory Cytokines, Stroke, TLR Agonists/Antagonists, TLRs.

## 1. INTRODUCTION

Brain injury from stroke represents the most common cause of death following

---

[*] **Corresponding author Maria Elsa Gambuzza:** Ministry of Health – Office of Messina, Via T. Cannizzaro, n. 88, 98100, Italy; Tel. +39 0659949384; Cell. 3476499803; Email: me.gambuzza@sanita.it

**Alberto Radaelli, Giuseppe Mancia, Carlo Ferrarese & Simone Beretta (Eds.)**

ischemic heart disease [1, 2], the leading cause of permanent adult physical disability, and the second cause of dementia in adults worldwide [3, 4], despite the considerable variability between countries and regions, partly explained by differences in environmental risk exposure, lifestyle, genetic predisposition, stroke management factors, and different statistical methods used [5]. Strokes is a heterogeneous group of vascular disorders that can be caused both by sudden and focal interruption of cerebral blood, that leads to ischemic brain damage, or by a cerebral vessel rupture, which causes hemorrhagic injury. Ischemic stroke can be thrombotic, when a blood clot, the so-called thrombus, is generated in an artery that supplies blood to the brain, or embolic, when a blood clot travels through the bloodstream to an artery in the brain. Hemorrhagic stroke refers to the two main types of intracerebral and subarachnoid hemorrhage. Despite the progresses made in improving the care of stroke patients, the therapeutic options for acute and post-acute stroke remain limited. Stroke-related focal and systemic inflammation has recently been shown to play an important role in cerebral ischemic and hemorrhagic injury, due to the significant interaction existing between the immune system and nervous system [6, 7]. In addition, systemic inflammatory status at the onset of ischemic or hemorrhagic strokes, has been shown to be a key determinant of mortality and long-term prognosis [7 - 9]. This inflammatory reaction is mediated by various molecules, such as chemokines and pro-inflammatory cytokines [10] produced by several immune cell types, glial cells and neurons [11]. The immune system has been classically divided into innate and adaptive immunity, with distinct roles and functions. In contrast to previous hypotheses considering the CNS as fully isolated from the immune system, most recent studies have shown that the CNS is in dynamic bidirectional communication with the peripheral immune system across the blood–brain barrier (BBB) [12]. As a result of the stroke, the well-balanced interaction between CNS and immune system can be affected, and a few minutes after ischemic events, innate immune responses become active, inducing both beneficial and adverse effects on the disease evolution. In fact they are capable of promoting both necrotic cell clearance (tissue repair), and the initiation and amplification of post-stroke inflammation, that further increases the extent of brain injury [13, 14]. According to Yin and Yang effects of innate immunity, unspecific immune suppression or activation can be harmful, whereas the most promising therapeutic approach could be represented by the specific inhibition of the detrimental effects of the immune response, without affecting the beneficial immune-mediated processes, mainly consisting in tissue regeneration [10]. Therefore, stroke-induced immune responses should be carefully modulated. Taking into consideration the complex events occurring before and post stroke, innate immune response could be manipulated by using immunotherapeutic compounds able to limit the stroke-induced damage and to stimulate repair processes caused by the injury.

## 2. INNATE IMMUNE CELLS AND THEIR REGULATION IN THE CNS

The innate immune system is considered as the first line of host defenses against invading microorganisms, malignant cells, and viruses. Innate defense mechanism is mediated by phagocytes, including basophils, dendritic cells, eosinophils, Langerhans cells, mast cells, monocytes, macrophages, and cytotoxic cells (neutrophils, and NK cells). In addition, most innate immune cells, such as dendritic cells, macrophages, Langerhans cells and B cells, mediate cellular immune responses by acting as antigen presenting cells and also producing cytokines involved in the activation, proliferation and growth of other immune cells. Despite the CNS is considered an immune-privileged site, it is continuously monitored by resident and blood-borne immune cells. Current data show that CNS and immune cells interact with each other in both physiological conditions and pathological events [15, 16]. Immune responses in healthy brain are mediated by resident immune cells, including parenchymal microglia, astrocytes and endothelial cells that contribute to maintain homeostasis and to provide neuronal protection [17 - 23]. Microglia are considered hematopoietic-derived brain-resident macrophages capable of self-renewal without requirement of replenishment, unlike other tissue-specific macrophages, which are initially released from the bone marrow as immature monocytes, also called bone marrow-derived cells (BMDCs), and recruited from the circulation after stroke [25]. Microglia are ramified brain macrophages, capable of responding appropriately to injury signals released by damaged cells through the production and release of cytokines that promote the phagocytic clearance of apoptotic cells and cellular debris and that attract other immune cells to the injury site in a stimulus-dependent way [24]. Pro- and anti-inflammatory cytokines can polarize microglia into two distinct activation states. In the pro-inflammatory status, they produce pro-inflammatory cytokines and show high ability of bacterial phagocytosis and degradation, also mediated by inducible nitric oxide synthase (iNOS) and reactive oxygen species (ROS) release [26]. In anti-inflammatory status, characterized by the release of anti-inflammatory mediators and type I interferons (I IFNs), microglia play a key role in tissue repair and remodeling [27]. However, microglial response can be different according to different stimuli. Following infections, microglial cells can be activated both by bacterial cell wall and viral capsid compounds and by microbial DNA, RNA, ATP, in addition to endogenous stimuli, including danger and stressor signals. Despite neurons, astrocytes, glial cells and microvascular endothelial cells of BBB, together with pericytes and extracellular matrix components, are in close proximity to each other to form a neurovascular unit [28, 29], CNS surveillance is exclusively performed by the innate immune cells, whereas the adaptive responses occur only under specific conditions [30]. In the CNS, innate immune cells constantly communicate each other and with numerous peripheral cell types, through cytokine-mediated mechanisms, in a so-called molecular crosstalk. Whereas in normal conditions the recruitment of BMDC in the CNS represents a marginal event [22, 23, 31], in several neurological conditions, including acute stroke [32], multiple sclerosis [33] and amyotrophic lateral sclerosis [34], this process acquires a more important role, which can be either beneficial or harmful [35].

Cerebral homeostasis allows oxygen and nutrients to be maintained at satisfactory levels [28]. The BBB is a tightly controlled membrane that mechanically separates the CNS from the circulation *via* specialized endothelial cells closely connected each other *via* tight and adherent junctions [36, 37].The BBB prevents therefore blood circulating molecules and peripheral cells from entering the CNS [38, 39]. Moreover, the BBB maintains a homeostatic balance within the CNS microenvironment able to guarantee optimal neuronal functions [40]. In addition, BBB contributes actively to the immune response in the CNS [41] by allowing a constant, although limited, transit of peripheral immune cells [42] and by limiting and controlling the fate of infiltrating cells [43]. Whereas under many circumstances, such as infections, chronic neurodegenerative diseases and acute ischemic/hemorrhagic stroke, the BBB limits the infiltration of peripheral immune cells like neutrophils, eosinophils, T lymphocytes, and monocytes, on the other end resident CNS immune cells attract inflammatory peripheral cells from the circulation and interact with them leading to an enhancement of the inflammatory response [38, 44]. Consequently, innate immune responses can be engaged in the CNS not only by resident microglia and astrocytes, which are innate immune cells resident exclusively in the brain, but also by CNS-infiltrating innate immune cells and other components of the innate immune system [45]. The most important functions of innate immune cells are the recognition and the response to pathogen- and damage-associated molecular patterns (PAMPs and DAMPs).

In many pathological conditions, such as neurodegenerative disorders, infections, and traumas, CNS cells come into contact with small molecular compounds represented by PAMPs or DAMPs [46]. The different PAMP and DAMP classes are recognized by specific pattern recognition receptors (PRRs), expressed either on the cell surface or within distinct intracellular compartments. At present, four different categories of PRR have been identified. These categories include transmembrane proteins such as the Toll-like receptors (TLRs), C-type lectin receptors (CLRs), cytoplasmic proteins, mainly represented by the retinoic acid-inducible gene (RIG)-I-like receptors (RLRs) and NOD-like receptors (NLRs) [47]. Among them, TLRs represent the most important class of PRRs that play a key role in inflammatory responses. Their high expression in CNS cells and their capability of responding to endogenous compounds released by damaged neurons suggest their direct involvement in the modulation of injury-related brain inflammation.

The activation of TLRs expressed on microglia, neurons, and astrocytes leads the CNS innate immune cells to produce specific cytokines that contribute to improve or increase the damage [48].

## 3. TLRS: STRUCTURE, ROLE AND EXPRESSION IN CNS

TLRs are type I transmembrane proteins characterized by an extracellular domain containing leucine-rich repeats (LRRs) and a cytoplasmic tail containing a conserved region called the Toll/IL-1 receptor (TIR) domain. TLRs are expressed on the outer cell membrane, in phagosomal/lysosomal or endosomal/lysosomal compartments and endoplasmic reticulum of many types of both innate immune, and non-immune cells, such as epithelial and endothelial cells [49 - 56]. TLRs recognize highly conserved exogenous and endogenous structural motifs, known as PAMPs, and DAMPs respectively. In contrast to PAMPs, that include different classes of microbial proteins, lipopolysaccharides, glycosaminoglycans, glycoproteins, RNA, and DNA, DAMPs include endogenous ligands, mainly represented by intracellular compounds released from damaged cells, oxidatively modified lipids, heat shock proteins and other soluble mediators, that activate TLR-mediated sterile inflammatory responses in many pathological processes, such as trauma, ischemia, cancer, and other settings of tissue damage [57]. To date, 10 human TLRs have been identified, with TLR1, TLR2, TLR4, TLR5, TLR6, and TLR11 localized on the cell surface, and TLR3, TLR7, TLR8, and TLR9 localized within endosomal/lysosomal compartments. Certain TLRs may require additional co-stimulatory proteins to be activated [57 - 63]. Each TLR can recognize most different compounds, lacking any structural similarity, and can interact with the specific ligands as homo or heterodimers. TLR2 acts as a heterodimer with either TLR1 or TLR6 to sense bacterial compounds, with TLR1/2 dimers to recognize triacylated lipopeptides and TLR2/6 diacylated lipopeptides [64]. Among TLR homodimers, TLR4 is mainly activated by LPS from gram negative bacteria [64], although it is also capable of binding F protein from respiratory syncytial virus and glycerophosphatidylinositol anchors from parasites, TLR5 binds bacterial flagellin, and TLR3 senses double-stranded RNA. TLR7/8 dimers recognize both single-stranded RNA and TLR9 homodimer senses CpG-rich hypomethylated DNA [64].

TLR signaling consists of at least two distinct TLR-mediated signaling pathways, depending on which of the two adapter molecules (MyD88 and TRIF) is involved: the MyD88-dependent pathway, that leads to inflammatory cytokine production, and the MyD88-independent and TRIF-dependent pathways, that is mainly associated with the production of type I IFNα/β [57]. TLR4 signaling occurs *via* both the MyD88 and TRIF-dependent pathways, TLR3 *via* TRIF-dependent pathway, whereas all other TLRs are mediated *via* the MyD88 pathway [57]. In the MyD88 dependent pathway, the TIR domain of TLRs combines with a TIR domain-containing adaptor MyD88 that in turn recruits IL-1 receptor-associated kinase-4 (IRAK-4). IRAK4 is subsequently activated by phosphorylation IRAK-1, that in turn combines with TRAF6, thereby activating the IKK complex and leading to activation of MAP kinases (JNK, p38 MAPK) and NF-κB. The activation of NF-κB triggers the production of pro-inflammatory cytokines, such as TNF-α, IL-1 and IL-12 [57]. In contrast, the MyD88-independent and TRIF-dependent signaling pathway leads to type I IFNs production, as result of IFN-regulatory factor (IRF)3 [65]. Type I IFNα/β, well known for their effects in viral infections, are also capable of counteracting inflammatory responses [66, 67]. In the CNS, multiple TLRs are dynamically expressed in a variety of both infiltrating and resident cell types and their expression profiles differ among the different cells [68 - 72] (Table **1**). Altogether, the TLRs expressed by the CNS immune cells are involved in different processes as induction and modulation of inflammatory response, brain cell injury and degeneration, neurogenesis and regulation of neuronal growth [19, 20, 45, 48, 72 - 76]. They are also involved in defense mechanisms against harmful pathogens and neurotoxic compounds, including "altered self" molecules and apoptotic cells [72]. Human microglia express all TLRs, which together endow the cells with potent inflammatory and/or phagocytic action. In contrast, astrocytes utilize a more limited TLR repertoire [69]. In many neurodegenerative processes, including stroke and Alzheimer's disease, specific TLRs expressed by microglia, astrocytes and oligodendrocytes may indirectly induce neuronal damage through the induction of pro-inflammatory cytokines [77]. Moreover, neurons themselves express a subset of TLRs capable of inducing neuronal degeneration in experimental models of stroke and Alzheimer's disease [77].

The TLRs expressed by the CNS cells may contribute to neuronal plasticity by enhancing neurogenesis. However, the loss of down regulation of TLR signaling, as well as their over stimulation by endogenous ligands, can induce adverse effects, through inflammatory and autoimmune responses. Therefore, the functional outcome of TLR-induced activation of CNS immune cells is the result of a correct balance between protective and harmful effects.

## 4. GENERAL CHARACTERISTICS AND IMMUNOLOGICAL ASPECTS OF STROKE

Stroke is a heterogeneous syndrome caused by the ischemia of the brain, with subsequent tissue damage [78]. The main cause of stroke-induced cell damage is represented by metabolic stress, due to decreased perfusion of resident cells, including neurons, which rapidly die, due to their high energy demand and lack of ATP storage [79, 80]. Both apoptosis and necrosis have been shown to be stroke-related processes, as also supported by *post-mortem* studies [81, 82]. Initial tissue injury induced by the ischemic damage leads to necrotic cell death, whose severity depends on the magnitude and duration of the interruption of blood supply to the brain. Prolonged brain ischemia, characterized by a reduced tissue oxygenation, induces the activation of anaerobic metabolism pathways, that in turn cause a dysfunction of the ATPase-dependent ion transport mechanisms. Consequently, the decrease in ATP level leads to a failure of the ionic pumps, that normally are able to maintain the ionic gradient across the neuronal membrane, and this in turn leads to a massive intracellular and mitochondrial calcium accumulation, elicited also by the formation of holes in the cell membrane, caused by reactive oxygen species (ROS) production [83]. These processes lead to a cell death mechanism defined as excitotoxicity, resulting from calcium-overload neurotoxicity, that induces the activation of enzymes that in turn degrade proteins, membranes and nucleic acids [84]. This leads to swelling and breakdown of cell organelles, irreversible damage of the plasma membrane and necrotic cell degeneration [85]. Necrosis mainly involves neurons, since they have a high metabolic rate and quickly suffer metabolic stress. However, neuronal death can also occur several hours or days after a stroke, through apoptotic pathways. More specifically, many neurons at the periphery of the ischemic region, the so-called "ischemic penumbra", show apoptosis. Both the intrinsic and extrinsic pathways of apoptosis can be triggered by brain ischemia [86, 87]. The intrinsic pathway is initiated by the mitochondrial release of cytochrome c and it appears to be associated to caspase-3 and -9 stimulation, leading to apoptosome formation. The extrinsic pathway is activated by the binding of FasL death ligand to Fas death receptor, leading to stimulation of caspase-8, which in turn causes neuronal apoptosis through the cleavage and activation of caspase-3. Recently, alternative forms of cell death mechanisms, involving newly discovered pathways that differ from apoptosis and/or necrosis, have shown to play an important role in stroke-induced neural damage. One of them is represented by the "necroptosis", a programmed form of necrosis, also described as a non-apoptotic "cellular suicide", occurring through a caspase-independent mechanism induced in response to pro-inflammatory compounds, such as TNF-α or Fas ligands [88]. A further type of death occurring in cerebral ischemia is represented by the autophagy, despite its role in ischemic neurons remains controversial [89, 90]. In addition to direct stroke-related insults occurring in the neuronal tissues closer to focal ischemia, increasing evidence shows that the cells of the surrounding penumbra are exposed to endogenous compounds originated from apoptotic or necrotic dying cells [91 - 93]. In this area, a potentially severe inflammatory environment is generated, mainly induced by reactive microglia and also enhanced by ROS generation, which further enhances inflammatory cytokine secretion [94]. Microglia activation induces inflammatory chemokine and cytokine production, including TNF-α [95] and interleukins [96]. In addition, an up-regulation of TNF-α receptor has been observed [97], suggesting that the production of TNF-α can act in an autocrine manner. The exact role played by TNF-α in the stroke-related damage is uncertain, since some studies have shown that it contributes to activate microglia, that in turn act protecting neurons from damage [98], whereas other studies have shown that an overexpression of TNF-α is detrimental to stroke outcome [99]. In an observational study, patients with chronic stroke treated with intrathecal administration of a TNF inhibitor showed neurological improvement [100], but this study seems to have methodological limitations that affect its validity [101]. However, the timing and the degree of inflammatory cytokine expression are important determinants of stroke outcome. In addition, further studies are needed to better characterize the effects of reducing the biological activities of pro-inflammatory cytokines, including IL-1 and TNF, by means of different and highly specific strategies involving the administration of neutralizing antibodies, soluble receptors, antagonist receptors, and protease inhibitors.

The initial stroke-induced neuroinflammation appears to be responsible for the disruption of BBB and for the peripheral immune cell recruitment, with a further production of inflammatory mediators that lead to a secondary ischemic brain damage, mainly characterized by cerebral edema, microvascular stasis, hypoperfusion and post-ischemic inflammation [102, 103]. This secondary ischemic brain damage, therefore, occurs mainly during restoration of blood flow by thrombolysis or mechanical recanalization [104], and it is mainly caused by peripheral immune cells that infiltrate the brain and that further amplify the inflammatory cascade [105]. Experimental stroke models support this hypothesis, showing how blocking the inflammatory cascade improves stroke outcome [106, 107]. Altogether, post-stroke events, including mainly post-ischemic inflammatory responses, that inhibit neuronal recovery [108, 109] and contribute to excitotoxicity, can lead to larger infarcts [110]. For up to 3 weeks after stroke also autoimmune responses can be induced, as shown by the detection of antibodies directed against brain antigens [111 - 114]. These autoimmune responses have shown a detrimental effect in murine models of experimental stroke [115, 116]. Both CNS and peripheral innate immune responses are activated by TLR-mediated pathways. Immediately following the infarct and neuronal damage, several DAMPs, including intracellular components, as well as hyaluronic acid [117, 118] and various HSPs [119, 120], are released by damaged cells. DAMPs are detected during the recovery phase of stroke by innate immune receptors, such as TLRs, also expressed by resident immune cells, like microglia, which in turn recruit others immune cells through the production of inflammatory mediators [121]. However, despite this, activated microglia represent also a major source of anti-inflammatory cytokines, like IL-10 and INF-β [122]. Neutrophils and macrophages reach the damaged tissue respectively within minutes and 24 h following brain ischemia, and remain for up to 15 days [123]. These immune cells show an enhanced phagocytic activity and potential capability of clearing cellular debris, further triggering inflammatory responses [124, 125]. Despite their dual action, their detrimental functions have shown to outweigh the beneficial effects [126, 127]. The recruitment of T cells appears to be a double edged sword, since cytotoxic T cells are capable of attacking both damaged and healthy cells, increasing then the infarct size. Moreover T helper 1 (Th1) cells further enhance inflammatory responses, through production of IL-2, IL-12, TNF-α and IFN-γ [128]. Th-2 and T-regs cells appear to play a beneficial role through the release of anti-inflammatory cytokines, including IL-10, able to reduce stroke-related injury [129 - 131].

**Table 1. Expression of TLR family members in CNS cells.**

| TLR expression | Microglia | Neurons | Astrocytes | Oligodendrocytes |
|---|---|---|---|---|
| TLR1 | + | - | - | - |
| TLR2 | + | - | + | + |
| TLR3 | + | + | + | + |
| TLR4 | + | - | - | - |
| TLR5 | + | - | - | - |
| TLR6 | + | - | - | - |
| TLR7 | + | + | - | - |
| TLR8 | + | + | - | - |
| TLR9 | + | + | + | - |

The symbol "+" indicates TLR expression; the "-" indicates lack of TLR expression.

Microglia express all TLRs identified to date, whereas astrocytes, oligodendrocytes and neurons express a more limited TLR repertoire in comparison.

## 5. ROLE OF TLRS IN ISCHEMIC EVENTS

Many studies have shown the direct involvement of specific TLRs, such as TLR2 and TLR4, in inflammation-induced deleterious effects during ischemia/reperfusion events associated with trauma and stroke. Cerebral ischemia leads to the release of several classes of DAMPs, that in turn induce the activation of specific TLRs expressed by microglia and astrocytes, and the production of pro-inflammatory cytokines that contribute to BBB disruption, with consequent recruitment of peripheral immune cells in the CNS [132]. During the focal cerebral ischemia, TLR2 protein appears to be up regulated in endothelial cells, neurons, and astrocytes, where it induces the release of pro-inflammatory and pro-apoptotic compounds, that contribute to the ischemic damage. In addition, TLR2 has been recently shown to mediate the recruitment of leukocyte and microglia in the site of ischemic damage, further promoting the neuronal death [132, 133], as also confirmed by results obtained by TLR2 inhibition "*in vivo*", that improves neuronal survival [132]. In a similar way, TLR4, that in cerebral ischemia is up regulated [74, 133], enhances the severity of ischemia-induced neuronal damage, by increasing neuroinflammation through the production of TNF-α and IL-6 [134 - 137] in addition to iNOS, COX2 and IFN-γ [138, 139]. Moreover, myeloid dendritic cells, activated by the endogenous TLR4 ligands represented by proteins 8 and 14 released by activated phagocytes, increase the recruitment of infiltrating myeloid cells and contribute to the maintenance of inflammation [133]. Among recruited immune cells, neutrophils and monocyte/macrophages play an important role, mainly mediated by TLR4 expression, as demonstrated by recent studies showing in TLR4-deficient mice a marked reduction of peri-hematoma inflammation [133]. Therefore, inhibition of TLR2 and TLR4, that have been shown to play a deleterious effect in stroke events, represents a promising therapeutic approach. TLR8 activation also shows detrimental effects due to enhancement of apoptotic and inflammatory responses after stroke, mainly mediated by T cells [140]. TLR8 stimulation has shown to enhance ischemic brain injury, and TLR8 up regulation in peripheral immune cells of patients affected by ischemic stroke appears to be significantly correlated with the prognosis of the patients [141], confirming the direct involvement of TLR8 in the inflammatory damage caused by cerebral ischemia and hypoxia.

In contrast, TLR3, located in intracellular endosomes, seems to play a beneficial role in counteracting inflammatory and autoimmune stroke-related responses. TLR3 is activated by double-stranded RNA (dsRNA) that can also result from endogenous products released by apoptotic and necrotic cells [142]. TLR3 has shown to be expressed at high levels by astrocytes and antigen-presenting cells, including dendritic cells, mast cells, monocytes, natural killer cells, and other immune cells, in addition to CNS immune cells, such as endothelial cells, neurons, microglia, astrocytes and oligodendrocytes [143]. TLR3-mediated signaling predominantly activates IRF3 to stimulate type I IFN production [67, 142]. Recent studies have shown that the pretreatment of mice with specific TLR3 ligands can reduce infarct volume following cerebral ischemia-reperfusion damage [144, 145]. TLR3 activation promote the release of a number of cytokines, including type I IFNs, which in addition to anti-viral properties, exhibits anti-inflammatory properties able to counteract the pro-inflammatory effects induced by TLR2 and TLR4 [146]. Nevertheless exaggerated or persistent

I IFN production in the CNS can induce the progression of neurodegenerative diseases [147].

## 6. TLR TARGETING AS A PROMISING THERAPY IN CEREBRAL ISCHEMIA

The expanding knowledge concerning the role of TLRs in neuroinflammatory events led to new potential therapeutic approaches based on TLR modulation [148]. Stroke-induced brain injury is further enhanced by the release of DAMPs, which activate TLRs, inducing a strong inflammatory response that in turn increases the neuronal damage. Among the different TLR antagonists developed by pharmaceutical companies, the most known are anti-TLR humanized and recombinant antibodies. Among these, the class of recombinant nanobodies, consisting in antigen-specific, single-domain, variable fragments of camelid heavy chain-only antibodies (VHH-based single variable domains) with very long complementarity-determining regions 3 (CDR3), have shown to be capable of inhibiting efficiently different protein antigens. Due to their small size (12 to 15 kDa), nanobodies have several additional advantages, compared to conventional antibodies, including their extreme stability towards changes in temperature and chemical environments, and resistance to extreme pH levels. Because of their reduced size, nanobodies can penetrate tissues and cells faster than the conventional antibodies, being also capable of crossing the BBB [149]. Other TLR antagonists are represented by mimetic molecules with short aminoacid sequences, able to prevent the interaction of prototype proteins with their partners. Among these, specific "decoy peptides" have shown to block selectively TLR signaling pathways, by the inhibition of TIR-TIR interactions *via* structural mimicry, due to three-dimensional fold similarities with TIR structures of specific TLRs [150]. Mimetic TLR inhibitors have been also developed to prevent homo- or hetero-dimerization of TLRs. Antagonistic molecules directed against intracellular TLRs are mainly represented by single-stranded DNA or RNA molecules. Among these, the aptamers, obtained by "*in vitro*" selection processes from pools of random oligonucleotide sequences, are capable of binding a wide range of antigens of biomedical interest with high grade of affinity and specificity also comparable to conventional antibodies. In particular, the aptamers obtained using immunoprecipitation strategy together with exponential enrichment

(SELEX) appear to selectively inhibit endosomal TLR-mediated pathways responsible for inappropriate or excessive inflammation [151, 152]. More recently, small RNA-selective interference compounds have been obtained by using predictive modeling methods [153] that represent important approaches allowing to obtain also interference RNA-based TLR modulators [154]. Altogether, the highly specific activation or inhibition of TLR responses with small TLR-targeting compounds represents an innovative and attractive approach in stroke therapy.

Since TLR3 stimulation has been shown to counteract neuroinflammation through the production of endogenous IFNβ, which has been shown to prevent inflammation and demyelination and to have also a neuroprotective activity, the administration of TLR3 agonists could represent the most promising immunotherapeutic TLR-targeting approach in stroke therapy [155]. The utilization of dsRNA with a minimum size of at least 50 base pairs, that has been shown to selectively activate the production of IFNs [156, 157], could therefore represent a new therapeutic option.

## CONCLUSION AND FUTURE DIRECTIONS

Despite several therapies have been proposed to counteract neuroinflammation following both hemorrhagic and ischemic strokes, none of them has been definitely proved to be effective. The strong TLR-mediated inflammatory response appears to worsen the course of the disease. Therefore, a selective inhibition of specific TLRs, such as TLR2 and TLR4, could represent a promising approach to prevent the progression of stroke-related damage. In contrast, TLR3 stimulation could improve stroke prognosis, because of its ability to enhance anti-inflammatory responses. Consequently, the modulation of specific TLR-mediated pathways, by using small molecules acting as TLR-agonists/antagonists, might represent an alternative and attractive approach in stroke therapy. A more comprehensive understanding about the role of the TLR signaling will allow to discover other potential targets for immunotherapy. TLRs are important modulators of the ischemic tolerance phenotype, as shown by TLR preconditioning studies with TLR ligands that are able to reduce cerebral ischemic injury [158]. More specifically, it has been shown that the inhibition of the

TLR4/NF-κB signaling pathway and the enhancement of the IRF-dependent signaling result in TLR ischemic tolerance. These studies suggest that ischemic tolerance mediated by TLRs represents an important target for the prevention and treatment of cerebral ischemia. In addition, other studies have shown that also ischemic post-conditioning with low doses of specific TLR ligands after cerebral ischemia can produce a protective effect [158]. Further studies on TLR ischemic tolerance will contribute to upgrade the development of next-generation therapeutic molecules.

## TAKE HOME MESSAGE:

Inflammation is a classical hallmark of stroke. Innate immune responses can promote or inhibit stroke-related damage. Manipulating TLR-mediated innate immune responses can counteract stroke-related inflammation. A deeper understanding of the role played by the TLR signaling in stroke events is essential for the development of new therapeutic options.

## CONFLICT OF INTEREST

The authors confirm that the author have no conflict of interest to declare for this publication.

## ACKNOWLEDGEMENTS

Declared none.

## REFERENCES

[1]     Chang KC, Lee HC, Tseng MC, Huang YC. Three-year survival after first-ever ischemic stroke is predicted by initial stroke severity: A hospital-based study. Clin Neurol Neurosurg 2010; 112(4): 296-301.
[http://dx.doi.org/10.1016/j.clineuro.2009.12.016] [PMID: 20106589]

[2]     Machado MF, Brucki SM, Nogueira CF, Rocha MS. Infectious disease is the most common cause of death among stroke patients: two-years of follow-up. Arq Neuropsiquiatr 2013; 71(6): 371-5.
[http://dx.doi.org/10.1590/0004-282X20130041] [PMID: 23828522]

[3]     Macrez R, Ali C, Toutirais O, *et al.* Stroke and the immune system: from pathophysiology to new therapeutic strategies. Lancet Neurol 2011; 10(5): 471-80.
[http://dx.doi.org/10.1016/S1474-4422(11)70066-7] [PMID: 21511199]

[4]     Jiang Y, Wei N, Lu T, Zhu J, Xu G, Liu X. Intranasal brain-derived neurotrophic factor protects brain

from ischemic insult *via* modulating local inflammation in rats. Neuroscience 2011; 172: 398-405.
[http://dx.doi.org/10.1016/j.neuroscience.2010.10.054] [PMID: 21034794]

[5]     Thrift AG, Cadilhac DA, Thayabaranathan T, *et al.* Global stroke statistics. Int J Stroke 2014; 9(1): 6-18.
[http://dx.doi.org/10.1111/ijs.12245] [PMID: 24350870]

[6]     Lopez AD, Mathers CD, Ezzati M, Jamison DT, Murray CJ. Global and regional burden of disease and risk factors, 2001: systematic analysis of population health data. Lancet 2006; 367(9524): 1747-57.
[http://dx.doi.org/10.1016/S0140-6736(06)68770-9] [PMID: 16731270]

[7]     McColl BW, Allan SM, Rothwell NJ. Systemic infection, inflammation and acute ischemic stroke. Neuroscience 2009; 158(3): 1049-61.
[http://dx.doi.org/10.1016/j.neuroscience.2008.08.019] [PMID: 18789376]

[8]     Lee Y, Lee S-R, Choi SS, Yeo H-G, Chang K-T, Lee HJ. Therapeutically targeting neuroinflammation and microglia after acute ischemic stroke. BioMed Res Intern Ed 2014; 9.
[http://dx.doi.org/10.1155/2014/297241]

[9]     Emsley HC, Hopkins SJ. Acute ischaemic stroke and infection: recent and emerging concepts. Lancet Neurol 2008; 7(4): 341-53.
[http://dx.doi.org/10.1016/S1474-4422(08)70061-9] [PMID: 18339349]

[10]    Xu X, Jiang Y. The Yin and Yang of innate immunity in stroke. BioMed Res Intern Review 2014; 8.
[http://dx.doi.org/10.1155/2014/807978]

[11]    Sairanen T, Carpén O, Karjalainen-Lindsberg ML, *et al.* Evolution of cerebral tumor necrosis factor-alpha production during human ischemic stroke. Stroke 2001; 32(8): 1750-8.
[http://dx.doi.org/10.1161/01.STR.32.8.1750] [PMID: 11486101]

[12]    Chamorro Á, Meisel A, Planas AM, Urra X, van de Beek D, Veltkamp R. The immunology of acute stroke. Nat Rev Neurol 2012; 8(7): 401-10.
[http://dx.doi.org/10.1038/nrneurol.2012.98] [PMID: 22664787]

[13]    Downes CE, Crack PJ. Neural injury following stroke: are Toll-like receptors the link between the immune system and the CNS? Br J Pharmacol 2010; 160(8): 1872-88.
[http://dx.doi.org/10.1111/j.1476-5381.2010.00864.x] [PMID: 20649586]

[14]    Yenari MA, Kauppinen TM, Swanson RA. Microglial activation in stroke: therapeutic targets. Neurotherapeutics 2010; 7(4): 378-91.
[http://dx.doi.org/10.1016/j.nurt.2010.07.005] [PMID: 20880502]

[15]    Huber AK, Duncker PC, Irani DN. Immune responses to non-tumor antigens in the central nervous system. Front Oncol 2014; 4: 328. [Review].
[http://dx.doi.org/10.3389/fonc.2014.00328] [PMID: 25431758]

[16]    Banks WA. The blood-brain barrier in neuroimmunology: Tales of separation and assimilation. Brain Behav Immun 2015; 44: 1-8.
[http://dx.doi.org/10.1016/j.bbi.2014.08.007] [PMID: 25172555]

[17]    Shastri A, Bonifati DM, Kishore U. Innate immunity and neuroinflammation. Mediators Inflamm 2013; 2013: 342931.
[http://dx.doi.org/10.1155/2013/342931]

[18]    Brenu EW, Staines DR, Baskurt OK, *et al.* Immune and hemorheological changes in chronic fatigue syndrome. J Transl Med 2010; 8: 1.
[http://dx.doi.org/10.1186/1479-5876-8-1] [PMID: 20064266]

[19]    Olson JK, Miller SD. Microglia initiate central nervous system innate and adaptive immune responses through multiple TLRs. J Immunol 2004; 173(6): 3916-24.
[http://dx.doi.org/10.4049/jimmunol.173.6.3916] [PMID: 15356140]

[20]    Bowman CC, Rasley A, Tranguch SL, Marriott I. Cultured astrocytes express toll-like receptors for bacterial products. Glia 2003; 43(3): 281-91.
[http://dx.doi.org/10.1002/glia.10256] [PMID: 12898707]

[21]    Peterson PK. Neuroinflammation and neurodegeneration. New York: Springer 2014.
[http://dx.doi.org/10.1007/978-1-4939-1071-7]

[22]    Lampron A, Elali A, Rivest S. Innate immunity in the CNS: redefining the relationship between the CNS and Its environment. Neuron 2013; 78(2): 214-32.
[http://dx.doi.org/10.1016/j.neuron.2013.04.005] [PMID: 23622060]

[23]    Lampron A, Pimentel-Coelho PM, Rivest S. Migration of bone marrow-derived cells into the central nervous system in models of neurodegeneration. J Comp Neurol 2013; 521(17): 3863-76.
[http://dx.doi.org/10.1002/cne.23463] [PMID: 23682015]

[24]    Soulet D, Rivest S. Microglia. Curr Biol 2008; 18(12): R506-8. b
[http://dx.doi.org/10.1016/j.cub.2008.04.047] [PMID: 18579087]

[25]    Selvarai UM, Ortega SB, Hu R. Preconditioning-induced CXCL12 upregulation minimizes leukocyte infiltration after stroke in ischemia-tolerant mice. J Cereb Blood Flow Metab 2016; pii: 0271678X16639327.
[http://dx.doi.org/10.1177/0271678X16639327] [PMID: 27006446]

[26]    Martinez FO, Sica A, Mantovani A, Locati M. Macrophage activation and polarization. Front Biosci 2008; 13: 453-61.
[http://dx.doi.org/10.2741/2692] [PMID: 17981560]

[27]    Boche D, Perry VH, Nicoll JA. Review: activation patterns of microglia and their identification in the human brain. Neuropathol Appl Neurobiol 2013; 39(1): 3-18. [Review].
[http://dx.doi.org/10.1111/nan.12011] [PMID: 23252647]

[28]    Muoio V, Persson PB, Sendeski MM. The neurovascular unit - concept review. Acta Physiol (Oxf) 2014; 210(4): 790-8.
[http://dx.doi.org/10.1111/apha.12250] [PMID: 24629161]

[29]    Zlokovic BV. The blood-brain barrier in health and chronic neurodegenerative disorders. Neuron 2008; 57(2): 178-201.
[http://dx.doi.org/10.1016/j.neuron.2008.01.003] [PMID: 18215617]

[30]    Rivest S. Regulation of innate immune responses in the brain. Nat Rev Immunol 2009; 9(6): 429-39. [Review].
[http://dx.doi.org/10.1038/nri2565] [PMID: 19461673]

[31]    Simard AR, Rivest S. Neuroprotective effects of resident microglia following acute brain injury. J Comp Neurol 2007; 504(6): 716-29.

[http://dx.doi.org/10.1002/cne.21469] [PMID: 17722035]

[32]  Schilling M, Strecker JK, Schäbitz WR, Ringelstein EB, Kiefer R. Effects of monocyte chemoattractant protein 1 on blood-borne cell recruitment after transient focal cerebral ischemia in mice. Neuroscience 2009; 161(3): 806-12.
[http://dx.doi.org/10.1016/j.neuroscience.2009.04.025] [PMID: 19374937]

[33]  Floris S, van der Goes A, Killestein J, *et al.* Monocyte activation and disease activity in multiple sclerosis. A longitudinal analysis of serum MRP8/14 levels. J Neuroimmunol 2004; 148(1-2): 172-7.
[http://dx.doi.org/10.1016/j.jneuroim.2003.11.005] [PMID: 14975598]

[34]  Vaknin I, Kunis G, Miller O, *et al.* Excess circulating alternatively activated myeloid (M2) cells accelerate ALS progression while inhibiting experimental autoimmune encephalomyelitis. PLoS One 2011; 6(11): e26921.
[http://dx.doi.org/10.1371/journal.pone.0026921] [PMID: 22073221]

[35]  Shechter R, Schwartz M. CNS sterile injury: just another wound healing? Trends Mol Med 2013; 19(3): 135-43.
[http://dx.doi.org/10.1016/j.molmed.2012.11.007] [PMID: 23279948]

[36]  Hermann DM, ElAli A. The abluminal endothelial membrane in neurovascular remodeling in health and disease. Sci Signal 2012; 5(236): re4. [Review].
[http://dx.doi.org/10.1126/scisignal.2002886] [PMID: 22871611]

[37]  Hawkins BT, Davis TP. The blood-brain barrier/neurovascular unit in health and disease. Pharmacol Rev 2005; 57(2): 173-85. [Review].
[http://dx.doi.org/10.1124/pr.57.2.4] [PMID: 15914466]

[38]  Wilson EH, Weninger W, Hunter CA. Trafficking of immune cells in the central nervous system. J Clin Invest 2010; 120(5): 1368-79.
[http://dx.doi.org/10.1172/JCI41911] [PMID: 20440079]

[39]  Pardridge WM. Blood-brain barrier drug targeting: the future of brain drug development. Mol Interv 2003; 3(2): 90-105, 51. [Review].
[http://dx.doi.org/10.1124/mi.3.2.90] [PMID: 14993430]

[40]  ElAli A, Thériault P, Rivest S. The role of pericytes in neurovascular unit remodeling in brain disorders. Int J Mol Sci 2014; 15(4): 6453-74.
[http://dx.doi.org/10.3390/ijms15046453] [PMID: 24743889]

[41]  Muldoon LL, Alvarez JI, Begley DJ, *et al.* Immunologic privilege in the central nervous system and the blood-brain barrier. J Cereb Blood Flow Metab 2013; 33(1): 13-21.
[http://dx.doi.org/10.1038/jcbfm.2012.153] [PMID: 23072749]

[42]  Carson MJ, Doose JM, Melchior B, Schmid CD, Ploix CC. CNS immune privilege: hiding in plain sight. Immunol Rev 2006; 213: 48-65.
[http://dx.doi.org/10.1111/j.1600-065X.2006.00441.x] [PMID: 16972896]

[43]  Ifergan I, Kébir H, Bernard M, *et al.* The blood-brain barrier induces differentiation of migrating monocytes into Th17-polarizing dendritic cells. Brain 2008; 131(Pt 3): 785-99.
[http://dx.doi.org/10.1093/brain/awm295] [PMID: 18156156]

[44]  Jin R, Yang G, Li G. Inflammatory mechanisms in ischemic stroke: role of inflammatory cells. J

Leukoc Biol 2010; 87(5): 779-89.
[http://dx.doi.org/10.1189/jlb.1109766] [PMID: 20130219]

[45]   Ransohoff RM, Brown MA. Innate immunity in the central nervous system. J Clin Invest 2012; 122(4): 1164-71.
[http://dx.doi.org/10.1172/JCI58644] [PMID: 22466658]

[46]   Kumar H, Kawai T, Akira S. Pathogen recognition by the innate immune system. Int Rev Immunol 2011; 30(1): 16-34. [Review].
[http://dx.doi.org/10.3109/08830185.2010.529976] [PMID: 21235323]

[47]   Kigerl KA, de Rivero Vaccari JP, Dietrich WD, Popovich PG, Keane RW. Pattern recognition receptors and central nervous system repair. Exp Neurol 2014; 258: 5-16.
[http://dx.doi.org/10.1016/j.expneurol.2014.01.001] [PMID: 25017883]

[48]   Hanamsagar R, Hanke ML, Kielian T. Toll-like receptor (TLR) and inflammasome actions in the central nervous system. Trends Immunol 2012; 33(7): 333-42. [Review].
[http://dx.doi.org/10.1016/j.it.2012.03.001] [PMID: 22521509]

[49]   Eriksson M, Meadows SK, Basu S, Mselle TF, Wira CR, Sentman CL. TLRs mediate IFN-gamma production by human uterine NK cells in endometrium. J Immunol 2006; 176(10): 6219-24.
[http://dx.doi.org/10.4049/jimmunol.176.10.6219] [PMID: 16670332]

[50]   Kaisho T, Akira S. Toll-like receptor function and signaling. J Allergy Clin Immunol 2006; 117(5): 979-87.
[http://dx.doi.org/10.1016/j.jaci.2006.02.023] [PMID: 16675322]

[51]   Yoshimoto T, Nakanishi K. Roles of IL-18 in basophils and mast cells. Allergol Int 2006; 55(2): 105-13.
[http://dx.doi.org/10.2332/allergolint.55.105] [PMID: 17075246]

[52]   Gerondakis S, Grumont RJ, Banerjee A. Regulating B-cell activation and survival in response to TLR signals. Immunol Cell Biol 2007; 85(6): 471-5.
[http://dx.doi.org/10.1038/sj.icb.7100097] [PMID: 17637697]

[53]   Sabroe I, Whyte MK. Toll-like receptor (TLR)-based networks regulate neutrophilic inflammation in respiratory disease. Biochem Soc Trans 2007; 35(Pt 6): 1492-5.
[http://dx.doi.org/10.1042/BST0351492] [PMID: 18031251]

[54]   Sutmuller R, Garritsen A, Adema GJ. Regulatory T cells and toll-like receptors: regulating the regulators. Ann Rheum Dis 2007; 66 (Suppl. 3): iii91-5.
[http://dx.doi.org/10.1136/ard.2007.078535] [PMID: 17934105]

[55]   Iwamura C, Nakayama T. Toll-like receptors in the respiratory system: their roles in inflammation. Curr Allergy Asthma Rep 2008; 8(1): 7-13.
[http://dx.doi.org/10.1007/s11882-008-0003-0] [PMID: 18377768]

[56]   Gibson FC III, Ukai T, Genco CA. Engagement of specific innate immune signaling pathways during Porphyromonas gingivalis induced chronic inflammation and atherosclerosis. Front Biosci 2008; 13: 2041-59. [Review].
[http://dx.doi.org/10.2741/2822] [PMID: 17981690]

[57]   Kawai T, Akira S. The role of pattern-recognition receptors in innate immunity: update on Toll-like

receptors. Nat Immunol 2010; 11(5): 373-84.
[http://dx.doi.org/10.1038/ni.1863] [PMID: 20404851]

[58]  Triantafilou M, Triantafilou K. Lipopolysaccharide recognition: CD14, TLRs and the LPS-activation cluster. Trends Immunol 2002; 23(6): 301-4. [Review].
[http://dx.doi.org/10.1016/S1471-4906(02)02233-0] [PMID: 12072369]

[59]  Blasius AL, Beutler B. Intracellular toll-like receptors. Immunity 2010; 32(3): 305-15.
[http://dx.doi.org/10.1016/j.immuni.2010.03.012] [PMID: 20346772]

[60]  Lehnardt S. Innate immunity and neuroinflammation in the CNS: the role of microglia in Toll-like receptor-mediated neuronal injury. Glia 2010; 58(3): 253-63.
[PMID: 19705460]

[61]  Bajramovic JJ. Regulation of innate immune responses in the central nervous system. CNS Neurol Disord Drug Targets 2011; 10(1): 4-24.
[http://dx.doi.org/10.2174/187152711794488610] [PMID: 21143142]

[62]  Holley MM, Zhang Y, Lehrmann E, Wood WH, Becker KG, Kielian T. TLR29 crosstalk dictates IL-12 family cytokine production in microglia. Glia 2012; 60: 29-42.
[http://dx.doi.org/10.1002/glia.21243] [PMID: 21901759]

[63]  Ousman SS, Kubes P. Immune surveillance in the central nervous system. Nat Neurosci 2012; 15(8): 1096-101.
[http://dx.doi.org/10.1038/nn.3161] [PMID: 22837040]

[64]  Liew FY, Xu D, Brint EK, ONeill LA. Negative regulation of toll-like receptor-mediated immune responses. Nat Rev Immunol 2005; 5(6): 446-58.
[http://dx.doi.org/10.1038/nri1630] [PMID: 15928677]

[65]  Oshiumi H, Matsumoto M, Funami K, Akazawa T, Seya T. TICAM-1, an adaptor molecule that participates in Toll-like receptor 3-mediated interferon-beta induction. Nat Immunol 2003; 4(2): 161-7.
[http://dx.doi.org/10.1038/ni886] [PMID: 12539043]

[66]  Taniguchi T, Ogasawara K, Takaoka A, Tanaka N. IRF family of transcription factors as regulators of host defense. Annu Rev Immunol 2001; 19: 623-55.
[http://dx.doi.org/10.1146/annurev.immunol.19.1.623] [PMID: 11244049]

[67]  Yamamoto M, Sato S, Hemmi H, *et al.* Role of adaptor TRIF in the MyD88-independent toll-like receptor signaling pathway. Science 2003; 301(5633): 640-3.
[http://dx.doi.org/10.1126/science.1087262] [PMID: 12855817]

[68]  Gambuzza M, Licata N, Palella E, *et al.* Targeting Toll-like receptors: emerging therapeutics for multiple sclerosis management. J Neuroimmunol 2011; 239(1-2): 1-12. [Review].
[http://dx.doi.org/10.1016/j.jneuroim.2011.08.010] [PMID: 21889214]

[69]  Gambuzza ME, Sofo V, Salmeri FM, Soraci L, Marino S, Bramanti P. Toll-like receptors in Alzheimers disease: a therapeutic perspective. CNS Neurol Disord Drug Targets 2014; 13(9): 1542-58.
[http://dx.doi.org/10.2174/1871527313666140806124850] [PMID: 25106635]

[70]  Gambuzza ME, Salmeri FM, Soraci L, *et al.* The role of toll-like receptors in chronic fatigue syndrome/myalgic encephalomyelitis: A new promising therapeutic approach? CNS Neurol Disord Drug Targets 2015; 14(7): 903-14.

[http://dx.doi.org/10.2174/1871527314666150325235247] [PMID: 25808894]

[71]    Gambuzza ME, Sofo V, Salmeri FM, Soraci L, Marino S, Bramanti P. A toll-like receptor 3-agonist as promising candidate in multiple sclerosis treatment. J Clin Cell Immunol 2015; 6: 339.
[http://dx.doi.org/10.4172/2155-9899.1000339]

[72]    Carty M, Bowie AG. Evaluating the role of Toll-like receptors in diseases of the central nervous system. Biochem Pharmacol 2011; 81(7): 825-37.
[http://dx.doi.org/10.1016/j.bcp.2011.01.003] [PMID: 21241665]

[73]    Aravalli RN, Peterson PK, Lokensgard JR. Toll-like receptors in defense and damage of the central nervous system. J Neuroimmune Pharmacol 2007; 2(4): 297-312.
[http://dx.doi.org/10.1007/s11481-007-9071-5] [PMID: 18040848]

[74]    Tang SC, Arumugam TV, Xu X, *et al.* Pivotal role for neuronal Toll-like receptors in ischemic brain injury and functional deficits. Proc Natl Acad Sci USA 2007; 104(34): 13798-803.
[http://dx.doi.org/10.1073/pnas.0702553104] [PMID: 17693552]

[75]    Jack CS, Arbour N, Manusow J, *et al.* TLR signaling tailors innate immune responses in human microglia and astrocytes. J Immunol 2005; 175(7): 4320-30.
[http://dx.doi.org/10.4049/jimmunol.175.7.4320] [PMID: 16177072]

[76]    Cooper MA, Yokoyama WM. Memory-like responses of natural killer cells. Immunol Rev 2010; 235(1): 297-305.
[http://dx.doi.org/10.1111/j.0105-2896.2010.00891.x] [PMID: 20536571]

[77]    Okun E, Griffioen KJ, Lathia JD, Tang S-C, Mattson MP, Arumugam TV. Toll-like receptors in neurodegeneration. Brain Res Brain Res Rev 2009; 59(2): 278-92.
[http://dx.doi.org/10.1016/j.brainresrev.2008.09.001] [PMID: 18822314]

[78]    Béjot Y, Osseby GV, Gremeaux V, *et al.* Changes in risk factors and preventive treatments by stroke subtypes over 20 years: a population-based study. J Neurol Sci 2009; 287(1-2): 84-8.
[http://dx.doi.org/10.1016/j.jns.2009.08.062] [PMID: 19766250]

[79]    Nishino H, Czurkó A, Fukuda A, *et al.* Pathophysiological process after transient ischemia of the middle cerebral artery in the rat. Brain Res Bull 1994; 35(1): 51-6.
[http://dx.doi.org/10.1016/0361-9230(94)90215-1] [PMID: 7953757]

[80]    Globus MY, Busto R, Martinez E, Valdés I, Dietrich WD. Ischemia induces release of glutamate in regions spared from histopathologic damage in the rat. Stroke 1990; 21(11) (Suppl.): III43-6.
[PMID: 2237984]

[81]    Love S, Barber R, Wilcock GK. Neuronal death in brain infarcts in man. Neuropathol Appl Neurobiol 2000; 26(1): 55-66.
[http://dx.doi.org/10.1046/j.1365-2990.2000.00218.x] [PMID: 10736067]

[82]    Sairanen T, Szepesi R, Karjalainen-Lindsberg ML, Saksi J, Paetau A, Lindsberg PJ. Neuronal caspase-3 and PARP-1 correlate differentially with apoptosis and necrosis in ischemic human stroke. Acta Neuropathol 2009; 118(4): 541-52.
[http://dx.doi.org/10.1007/s00401-009-0559-3] [PMID: 19529948]

[83]    Levraut J, Iwase H, Shao ZH, Vanden Hoek TL, Schumacker PT. Cell death during ischemia: relationship to mitochondrial depolarization and ROS generation. Am J Physiol Heart Circ Physiol

2003; 284(2): H549-58.
[http://dx.doi.org/10.1152/ajpheart.00708.2002] [PMID: 12388276]

[84]    Dong XX, Wang Y, Qin ZH. Molecular mechanisms of excitotoxicity and their relevance to pathogenesis of neurodegenerative diseases. Acta Pharmacol Sin 2009; 30(4): 379-87.
[http://dx.doi.org/10.1038/aps.2009.24] [PMID: 19343058]

[85]    Choi K, Kim J, Kim GW, Choi C. Oxidative stress-induced necrotic cell death *via* mitochondira-dependent burst of reactive oxygen species. Curr Neurovasc Res 2009; 6(4): 213-22.
[http://dx.doi.org/10.2174/156720209789630375] [PMID: 19807658]

[86]    Broughton BR, Reutens DC, Sobey CG. Apoptotic mechanisms after cerebral ischemia. Stroke 2009; 40(5): e331-9.
[http://dx.doi.org/10.1161/STROKEAHA.108.531632] [PMID: 19182083]

[87]    Iadecola C, Anrather J. The immunology of stroke: from mechanisms to translation. Nat Med 2011; 17(7): 796-808.
[http://dx.doi.org/10.1038/nm.2399] [PMID: 21738161]

[88]    Fayaz SM, Suvanish Kumar VS, Rajanikant GK. Necroptosis: who knew there were so many interesting ways to die? CNS Neurol Disord Drug Targets 2014; 13(1): 42-51.
[http://dx.doi.org/10.2174/18715273113126660189] [PMID: 24152329]

[89]    Degterev A, Huang Z, Boyce M, *et al.* Chemical inhibitor of nonapoptotic cell death with therapeutic potential for ischemic brain injury. Nat Chem Biol 2005; 1(2): 112-9.
[http://dx.doi.org/10.1038/nchembio711] [PMID: 16408008]

[90]    Adhami F, Liao G, Morozov YM, *et al.* Cerebral ischemia-hypoxia induces intravascular coagulation and autophagy. Am J Pathol 2006; 169(2): 566-83.
[http://dx.doi.org/10.2353/ajpath.2006.051066] [PMID: 16877357]

[91]    Bredesen DE, Rao RV, Mehlen P. Cell death in the nervous system. Nature 2006; 443(7113): 796-802.
[http://dx.doi.org/10.1038/nature05293] [PMID: 17051206]

[92]    Blomgren K, Leist M, Groc L. Pathological apoptosis in the developing brain. Apoptosis 2007; 12(5): 993-1010.
[http://dx.doi.org/10.1007/s10495-007-0754-4] [PMID: 17453164]

[93]    Degterev A, Yuan J. Expansion and evolution of cell death programmes. Nat Rev Mol Cell Biol 2008; 9(5): 378-90.
[http://dx.doi.org/10.1038/nrm2393] [PMID: 18414491]

[94]    Giulian D, Vaca K. Inflammatory glia mediate delayed neuronal damage after ischemia in the central nervous system. Stroke 1993; 24(12) (Suppl.): I84-90.
[PMID: 8249026]

[95]    Lambertsen KL, Meldgaard M, Ladeby R, Finsen B. A quantitative study of microglial-macrophage synthesis of tumor necrosis factor during acute and late focal cerebral ischemia in mice. J Cereb Blood Flow Metab 2005; 25(1): 119-35.
[http://dx.doi.org/10.1038/sj.jcbfm.9600014] [PMID: 15678118]

[96]    Block F, Peters M, Nolden-Koch M. Expression of IL-6 in the ischemic penumbra. Neuroreport 2000; 11(5): 963-7.

[http://dx.doi.org/10.1097/00001756-200004070-00013] [PMID: 10790864]

[97]   Lambertsen KL, Clausen BH, Fenger C, *et al.* Microglia and macrophages express tumor necrosis factor receptor p75 following middle cerebral artery occlusion in mice. Neuroscience 2007; 144(3): 934-49.
[http://dx.doi.org/10.1016/j.neuroscience.2006.10.046] [PMID: 17161916]

[98]   Lambertsen KL, Clausen BH, Babcock AA, *et al.* Microglia protect neurons against ischemia by synthesis of tumor necrosis factor. J Neurosci 2009; 29(5): 1319-30.
[http://dx.doi.org/10.1523/JNEUROSCI.5505-08.2009] [PMID: 19193879]

[99]   Pettigrew LC, Kindy MS, Scheff S, *et al.* Focal cerebral ischemia in the TNFalpha-transgenic rat. J Neuroinflammation 2008; 5: 47.
[http://dx.doi.org/10.1186/1742-2094-5-47] [PMID: 18947406]

[100]  Tobinick E, Kim NM, Reyzin G, Rodriguez-Romanacce H, DePuy V. Selective TNF inhibition for chronic stroke and traumatic brain injury: an observational study involving 629 consecutive patients treated with perispinal etanercept. CNS Drugs 2012; 26(12): 1051-70.
[http://dx.doi.org/10.1007/s40263-012-0013-2] [PMID: 23100196]

[101]  Page SJ. Selective TNF inhibition for chronic stroke and traumatic brain injury: an observational study involving 629 consecutive patients treated with perispinal etanercept. CNS Drugs 2013; 27(5): 395-7.
[http://dx.doi.org/10.1007/s40263-013-0057-y] [PMID: 23580176]

[102]  Danton GH, Dietrich WD. Inflammatory mechanisms after ischemia and stroke. J Neuropathol Exp Neurol 2003; 62(2): 127-36.
[http://dx.doi.org/10.1093/jnen/62.2.127] [PMID: 12578222]

[103]  Emsley HC, Tyrrell PJ. Inflammation and infection in clinical stroke. J Cereb Blood Flow Metab 2002; 22(12): 1399-419.
[http://dx.doi.org/10.1097/01.WCB.0000037880.62590.28] [PMID: 12468886]

[104]  Pan J, Li X, Peng Y. Remote ischemic conditioning for acute ischemic stroke: dawn in the darkness. Rev Neurosci 2016; 27(5): 501-10. pii:/j/revneuro.ahead-of-print/revneuro-2015-0043/revneuro-2015-0043.xml.
[http://dx.doi.org/10.1515/revneuro-2015-0043] [PMID: 26812782]

[105]  Werner C, Engelhard K. Pathophysiology of traumatic brain injury. Br J Anaesth 2007; 99(1): 4-9. [Review].
[http://dx.doi.org/10.1093/bja/aem131] [PMID: 17573392]

[106]  Han HS, Yenari MA. Cellular targets of brain inflammation in stroke. Curr Opin Investig Drugs 2003; 4(5): 522-9.
[PMID: 12833644]

[107]  Becker K, Kindrick D, Relton J, Harlan J, Winn R. Antibody to the alpha4 integrin decreases infarct size in transient focal cerebral ischemia in rats. Stroke 2001; 32(1): 206-11.
[http://dx.doi.org/10.1161/01.STR.32.1.206] [PMID: 11136938]

[108]  Roth EJ, Lovell L, Harvey RL, Heinemann AW, Semik P, Diaz S. Incidence of and risk factors for medical complications during stroke rehabilitation. Stroke 2001; 32(2): 523-9.
[http://dx.doi.org/10.1161/01.STR.32.2.523] [PMID: 11157192]

[109] Vargas M, Horcajada JP, Obach V, *et al.* Clinical consequences of infection in patients with acute stroke: is it prime time for further antibiotic trials? Stroke 2006; 37(2): 461-5. [http://dx.doi.org/10.1161/01.STR.0000199138.73365.b3] [PMID: 16385093]

[110] Reith J, Jørgensen HS, Pedersen PM, *et al.* Body temperature in acute stroke: relation to stroke severity, infarct size, mortality, and outcome. Lancet 1996; 347(8999): 422-5. [http://dx.doi.org/10.1016/S0140-6736(96)90008-2] [PMID: 8618482]

[111] Bornstein NM, Aronovich B, Korczyn AD, Shavit S, Michaelson DM, Chapman J. Antibodies to brain antigens following stroke. Neurology 2001; 56(4): 529-30. [http://dx.doi.org/10.1212/WNL.56.4.529] [PMID: 11222800]

[112] Gromadzka G, Zielińska J, Ryglewicz D, Fiszer U, Członkowska A. Elevated levels of anti-heat shock protein antibodies in patients with cerebral ischemia. Cerebrovasc Dis 2001; 12(3): 235-9. [http://dx.doi.org/10.1159/000047709] [PMID: 11641589]

[113] Dambinova SA, Khounteev GA, Izykenova GA, Zavolokov IG, Ilyukhina AY, Skoromets AA. Blood test detecting autoantibodies to N-methyl-D-aspartate neuroreceptors for evaluation of patients with transient ischemic attack and stroke. Clin Chem 2003; 49(10): 1752-62. [http://dx.doi.org/10.1373/49.10.1752] [PMID: 14500616]

[114] Gee JM, Kalil A, Thullbery M, Becker KJ. Induction of immunologic tolerance to myelin basic protein prevents central nervous system autoimmunity and improves outcome after stroke. Stroke 2008; 39(5): 1575-82. [http://dx.doi.org/10.1161/STROKEAHA.107.501486] [PMID: 18323496]

[115] Hurn PD, Subramanian S, Parker SM, *et al.* T- and B-cell-deficient mice with experimental stroke have reduced lesion size and inflammation. J Cereb Blood Flow Metab 2007; 27(11): 1798-805. [http://dx.doi.org/10.1038/sj.jcbfm.9600482] [PMID: 17392692]

[116] Rosenzweig HL, Lessov NS, Henshall DC, Minami M, Simon RP, Stenzel-Poore MP. Endotoxin preconditioning prevents cellular inflammatory response during ischemic neuroprotection in mice. Stroke 2004; 35(11): 2576-81. [http://dx.doi.org/10.1161/01.STR.0000143450.04438.ae] [PMID: 15375302]

[117] Termeer C, Benedix F, Sleeman J, *et al.* Oligosaccharides of Hyaluronan activate dendritic cells *via* toll-like receptor 4. J Exp Med 2002; 195(1): 99-111. [http://dx.doi.org/10.1084/jem.20001858] [PMID: 11781369]

[118] Karikó K, Ni H, Capodici J, Lamphier M, Weissman D. mRNA is an endogenous ligand for Toll-like receptor 3. J Biol Chem 2004; 279(13): 12542-50. [http://dx.doi.org/10.1074/jbc.M310175200] [PMID: 14729660]

[119] Ohashi K, Burkart V, Flohé S, Kolb H. Cutting edge: heat shock protein 60 is a putative endogenous ligand of the toll-like receptor-4 complex. J Immunol 2000; 164(2): 558-61. [http://dx.doi.org/10.4049/jimmunol.164.2.558] [PMID: 10623794]

[120] Asea A, Rehli M, Kabingu E, *et al.* Novel signal transduction pathway utilized by extracellular HSP70: role of toll-like receptor (TLR) 2 and TLR4. J Biol Chem 2002; 277(17): 15028-34. [http://dx.doi.org/10.1074/jbc.M200497200] [PMID: 11836257]

[121] Gelderblom M, Leypoldt F, Steinbach K, *et al.* Temporal and spatial dynamics of cerebral immune cell

accumulation in stroke. Stroke 2009; 40(5): 1849-57.
[http://dx.doi.org/10.1161/STROKEAHA.108.534503] [PMID: 19265055]

[122] Tarassishin L, Suh HS, Lee SC, Lee SC. Interferon regulatory factor 3 plays an anti-inflammatory role in microglia by activating the PI3K/Akt pathway. J Neuroinflammation 2011; 8: 187.
[http://dx.doi.org/10.1186/1742-2094-8-187] [PMID: 22208359]

[123] Weston RM, Jones NM, Jarrott B, Callaway JK. Inflammatory cell infiltration after endothelin--induced cerebral ischemia: histochemical and myeloperoxidase correlation with temporal changes in brain injury. J Cereb Blood Flow Metab 2007; 27(1): 100-14.
[http://dx.doi.org/10.1038/sj.jcbfm.9600324] [PMID: 16736051]

[124] Petry KG, Boiziau C, Dousset V, Brochet B. Magnetic resonance imaging of human brain macrophage infiltration. Neurotherapeutics 2007; 4(3): 434-42.
[http://dx.doi.org/10.1016/j.nurt.2007.05.005] [PMID: 17599709]

[125] Yilmaz G, Granger DN. Cell adhesion molecules and ischemic stroke. Neurol Res 2008; 30(8): 783-93.
[http://dx.doi.org/10.1179/174313208X341085] [PMID: 18826804]

[126] Ceulemans AG, Zgavc T, Kooijman R, Hachimi-Idrissi S, Sarre S, Michotte Y. The dual role of the neuroinflammatory response after ischemic stroke: modulatory effects of hypothermia. J Neuroinflammation 2010; 7: 74.
[http://dx.doi.org/10.1186/1742-2094-7-74] [PMID: 21040547]

[127] Phillips JB, Williams AJ, Adams J, Elliott PJ, Tortella FC. Proteasome inhibitor PS519 reduces infarction and attenuates leukocyte infiltration in a rat model of focal cerebral ischemia. Stroke 2000; 31(7): 1686-93.
[http://dx.doi.org/10.1161/01.STR.31.7.1686] [PMID: 10884474]

[128] Yilmaz G, Arumugam TV, Stokes KY, Granger DN. Role of T lymphocytes and interferon-gamma in ischemic stroke. Circulation 2006; 113(17): 2105-12.
[http://dx.doi.org/10.1161/CIRCULATIONAHA.105.593046] [PMID: 16636173]

[129] Pelidou SH, Kostulas N, Matusevicius D, Kivisäkk P, Kostulas V, Link H. High levels of IL-10 secreting cells are present in blood in cerebrovascular diseases. Eur J Neurol 1999; 6(4): 437-42.
[http://dx.doi.org/10.1046/j.1468-1331.1999.640437.x] [PMID: 10362896]

[130] Liesz A, Suri-Payer E, Veltkamp C, *et al.* Regulatory T cells are key cerebroprotective immunomodulators in acute experimental stroke. Nat Med 2009; 15(2): 192-9.
[http://dx.doi.org/10.1038/nm.1927] [PMID: 19169263]

[131] Grilli M, Barbieri I, Basudev H, *et al.* Interleukin-10 modulates neuronal threshold of vulnerability to ischaemic damage. Eur J Neurosci 2000; 12(7): 2265-72.
[http://dx.doi.org/10.1046/j.1460-9568.2000.00090.x] [PMID: 10947805]

[132] Hayward JH, Lee SJ. A decade of research on TLR2 discovering its pivotal role in glial activation and neuroinflammation in neurodegenerative diseases. Exp Neurobiol 2014; 23(2): 138-47.
[http://dx.doi.org/10.5607/en.2014.23.2.138] [PMID: 24963278]

[133] Ziegler G, Harhausen D, Schepers C, *et al.* TLR2 has a detrimental role in mouse transient focal cerebral ischemia. Biochem Biophys Res Commun 2007; 359(3): 574-9.

[http://dx.doi.org/10.1016/j.bbrc.2007.05.157] [PMID: 17548055]

[134]   Yang QW, Li JC, Lu FL, *et al.* Upregulated expression of toll-like receptor 4 in monocytes correlates with severity of acute cerebral infarction. J Cereb Blood Flow Metab 2008; 28(9): 1588-96.
[http://dx.doi.org/10.1038/jcbfm.2008.50] [PMID: 18523439]

[135]   Jayaraman T, Paget A, Shin YS, *et al.* TNF-alpha-mediated inflammation in cerebral aneurysms: a potential link to growth and rupture. Vasc Health Risk Manag 2008; 4(4): 805-17. [Review].
[http://dx.doi.org/10.2147/VHRM.S2700] [PMID: 19065997]

[136]   Boonstra A, Rajsbaum R, Holman M, *et al.* Macrophages and myeloid dendritic cells, but not plasmacytoid dendritic cells, produce IL-10 in response to MyD88- and TRIF-dependent TLR signals, and TLR-independent signals. J Immunol 2006; 177(11): 7551-8.
[http://dx.doi.org/10.4049/jimmunol.177.11.7551] [PMID: 17114424]

[137]   Dagvadorj J, Naiki Y, Tumurkhuu G, *et al.* Interleukin-10 inhibits tumor necrosis factor-alpha production in lipopolysaccharide-stimulated RAW 264.7 cells through reduced MyD88 expression. Innate Immun 2008; 14(2): 109-15.
[http://dx.doi.org/10.1177/1753425908089618] [PMID: 18713727]

[138]   Caso JR, Pradillo JM, Hurtado O, Lorenzo P, Moro MA, Lizasoain I. Toll-like receptor 4 is involved in brain damage and inflammation after experimental stroke. Circulation 2007; 115(12): 1599-608.
[http://dx.doi.org/10.1161/CIRCULATIONAHA.106.603431] [PMID: 17372179]

[139]   Caso JR, Pradillo JM, Hurtado O, Leza JC, Moro MA, Lizasoain I. Toll-like receptor 4 is involved in subacute stress-induced neuroinflammation and in the worsening of experimental stroke. Stroke 2008; 39(4): 1314-20.
[http://dx.doi.org/10.1161/STROKEAHA.107.498212] [PMID: 18309167]

[140]   Tang SC, Yeh SJ, Li YI, *et al.* Evidence for a detrimental role of TLR8 in ischemic stroke. Exp Neurol 2013; 250: 341-7.
[http://dx.doi.org/10.1016/j.expneurol.2013.10.012] [PMID: 24196452]

[141]   Cavassani KA, Ishii M, Wen H, *et al.* TLR3 is an endogenous sensor of tissue necrosis during acute inflammatory events. J Exp Med 2008; 205(11): 2609-21.
[http://dx.doi.org/10.1084/jem.20081370] [PMID: 18838547]

[142]   Brea D, Sobrino T, Rodríguez-Yáñez M, *et al.* Toll-like receptors 7 and 8 expression is associated with poor outcome and greater inflammatory response in acute ischemic stroke. Clin Immunol 2011; 139(2): 193-8.
[http://dx.doi.org/10.1016/j.clim.2011.02.001] [PMID: 21354862]

[143]   Gambuzza ME, Sofo V, Salmeri FM, Soraci L, Marino S, Bramanti P. A Toll-Like Receptor 3-Agonist as Promising Candidate in Multiple Sclerosis Treatment. J Clin Cell Immunol 2015; 6: 339.
[http://dx.doi.org/10.4172/2155-9899.1000339]

[144]   Packard AE, Hedges JC, Bahjat FR, *et al.* Poly-IC preconditioning protects against cerebral and renal ischemia-reperfusion injury. J Cereb Blood Flow Metab 2012; 32(2): 242-7.
[http://dx.doi.org/10.1038/jcbfm.2011.160] [PMID: 22086194]

[145]   Pan LN, Zhu W, Li C, Xu XL, Guo LJ, Lu Q. Toll-like receptor 3 agonist Poly I:C protects against simulated cerebral ischemia *in vitro* and *in vivo*. Acta Pharmacol Sin 2012; 33(10): 1246-53.

[http://dx.doi.org/10.1038/aps.2012.122] [PMID: 22983393]

[146] Hua LL, Kim MO, Brosnan CF, Lee SC. Modulation of astrocyte inducible nitric oxide synthase and cytokine expression by interferon beta is associated with induction and inhibition of interferon gamma-activated sequence binding activity. J Neurochem 2002; 83(5): 1120-8.
[http://dx.doi.org/10.1046/j.1471-4159.2002.01226.x] [PMID: 12437583]

[147] Hofer MJ, Campbell IL. Type I interferon in neurological disease-the devil from within. Cytokine Growth Factor Rev 2013; 24(3): 257-67.
[http://dx.doi.org/10.1016/j.cytogfr.2013.03.006] [PMID: 23548179]

[148] Lok KZ, Basta M, Manzanero S, Arumugam TV. Intravenous immunoglobulin (IVIg) dampens neuronal toll-like receptor-mediated responses in ischemia. J Neuroinflammation 2015; 12: 73.
[http://dx.doi.org/10.1186/s12974-015-0294-8] [PMID: 25886362]

[149] Hassanzadeh-Ghassabeh G, Devoogdt N, De Pauw P, Vincke C, Muyldermans S. Nanobodies and their potential applications. Nanomedicine (Lond) 2013; 8(6): 1013-26.
[http://dx.doi.org/10.2217/nnm.13.86] [PMID: 23730699]

[150] Couture LA, Piao W, Ru LW, Vogel SN, Toshchakov VY. Targeting Toll-like receptor (TLR) signaling by Toll/interleukin-1 receptor (TIR) domain-containing adapter protein/MyD88 adapter-like (TIRAP/Mal)-derived decoy peptides. J Biol Chem 2012; 287(29): 24641-8.
[http://dx.doi.org/10.1074/jbc.M112.360925] [PMID: 22648407]

[151] Chang YC, Kao WC, Wang WY, Wang WY, Yang RB, Peck K. Identification and characterization of oligonucleotides that inhibit Toll-like receptor 2-associated immune responses. FASEB J 2009; 23(9): 3078-88.
[http://dx.doi.org/10.1096/fj.09-129312] [PMID: 19406842]

[152] Lundin KE, Gissberg O, Smith CI. Oligonucleotide therapies: The past and the present. Hum Gene Ther 2015; 26(8): 475-85.
[http://dx.doi.org/10.1089/hum.2015.070] [PMID: 26160334]

[153] Castel SE, Martienssen RA. RNA interference in the nucleus: roles for small RNAs in transcription, epigenetics and beyond. Nat Rev Genet 2013; 14(2): 100-12.
[http://dx.doi.org/10.1038/nrg3355] [PMID: 23329111]

[154] Gambuzza ME, Soraci L, Sofo V, Marino S, Bramanti P. A New Era for Immunotherapeutic approaches in multiple sclerosis treatment. J Clin Trials 2016; 6: 1.
[http://dx.doi.org/10.4172/2167-0870.1000253]

[155] Wang P-F, Fang H, Chen J, Lin S, Liu Y, Xiong X-Y, *et al.* Polyinosinic-polycytidylic acid has therapeutic effects against cerebral ischemia/reperfusion injury through the downregulation of tlr4 signaling *via* TLR3. J Immunol 2014. published online 11 April 2014; http://www.jimmunol.org/content/early/2014/04/11/jimmunol.1303108

[156] Liu L, Botos I, Wang Y, *et al.* Structural basis of toll-like receptor 3 signaling with double-stranded RNA. Science 2008; 320(5874): 379-81.
[http://dx.doi.org/10.1126/science.1155406] [PMID: 18420935]

[157] Carter WA. Double-stranded ribonucleic acids with rugged physico-chemical structure and highly specific biologic activity. Unites States patent WO2011059505, 2014.

[158]  Wang P-F, Xiong X-Y, Chen J, Wang Y-C, Duan W, Yang Q-W. Function and mechanism of toll-like receptors in cerebral ischemic tolerance: from preconditioning to treatment. J Neuroinflammation 2015; 12: 80.
[http://dx.doi.org/10.1186/s12974-015-0301-0] [PMID: 25928750]

# CHAPTER 4

# Intracerebral Bleeding and Oral Anticoagulant Therapies: Clinical Relevance and Management

**Monica Carpenedo**[*]

*Hematology and Transplant Unit, San Gerardo Hospital, Monza, Italy*

**Abstract:** Vitamin K antagonists such as warfarin and acenocumarol are the most widely used oral anticoagulants. Their clinical indications include both stroke prevention and prophylaxis and treatment of venous thromboembolism. Intracerebral hemorrhage (ICH) is the most important side effect of anticoagulant therapy accounting for almost 20% of all ICH. Non vitamin K anticoagulants or direct oral anticoagulants (DOACs) have been recently introduced in clinical practice due to their practical advantages over VKA. They are at least as effective as warfarin in the management of thromboembolic diseases and in the thromboprophylaxis of non-valvular atrial fibrillation, moreover, they have a more favorable safety profile. The present chapter will focus on vitamin K antagonists and DOACs mechanisms of action, on their pharmacokinetics and pharmacodynamics, and on the relative risk of bleeding during treatment.

**Keywords:** Anticoagulation reversal, Anticoagulants, Bleeding risk, Intracerebral hemorrhage.

Anticoagulant drugs are the cornerstone of prevention and treatment of thromboembolic diseases. Vitamin K anticoagulants (VKA) have been used for over six decades [1 - 3] in patients with atrial fibrillation, in patients with mechanical valve prosthesis and in patients with venous thrombosis.

Novel target-specific oral anticoagulants, known as "direct oral anticoagulants" (DOACs) or "non - vitamin K oral anticoagulants" (NOACs) have become

---

[*] **Corresponding author Monica Carpenedo:** Hematology and Transplant Unit, San Gerardo Hospital, Monza, Italy; Tel: +390392332394; Fax: +390392332539; Email: m.carpenedo@hsgerardo.org

**Alberto Radaelli, Giuseppe Mancia, Carlo Ferrarese & Simone Beretta (Eds.)**

available for various indications in the last few years, and their use is rapidly spreading. The number of patients receiving anticoagulant drugs is expected to double by 2050, because of aging and because of the increasing indications for their use.

Prospective controlled trials have demonstrated that in atrial fibrillation DOAC are associated with a similar or even increased reduction of thromboembolic events compared with VKA [4 - 8]. Furthermore, major bleeding complications, such as intracranial hemorrhage and fatal bleeding, occur less frequently with DOAC than with VKA. Nonetheless, concerns regarding the absence of specific reversal agents in case of life-threatening bleeding exist and guidelines for the management of bleeding complications are actually based on pathophysiological rationales and pre-clinical studies.

This chapter will focus on the following sections:

1. VKA-associated cerebral hemorrhages
2. DOACs for stroke prevention: update on intracranial bleeding risk
3. Reversal of DOACs activity and management of bleeding complications

## 1. VKA-ASSOCIATED CEREBRAL HEMORRHAGES

Anticoagulant-associated intracerebral hemorrhages (ICH) have been reported accounting for almost 20% of all ICHs, most of them being VKA-ICHs [9 - 11]. Nowadays, it remains unclear whether VKA should be considered as a cause or as a risk factor for ICH. Both experimental and clinical observations have demonstrated that VKA-ICHs are more severe than other ICHs, although the mechanism by which VKA worsen the severity of ICH is not completely understood [12, 13].

### 1.1. Warfarin: Mechanism of Action and Main Characteristics

Despite the availability of newer drugs, warfarin is still the most widely used oral anticoagulant. From a chemical point of view, warfarin is a racemic mixture of enantiomers, with the S enantiomer being recognized as the most effective of the racemic mixture. Warfarin acts as a powerful inhibitor of the vitamin K epoxide reductase (VKORC1), a liver enzyme required for the synthesis of many coagulation factors such as FVII, FII, FIX, FX and the natural anticoagulant protein C and protein S (Fig. **1**) [14].

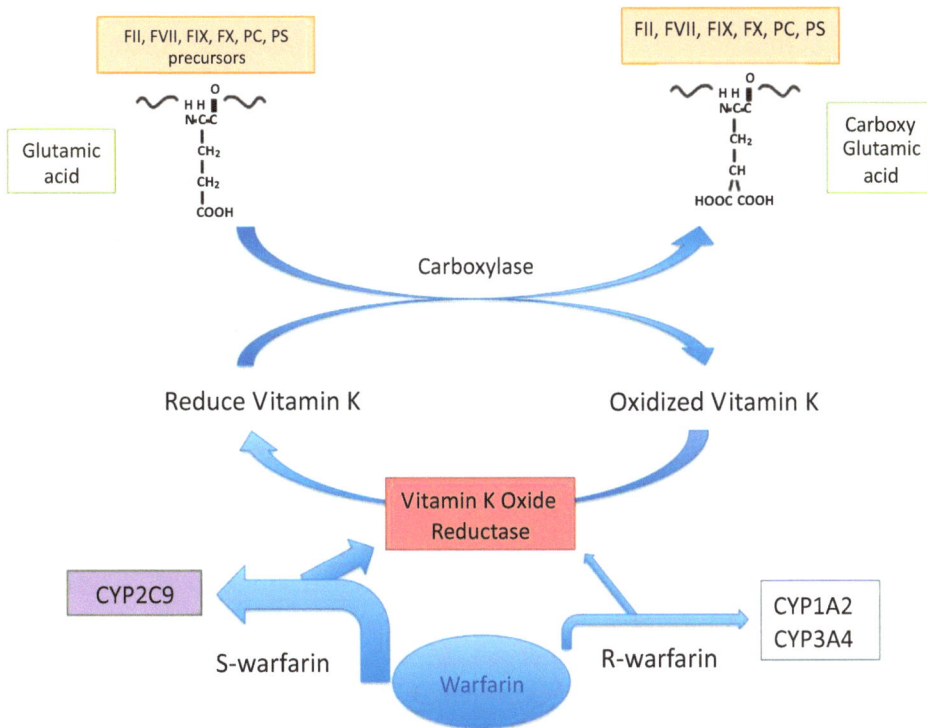

**Fig. (1).** Mechanism of action of warfarin: it inhibits the synthesis of vitamin K dependent coagulation factors acting on VKORC1, and it is metabolized by liver cytochromes.

VKAs produce their anticoagulant effect by interfering with the cyclic interconversion of vitamin K and its 2,3 epoxide (vitamin K epoxide), thereby modulating the beta-carboxylation of glutamate residues (Gla) on the N-terminal regions of vitamin K-dependent proteins. The vitamin K-dependent coagulation factors II, VII, IX, and X require beta-carboxylation for their procoagulant activity, and treatment with VKAs results in the hepatic production of partially carboxylated and decarboxylated proteins with reduced coagulant activity. Carboxylation is required for a calcium-dependent conformational change in coagulation proteins that promotes binding to cofactors on phospholipid surfaces. In addition, the VKAs inhibit carboxylation of the regulatory anticoagulant proteins C and S.

Racemic warfarin has a half-life of 36 to 42 hours, it circulates bound to plasma proteins and accumulates in the liver where the S enantiomer is metabolically transformed by different pathways involving the CYP2C9 enzyme of the cytochrome P450 system and to a lesser extent by CYP3A4.

Despite their well-documented effectiveness, warfarin and other VKA such as acenocoumarol, phenprocoumon and fluindione exhibit considerable variability in their anticoagulant activity, influenced by a number of factors including food intake, concomitant medications and mainly genetic factors. A number of point mutations in the gene encoding for the CYP2C9 have been identified, the most common being CYP2C9*2 and CYP2C9*3. These polymorphisms are associated with a reduced ability to metabolize S-warfarin, leading therefore to a reduction in its clearance and to an increased half-life of S-warfarin with a higher risk of bleeding [15]. In addition, mutations in the gene encoding for VKORC1 have been identified that are responsible for different sensitivities to the inhibitory effect of warfarin thus affecting its pharmacodynamics [16]. These mutations occur with different frequencies in various ethnic population and account, at least in part, for the difference in warfarin dose required to maintain a therapeutic international normalized ratio (INR).

The antithrombotic effect of warfarin requires some days of treatment to be evident, depending on the reduction of prothrombin (factor II) levels, whose half-life is 60 to 72 h [17]. For this reason, it is necessary to add a parenteral anticoagulant (*i.e.* unfractionated heparin or low molecular weight heparin or fondaparinux) until the PT-INR is prolonged.

## 1.2. Monitoring Warfarin, and Risk of Intracerebral Bleeding

Prothrombin time (PT) monitoring is required in patients treated with VKA. Since 1982 a calibration model has been introduced to standardize the results by converting the PT ratio into a value named International Normalized Ratio (INR), as follows [18]:

$$INR=(PTmeasured/PTmean)^{International\ sensitivity\ index}$$

This approach reduced the variability among different laboratories because of the different sensitivities of thromboplastin reagents used. Warfarin therapy has a narrow therapeutic range, which varies due to the clinical condition (for thromboembolic prophylaxis and venous thromboembolism INR 2.0–3.0; for mechanical heart valve, INR 2.5–3.5) [19].

Risk of major bleeding can be deduced by comparing the times when patients are above *vs* within the therapeutic range of INR [20, 21]. A strong relationship in fact has been observed between Time in Therapeutic Range (TTR) and the rates of bleeding [22, 23]. The percentage of correct INRs or TTR is highly dependent on the quality of dose management: non randomized, retrospective studies have reported a better outcome when anticoagulant therapy was managed by an Anticoagulation Management Service or an Anticoagulant Clinic. Independent predictors of a lower risk were age >70 years, the absence of chronic diseases, and male gender. On the other hand, congestive heart failure, diabetes, and a target range for INR ≥ 3.0 were associated with an increased risk of bleeding [24].

The incidence of ICH is higher when INR is ≥4 [25]. Nonetheless, the majority of VKA-associated ICHs occur when INR values are within the therapeutic range, the overall incidence of ICHs being 0.03 to 3.7% annually [26].

It has been demonstrated that the use of VKA did not influence the anatomic distribution of ICHs. The impact of VKA on ICH volume differed according to ICH location: in non-lobar ICH, VKA use was associated with larger ICH [11]. These results suggest that VKAs should not be regarded as a primary cause of ICH but other factors need to be taken into account like the underlying vessel disease. Despite a reported lower risk of intracranial bleeding, the impact of the newer anticoagulant drugs on the anatomic distribution and volume of ICHs need to be further elucidated.

## 1.3. Reversal of VKA Effect and Management of VKA-Associated ICH

Around 20% of all ICHs occur in patients taking VKA, with the incidence of VKA-ICH increasing as the population gets older. The 3-month case fatality of this condition is high, almost 50% [27]. One-third of ICH patients develop a significant hematoma expansion, which occurs more frequently in VKA treated patients.

Since VKA effect is due to reduced availability of vitamin K coagulant factors (*i.e.* II, VII, IX and X), reversal strategies are based on the replenishment of vitamin K-dependent factors to normalize hemostasis and avoid hematoma expansion. Treatment options include vitamin K, fresh frozen plasma (FFP), prothrombin complex concentrate (PCC) but also recombinant activated FVII (aFVII).

Evidence from patients with major VKA-associated bleeding (predominantly gastrointestinal hemorrhage) demonstrates that PCC normalizes the INR more quickly than FFP, it reduces the need for red blood cell transfusion, and it does not lead to an increase in adverse events. Although PCC is more expensive, it has practical advantages including a more rapid administration, smaller infusion volumes, and no need for ABO blood type matching.

### 1.3.1. Vitamin K

The infusion of PCC or FFP leads to a rapid replacement of vitamin K-dependent factors. However, their anti-hemorrhagic effect is only transient, due to the relative short half-life of FVII (6 h) and of other coagulation factors (36-48 h) when compared to that of VKAs (20-60 h). Sustained reversal of VKA requires the use of vitamin K1 (phytonadione). Vitamin K is available in subcutaneous (SC), oral, and intravenous (IV) formulations. The intravenous administration of vitamin K is more rapid and demonstrates a greater consistency in reversing anticoagulation (the effect being evident within 2-4 h) [28, 29].

Current ACCP (American College of Chest Physicians) guidelines recommend rapid administration of PCC along with concomitant slow (over 30 min) infusion of 5-10 mg of IV vitamin K [19]. A threefold reduction in the 7-day mortality of these patients has been demonstrated when both PCC and vitamin K were given within 8 h of presentation of bleeding [30].

### 1.3.2. FFP (Fresh Frozen Plasma)

On average, 1 unit of plasma contains a little less than 1 IU/mL of each clotting factor. The necessary steps required to prepare and infuse plasma are nevertheless time consuming and represent a considerable delay in treatment with significant potential impacts on the mortality and on the long-term outcomes of these patients. In fact, in the first 24 hours, a 20% decrease in INR reversal has been demonstrated for each 30-min delay in the administration of the first dose of plasma [31].

In a patient with INR >5 a rapid transfusion of 20–30 mL/kg of plasma (assuming factor concentrations 1 IU/mL) is necessary to increase clotting factors by 30–50%. In an 80-kg-weight patient, it means that a plasma volume of 1600–2400 mL (5–8 units) is needed. These large volumes represent a risk as they can produce a circulatory overload, especially in patients with volume limitations secondary to a compromised cardiac or renal function. Moreover, plasma infusion can increase the incidence of transfusion-related acute lung injury (TRALI) in critically ill patients. It has also to be remembered that FFP has the potential to transmit infectious diseases such as hepatitis B and/or C viruses and HIV.

### 1.3.3. About PCC (Prothrombin Complex Concentrates)

The available formulations of PCC contain varying concentrations of factors II, VII, IX and X. There are two types of PCC. The first available product is a non-activated 3 factors PCC, with significant concentrations of FII, FIX and FX but with only a minor concentration of FVII. The second product is a non-activated 4 factors PCC and it contains significant concentrations of all vitamin K dependent factors (FII, FVII, FIX, FX but also PC and PS). 4 factors PCC has been recently licensed by FDA for urgent VKA reversal.

The volume of PCC required to antagonize the effect of VKAs is smaller than that of FFP (median of 99.4 ml of 4F-PCC *versus* 8135 ml ml of FFP) and can be transfused over a shorter period of time. Complete and rapid correction of the INR to values <1.5 occurs within 10–30 min [32].

The INR should be re-evaluated 30 min after the administration of PCC. An additional dose is necessary in case of a consistently prolonged INR (>1.5). In this case, the presence of a low level of fibrinogen has to be excluded. In presence of ICH different scientific organizations nowadays endorse PCC use to antagonize VKA related anticoagulant effect [19, 33 - 35]. Summary of management of VKA-related ICH are listed in Table **1**.

**Table 1. Summary of management of VKA associated ICH.**

| Lab investigation | Reversal |
|---|---|
| PT-INR at presentation | Hold VKA |
| PT-INR after 15-30 min after PCC administration | Vitamin K 10 mg, slow ev infusion |
| | if INR 2-4 use 25 U/kg of 3F-PCC or 4F-PCC |
| | if INR 4-6 use 35 U/kg of 3F-PCC or 4F-PCC |
| | if INR>6 use 50 U/kg of 3F-PCC or 4F-PCC |

## 2. NON VITAMIN K ANTICOAGULANTS ASSOCIATED CEREBRAL HEMORRHAGES

Non-vitamin K anticoagulants or direct oral anticoagulants (DOACs) have been recently adopted in clinical practice due to their practical advantages over VKA. They are at least as effective as warfarin in the management of thromboembolic diseases and in the thromboprophylaxis of non-valvular atrial fibrillation, with a reported more favorable safety profile. They are also reported to have fewer drug-drug and drug-food interactions and have been licensed for use without the need for routine monitoring of the anticoagulant effect. Nonetheless a major concern regarding DOACs is the lack of a readily available antidote to reverse their effect in case of life-threatening bleeding or in case of emergency surgery.

### 2.1. DOACs Pharmacology

Direct oral anticoagulants bind directly to their target enzyme and block substrate interactions (Fig. **2**).

#### *2.1.1. Dabigatran*

Dabigatran etexilate is a pro-drug, with an oral bioavailability of about 6%, which is rapidly hydrolyzed to the active compound, dabigatran, by esterase within the gastrointestinal mucosa, liver and plasma.

Peak concentrations occur within 1 to 3 hours and its half-life is 14 to 17 hours. It is eliminated mainly *via* the kidneys, with 80% of the drug being excreted unchanged in the urine. Dabigatran exhibits predictable pharmacokinetic and pharmacodynamics with little interaction with food. Drug-drug interactions are limited. Nevertheless, the concomitant use of potent P-glycoprotein inhibitors, such as, quinidine, is contraindicated. Dabigatran acts binding directly to the active sites of both clot-bound and free thrombin, thus inhibiting the conversion of fibrinogen to fibrin and the thrombin mediated platelet activation [36].

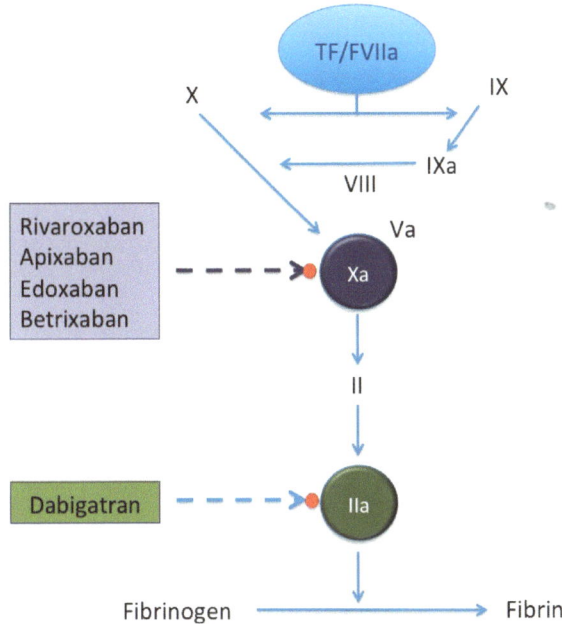

**Fig. (2).** Direct oral anticoagulants and their targets.

## 2.1.2. Rivaroxaban

Rivaroxaban is a direct factor Xa inhibitor with an oral bioavailability of more than 80%. Peak concentrations occur within 2 to 3 hours after administration. Its half-life is about 7 to 11 hours. Rivaroxaban is eliminated by the kidneys and in the feces. One third of the administered drug is cleared by the kidneys, one third is metabolized by the liver *via* CYP3A4-dependent and CYP3A4-independent pathways and then excreted in the feces, and one third is metabolized to inactive metabolites, which are then excreted by the kidneys (66%). The pharmacokinetic and pharmacodynamic profiles of rivaroxaban are predictable and dose-dependent and are not influenced by age, gender, or body weight. Concomitant use of potent inhibitors of both CYP3A4 and P-glycoprotein, such as ketoconazole or ritonavir, is contraindicated because they increase plasma drug concentrations [37].

## 2.1.3. Apixaban

Apixaban is an oral direct factor Xa inhibitor administered as active drug with an oral bioavailability of more than 45%. Like rivaroxaban, apixaban inhibits both free and clot-associated factor Xa activity [38]. In healthy volunteers plasmatic levels of apixaban reach peak concentrations 3 hours after oral administration. Its half-life is 8 - 14 hours. Apixaban is eliminated *via* multiple pathways, including oxidative metabolism, renal and intestinal routes. Apixaban has the smallest degree of renal excretion (only 25%) compared to dabigatran and rivaroxaban. Concomitant use of potent inhibitors of CYP3A4, such as ketoconazole or ritonavir, is contraindicated because they increase plasma drug concentrations.

## 2.1.4. Edoxaban

Edoxaban is an active drug with an oral bioavailability of at least 50% and it is rapidly absorbed from the gastrointestinal tract. Its plasma concentration peaks 1 to 2 hours after oral administration. Elimination follows a biphasic pattern, its half-life being approximately 10 - 14 hours [39]. Approximately 35% of the total administered oral dose is excreted *via* the kidneys, the other part being eliminated in the feces. A lower proportion (35%) of Edoxaban is eliminated by the kidneys compared to Dabigatran and Rivaroxaban. A very limited proportion of edoxaban (about 4%) is metabolized by cytochrome P450. The most important pharmacokinetic parameters of DOACs are listed in Table **2**.

**Table 2. Characteristics of thrombin inhibitor and factor Xa inhibitors.**

|  | **Dabigatran Etexilate** | **Rivaroxaban** | **Apixaban** | **Edoxaban** |
|---|---|---|---|---|
| Target | Factor IIa | Factor Xa | Factor Xa | Factor Xa |
| Prodrug | Yes | No | No | No |
| Bioavailability | 5% | 80% | 45% | 45-50% |
| Time to peak | 2 hours | 3 hours | 3 hours | 1-2 hours |
| Half-life | 15 hours | 10 hours | 12 hours | 10 hours |
| Metabolism through cytochrome P450 | No | Yes(30%) | Yes (15%) | Yes (3%) |
| Efflux transporter P-gp | Yes | Yes | Yes | Yes |
| Renal excretion | 80% | 65% | 25% | 35% |

(Table 2) contd.....

| | Dabigatran Etexilate | Rivaroxaban | Apixaban | Edoxaban |
|---|---|---|---|---|
| Dosing | Twice a day | Once a day | Twice a day | Once a day |
| Reversal by hemodialysis | Yes | No | No | No |
| Antidote | Idarucizumab | Andexanet | Andexanet | Andexanet |

## 2.2. DOACs Indications, Main Efficacy and Safety Data

The introduction of several novel oral anticoagulant drugs has recently transformed the clinical practice of oral anticoagulant therapy. Currently approved agents for prevention of strokes in non valvular atrial fibrillation (NVAF), and for prevention and treatment of venous thromboembolism include dabigatran, rivaroxaban, apixaban and edoxaban.

The most important advantages of these direct anticoagulants are:

• more predictable PK/PD profile
• reduced susceptibility to food and drug interactions
• predictable anticoagulant effect, not requested routine coagulation monitoring (which is mandatory with warfarin)
• relative rapid onset and offset of action
• no need of bridging therapies such as heparin in patients requiring surgery or interventions

Safety and efficacy of DOACs have been established in several large phase 3 clinical trials, both in NVAF and in venous thromboembolism areas.

In NVAF DOACs resulted to be not inferior or superior when compared to warfarin, with similar or lower levels of major bleeding [4 - 7].

A meta-analysis, comparing DOACs with warfarin in more than 70000 NVAF patients, showed a 19% larger reduction in stroke or systemic embolic risk with DOACs (relative risk 0.81; 95%CI 0.38-0.64; p< 0.001) [40]. Moreover in patients treated with DOACs intracranial hemorrhage was reduced by 52% (RR 0.48; 95%CI 0.39-0.59; p< 0.001) and all-cause mortality by 10% with respect to warfarin (RR 0.90; 95%CI 0.85-0.95; p=0.003). In patients treated with DOACs nevertheless an increased risk of gastrointestinal bleeding was observed (RR 1.25;

95%CI 1.01-1.55; p=0.04).

The use of VKA and the advanced age are both strong predictive factors for intracranial bleeding [25]. At this regard, it has to be emphasized that the reduction of intracranial bleeding observed with DOACs in the general population is present also in the elderly [41]. In the elderly population, DOACs demonstrated a reduction of the thrombotic risk which was similar to VKA. In elderly people an increased risk of gastrointestinal bleeding was reported only for Dabigatran [41].

## 2.3. DOACs Monitoring

Although DOACs do not require monitoring in routine clinical practice, the laboratory measurements of their anticoagulant effects may be useful in some clinical situations such as active bleeding and ICH. Routine coagulation assays such as PT and the activated partial thromboplastin time (aPTT) are affected to a variable extent by the different DOACs. Due to their short half-life, plasma concentrations of these drugs show large variability. Therefore, to correctly interpret a coagulation assay, it is necessary to know exactly the time of the last administration of the drug. As their maximal plasma concentration and maximal anticoagulant activity will occur approximately 1–4 hours after their oral intake [42], they will demonstrate a much larger impact on the coagulation at this time (peak) [43]. Qualitative (activated partial thromboplastin time for Dabigatran and prothrombin time for Rivaroxaban) and specific, quantitative (diluted thrombin time for Dabigatran, chromogenic anti-Xa assay for factor Xa inhibitors) laboratory assays to monitor the pharmacodynamic effect of DOACs are available that may help in case of emergency surgery or bleeding complications.

### 2.3.1. Monitoring of Dabigatran

Dabigatran plasma concentration shows a curvilinear relation with aPTT: therefore as the concentration of Dabigatran increases aPTT values reach a plateau. This relationship makes aPTT unsuitable for quantifying Dabigatran concentrations. On the other hand, therapeutic concentrations of Dabigatran will typically prolong aPTT [42]. Even though aPTT has important limitations and is not suited for a quantitative assessment of Dabigatran effect, due to its widespread use, easy accessibility and low cost, aPTT can be useful in providing rapid qualitative information in emergency situations. If a sensitive assay is used, a prolonged aPTT (*i.e.*, >2 times the upper limit of normal) indicates the presence of Dabigatran in the plasma and this is associated with an increased bleeding risk [44].

Dabigatran showed an exponential, concentration-dependent prolongation of PT, but without any reliable linear correlation with PT. Therefore, PT and INR should not be used to monitor the effect of Dabigatan [45].

The thrombin time (TT) is very sensitive to Dabigatran activity [42]; therefore, a normal TT may be used to rule out the presence of therapeutic levels of Dabigatran. The diluted TT (dTT), on the other hand, shows a linear relation with plasma levels of Dabigatran and has a good reproducibility. The dTT eliminates the issue of the oversensitivity of the conventional TT. This test has now become commercially available: the test procedure is simple, rapid and employs standard analyzers [46].

Other useful tests are the ecarin clotting time (ECT) and ecarin chromogenic assay. Nevertheless these tests are currently not standardized and they are not available in most laboratories.

### 2.3.2. Monitoring of Direct Xa Inhibitors

Therapeutic concentrations of Rivaroxaban prolong PT. However, PT clotting time is not a reliable index of Rivaroxaban function as it is influenced by the different sensitivities of the reagents used [47]. Dilute PT (dPT) due to inter-assay variability is also unsuiTable aPTT whose dose-dependent prolongation is not linearly related to the increasing plasma levels of rivaroxaban should not be used to assess the effects of Rivaroxaban, Apixaban and Edoxaban.

The most specific tests to monitor direct Xa inhibitors effects are based on the cleavage of synthetic chromogenic substrates. These assays are superior to the classic clot formation-based coagulation assays. Specific anti-Xa assays (aXa) with appropriate calibrators tweaked for the monitoring of Rivaroxaban or Apixaban have now been developed and introduced into clinical practice. These new anti-Xa chromogenic assays are still not widely available and may not be available in emergency units [48, 49]. Because of the lack of experience with these assays, there are no concentration ranges that have been associated with an increased risk of bleeding nor are cut-off concentrations known below which invasive procedures can be performed without additional bleeding risk.

In summary to monitor the pharmacodynamic effect of DOACs general, qualitative (activated partial thromboplastin time for Dabigatran and prothrombin time for Rivaroxaban) and specific, quantitative (diluted thrombin time for Dabigatran, chromogenic anti-Xa assay for factor Xa inhibitors) laboratory assays are available that may help clinical decision making in case of emergency surgery or bleeding complications.

## 2.4. DOACs Reversal and Management of Life Threatening Bleeding

Since DOACs appearance in clinical practice a major drawback was the absence of an effective antidote to treat severe bleeding. Despite suggested different strategies in case of bleeding [43, 50 - 52] official guidelines on DOACs reversal are lacking. Recently, a specific antidote has become available for Dabigatran, which has been approved by the FDA and EMA.

### 2.4.1. General Principles for Managing Bleeding Related to Anticoagulants

The approach and treatment of major bleeding and in particular of ICH requires a dedicated and trained team of clinicians. Anticoagulation procedures, in fact, increase the thrombotic risk in part because of the prothrombotic condition for which anticoagulation was initially prescribed, in part because of the procoagulant effect of the administered drug that may activate the coagulation cascade.

The general principles of management of anticoagulant-related bleeding are listed in Table **3**.

### 2.4.2. Traditional Reversal Agents

The available data on DOACs reversal with fresh frozen plasma (FFP) or with prothrombin complex concentrates (PCCs) are limited and obtained in a small number of case reports, or studies employing animals or healthy volunteers. However, in the absence of a true antidote for any specific DOAC, PCCs should be considered a cornerstone of the management of life-threatening bleeding in these patients.

**Table 3. General principle of management of anticoagulant-related bleeding.**

| General principles | |
|---|---|
|      Stop anticoagulation | |
|      Hemodynamic and hemostatic resuscitation | |
|          * volume replacement | |
|          * local hemostatic measures | |
|      Check coagulation tests, platelet count, fibrinogen | |
|      Check renal function | |
|      Blood product | |
|          * coagulation factors (PCC) | |
|          * platelet transfusion if indicated | |
|      Massive transfusion protocol if uncontrollable bleeding | |
| **Specific measure** | |
|      VKA/Oral Xa inhibitors: PCC | |
|      dabigatran: activated PCC, hemodialysis | |
|      Specific reversal agents when available (idarucizumab, andexanet) | |
| | |
| **Adjunctive measures** | |
|      Consider antifibrinolytics (tranexamic acid) | |

## *2.4.2.1. Dabigatran Reversal*

For mild or moderate bleeding or less urgent surgery in a patient taking Dabigatran, cessation of the drug intake may be sufficient as a first measure, because of the short half-life of the drug (about 12 hours). It is however mandatory to check renal function, because renal impairment significantly increases the plasma half-life of the drug.

Fresh frozen plasma (FFP) contains all coagulation factors but there are no data from human studies on the administration of FFP in case of Dabigatran-associated bleeding. In a mice model of Dabigatran-associated ICH, the administration of FFP decreased the volume of intracerebral hemorrhage but this had no effect on mortality [53]. Moreover, one has to consider that FFP administration could produce some side effects *i.e.* allergic reactions, infections and transfusion-related acute lung injury [42, 54].

The available PCC concentrates are:

- 3-factors PCC: factors II, IX, X
- 4-factors PCC: factors II, VII, IX, X
- activated PCC (aPCC) or Factor Eight Inhibitor Bypassing Agent (FEIBA ®): factor II,IX,X, protein C and activated factor VII

In an animal model of Dabigatran-related bleeding PCC administration produced a progressive reduction in blood loss even in absence of aPTT changes. When administered to healthy volunteers treated with Dabigatran, PCC (50 U/kg) had no effect on aPTT, TT and ecarin clotting time prolongation [55]. It seems therefore that laboratory parameters do not represent an appropriate end point in clinical studies.

Recombinant activated factor VII (rFVIIa) is a well-known pro-hemostatic agent. It promotes hemostasis by activating the extrinsic pathway, generating FXa and FIXa. It has been developed to treat congenital FVIII deficiency or to treat patients with acquired FVIII deficiency. Nevertheless, there are no human studies proving a beneficial effect of rFVIIa in patients receiving Dabigatran [56, 57]. In animal studies, rFVIIa resulted to be not effective in reducing intracerebral hematoma [53]. Moreover, FVIIa has potential prothrombotic effect.

When added to Dabigatran, activated charcoal resulted to absorb more than 99% of the drug. Therefore, it may be effective in reducing Dabigatran absorption following a recent ingestion that is 1–2 h after the last intake of Dabigatran.

Due to its limited (35%) binding to plasma protein, Dabigatran can be hemodialyzed in case of life-threatening bleeding or in case of overdose or before emergency surgery. Hemodialysis can be particularly useful in patients with renal impairment. A study including patients on hemodialysis receiving a single dose of Dabigatran showed, in fact, a removal of 62 to 68% of active Dabigatran after 2 to 4 h [58]. There are no published data on the use of antifibrinolytic agents in case of DOACs related bleeding. However, because of their demonstrated safety profile and of their efficacy in trauma related blood loss, their use in case of life-threatening bleeding caused by DOACs has to be considered.

### 2.4.2.2. Factor Xa Inhibitors Reversal

Due to the short half-life of factor Xa inhibitors, discontinuation of the drug might be enough in clinical situations where there is time to wait for spontaneous clearance.

In healthy volunteers receiving Rivaroxaban, PCC administration shortened PT prolongation and normalized endogenous thrombin potential. At high doses (50 U/kg), PCC administration reversed PT prolongation [55]. Animal studies support the pro-hemostatic effects of PCCs in bleeding models [59, 60] but it remains to be demonstrated whether PCC also improves outcome in case of bleeding in humans. In plasma of healthy volunteers treated with Rivaroxaban or Apixaban [42, 61] activated 4 factors PCC has been shown to correct all thrombin related parameters. In the same way, aPCC corrects PT, aPTT and factor Xa activity of Edoxaban-spiked plasma [62]. It has to be underlined nevertheless that these laboratory results cannot be automatically translated into clinical practice. Some authors suggest to use an initial dose of 50 UI/kg of PCC in case of life-threatening bleeding, to be repeated (25 UI/kg) if needed [43] and an initial dose of 50 UI/kg of aPCC, to be repeated if needed (max 200 u/kg/d). Until now, despite a considerable discussion about their advantages or disadvantages, it has not been established if 4 factor PCC is better than 3 factor PCC. The use of both PCCs is anyway supported by preclinical evidence [63, 64].

There are no data to support the use of FFP to reverse Rivaroxaban and Apixaban-induced bleeding. In cases of overdose of Apixaban and potentially also of Rivaroxaban, administration of activated charcoal may be useful, but so far there are no clinical data to support this. Hemodialysis is unlikely to be effective in case of treatment with FXa inhibitors, since all FXa inhibitors have a high degree of protein binding [54].

In an animal study, rFVIIa did not reverse bleeding and only partially corrected laboratory coagulation abnormalities induced by rivaroxaban [54, 65].

### 2.4.3. Novel Reversal Strategies

At the moment, agents with a specific activity against DOACs are: Idarucizumab the first to antagonize Dabigatran effect that have been approved by both FDA and EMA; Andexanet alfa that antagonizes the effect of all Xa inhibitors. Andexanet alfa is currently under investigation.

#### 2.4.3.1. Idarucizumab

Idarucizumab is a humanized monoclonal antibody fragment [Fab] that binds specifically to Dabigatran. Idarucizumab shows a 350 times greater affinity for Dabigatran than for thrombin and it does not bind to thrombin substrates. Therefore, functionally it does not resemble thrombin [66]. Idarucizumab reaches peak plasma levels rapidly, but its concentration decreases to 5% of the peak level within 4 hours due to renal removal. In order to be completely effective, Idarucizumab has to be dosed in 1:1 ratio with Dabigatran.

A phase 3 trial is ongoing to evaluate the reversal effect of Idarucizumab on the anticoagulant activity of Dabigatran in patients with uncontrolled bleeding or who require emergency surgery or procedures (REVERSE AD trial). The interim analysis of 90 patients has been recently published [67]. In this interim analysis 51 patients were enrolled in group A (uncontrolled bleeding) and 39 in group B (requiring emergency surgery or procedures). The mean patient age was 76.5 years. Ninety percent of the patients were receiving Dabigatran for stroke prevention because of atrial fibrillation. A total of 18 patients in group A had intracranial hemorrhage, 20 had gastrointestinal bleeding, 9 had traumatic bleeding, and 11 had bleeding for other causes. Sixteen patients in group A were hemodynamically unsTable Idarucizumab normalized the test in 88% to 98% of the patients within minutes. Concentrations of unbound Dabigatran remained 20 ng/mL at 24 hours in 79% of the patients. Among 35 patients in group A hemostasis was restored after 11.4 hours. Among 36 patients in group B normal intraoperative hemostasis was reported in 33 patients. Mildly or moderately abnormal hemostasis was reported in 2 and 1 patients, respectively. One thrombotic event occurred within 72 hours after Idarucizumab administration in a patient whom anticoagulant treatment was not restored. In this study, 18 deaths occurred (20%). This high number of deaths may be due to the relatively old age of the patients and to their comorbidities [68]. In this study, only 18 patients in group A had intracerebral hemorrhage, and no patients in group B required emergent surgery for cerebral bleeding. Further studies in neurosurgical patients with intracerebral hemorrhage are therefore needed.

### *2.4.3.2. Andexanet Alfa*

Andexanet alfa is a recombinant modified decoy of factor Xa. Andexanet is catalytically inactive but it binds with high affinity to factor Xa inhibitors on the active site thereby restoring the activity of endogenous factor Xa [69].

In preliminary studies in animals, Andexanet alfa was able to reverse the action of direct factor Xa inhibitors in a dose dependent manner. In healthy subjects Andexanet alfa has been shown to antagonize the anti Xa activity of both Apixaban and Rivaroxaban (5 mg twice daily, taken for 11 doses) [69, 70]. Recently, a randomized placebo controlled double-blind phase 3 trial on the efficacy of Andexanet alfa in reversing Apixaban- (ANNEXA-A study) and Rivaroxaban-(ANNEXA-R study) effects in older healthy volunteers (50 to 75 years) has been published [71].

In this trial the anti-factor Xa activity of Apixaban was reduced by 94% while in the placebo group it was reduced by only 21% (p<0.001). The same was observed for Rivaroxaban. Anti- factor Xa activity was rapidly reduced (within 2 to 5 minutes) after the endovenous administration of Andexanet, and the effect persisted for 2 hours after the infusion.

At the present time, more efficacy and safety trials on Andexanet alfa are required.

## CONCLUSION

Novel oral anticoagulants offer substantial clinical advantages over warfarin: they have predictable pharmacokinetic and pharmacodynamic profiles, they are given in a fixed dose and they show only minor drug and food interactions. Bleeding is the most common adverse side effect associated with therapeutic anticoagulation. Warfarin-associated ICHs occur most commonly within the conventional INR range of 2 to 3.5. In these cases it is important to have reliable and cost-effective treatments that reduce bleeding and therefore morbidity and mortality. Emergency units moreover should prepare clear protocols for the treatment of patients with anticoagulant-associated ICH. For VKA related ICHs the recommended treatment is administration of vitamin K together with the administration of 3 or 4-factor PCCs, or FFP. In case of ICH in patients taking DOACs vitamin K is not indicated and the use of PCCS, FFP or rFVIIa requires further studies. The reversal of anticoagulation with specific, rapidly acting antidotes (Idarucizumab, Andexanet) is indicated in case of emergency.

## TAKE HOME MESSAGES:

- Despite the recent introduction of direct oral anticoagulants in different clinical settings, vitamin K antagonists remain the mainstay of anticoagulant treatment in many patients.
- Direct oral anticoagulants are effective and well tolerated drugs, with a safer bleeding profile than traditional oral vitamin K antagonists.
- Bleeding is the most common adverse effect associated with the use of DOACs and VKA, and ICH is one of the worst bleeding complication that can occur even when the therapeutic target of INR (warfarin) is respected.
- In case of ICH in a VKA-treated patient, the patient should receive PCCs or FFP and vitamin K as soon as possible, together with the general procedures needed in the emergency situations (hemodynamic and hemostatic resuscitation procedures, check blood parameters, massive bleeding protocol if needed).
- In case of ICH in a DOAC-treated patient, the general emergency procedures should be started as soon as possible, but the role of FFP, PCC, rFVII is not well standardized and not so clear at the moment. The recent introduction of a specific antidote for one of the available DOACs and the imminent arrival of

other antidotes will offer a rapid and effective restoration of hemostasis in the emergency setting.

## CONFLICT OF INTEREST

The author confirms that the author has no conflict of interest to declare for this publication.

## ACKNOWLEDGEMENTS

Declared none.

## REFERENCES

[1]     Wysowski DK, Nourjah P, Swartz L. Bleeding complications with warfarin use: a prevalent adverse effect resulting in regulatory action. Arch Intern Med 2007; 167(13): 1414-9.
        [http://dx.doi.org/10.1001/archinte.167.13.1414] [PMID: 17620536]

[2]     Veltkamp R, Rizos T, Horstmann S. Intracerebral bleeding in patients on antithrombotic agents. Semin Thromb Hemost 2013; 39(8): 963-71.
        [http://dx.doi.org/10.1055/s-0033-1357506] [PMID: 24114010]

[3]     Go AS, Hylek EM, Phillips KA, *et al.* Prevalence of diagnosed atrial fibrillation in adults: national implications for rhythm management and stroke prevention: the AnTicoagulation and Risk Factors in Atrial Fibrillation (ATRIA) Study. JAMA 2001; 285(18): 2370-5.
        [http://dx.doi.org/10.1001/jama.285.18.2370] [PMID: 11343485]

[4]     Connolly SJ, Ezekowitz MD, Yusuf S, *et al.* Dabigatran *versus* warfarin in patients with atrial fibrillation. N Engl J Med 2009; 361(12): 1139-51.
        [http://dx.doi.org/10.1056/NEJMoa0905561] [PMID: 19717844]

[5]     Patel MR, Mahaffey KW, Garg J, *et al.* Rivaroxaban *versus* warfarin in nonvalvular atrial fibrillation. N Engl J Med 2011; 365(10): 883-91.
        [http://dx.doi.org/10.1056/NEJMoa1009638] [PMID: 21830957]

[6]     Granger CB, Alexander JH, McMurray JJ, *et al.* Apixaban *versus* warfarin in patients with atrial fibrillation. N Engl J Med 2011; 365(11): 981-92.
        [http://dx.doi.org/10.1056/NEJMoa1107039] [PMID: 21870978]

[7]     Giugliano RP, Ruff CT, Braunwald E, *et al.* Edoxaban *versus* warfarin in patients with atrial fibrillation. N Engl J Med 2013; 369(22): 2093-104.
        [http://dx.doi.org/10.1056/NEJMoa1310907] [PMID: 24251359]

[8]     Verheugt FW, Granger CB. Oral anticoagulants for stroke prevention in atrial fibrillation: current status, special situations, and unmet needs. Lancet 2015; 386(9990): 303-10.
        [http://dx.doi.org/10.1016/S0140-6736(15)60245-8] [PMID: 25777666]

[9]     Flaherty ML, Kissela B, Woo D, *et al.* The increasing incidence of anticoagulant-associated intracerebral hemorrhage. Neurology 2007; 68(2): 116-21.

[http://dx.doi.org/10.1212/01.wnl.0000250340.05202.8b] [PMID: 17210891]

[10]    Lovelock CE, Molyneux AJ, Rothwell PM. Change in incidence and aetiology of intracerebral haemorrhage in Oxfordshire, UK, between 1981 and 2006: a population-based study. Lancet Neurol 2007; 6(6): 487-93.
[http://dx.doi.org/10.1016/S1474-4422(07)70107-2] [PMID: 17509483]

[11]    Dequatre-Ponchelle N, Hénon H, Pasquini M, *et al.* Vitamin K antagonists-associated cerebral hemorrhages: what are their characteristics? Stroke 2013; 44(2): 350-5.
[http://dx.doi.org/10.1161/STROKEAHA.112.672303] [PMID: 23287784]

[12]    Flaherty ML, Haverbusch M, Sekar P, *et al.* Location and outcome of anticoagulant-associated intracerebral hemorrhage. Neurocrit Care 2006; 5(3): 197-201.
[http://dx.doi.org/10.1385/NCC:5:3:197] [PMID: 17290088]

[13]    Cucchiara B, Messe S, Sansing L, Kasner S, Lyden P. Hematoma growth in oral anticoagulant related intracerebral hemorrhage. Stroke 2008; 39(11): 2993-6.
[http://dx.doi.org/10.1161/STROKEAHA.108.520668] [PMID: 18703803]

[14]    Ansell J, Hirsh J, Hylek E, *et al.* Pharmacology and management of the vitamin K antagonists: American college of chest physicians evidence-based clinical practice guidelines (8th Edition) Chest 2008; 133(6 Suppl): 160S-98S.
[http://dx.doi.org/10.1378/chest.08-0670] [PMID: 18574265]

[15]    Aithal GP, Day CP, Kesteven PJ, Daly AK. Association of polymorphisms in the cytochrome P450 CYP2C9 with warfarin dose requirement and risk of bleeding complications. Lancet 1999; 353(9154): 717-9.
[http://dx.doi.org/10.1016/S0140-6736(98)04474-2] [PMID: 10073515]

[16]    DAndrea G, DAmbrosio RL, Di Perna P, *et al.* A polymorphism in the VKORC1 gene is associated with an interindividual variability in the dose-anticoagulant effect of warfarin. Blood 2005; 105(2): 645-9.
[http://dx.doi.org/10.1182/blood-2004-06-2111] [PMID: 15358623]

[17]    Wessler S, Gitel SN. Warfarin. From bedside to bench. N Engl J Med 1984; 311(10): 645-52.
[http://dx.doi.org/10.1056/NEJM198409063111007] [PMID: 6472343]

[18]    Kirkwood TB. Calibration of reference thromboplastins and standardisation of the prothrombin time ratio. Thromb Haemost 1983; 49(3): 238-44.
[PMID: 6879511]

[19]    Holbrook A, Schulman S, Witt DM, *et al.* Evidence-based management of anticoagulant therapy: antithrombotic therapy and prevention of thrombosis, 9th ed: American College of Chest Physicians evidence-based clinical practice guidelines. Chest 2012; 141(2 Suppl): e152S-84.
[http://dx.doi.org/10.1378/chest.11-2295] [PMID: 22315259]

[20]    Cannegieter SC, Rosendaal FR, Wintzen AR, van der Meer FJ, Vandenbroucke JP, Briët E. Optimal oral anticoagulant therapy in patients with mechanical heart valves. N Engl J Med 1995; 333(1): 11-7.
[http://dx.doi.org/10.1056/NEJM199507063330103] [PMID: 7776988]

[21]    Optimal oral anticoagulant therapy in patients with nonrheumatic atrial fibrillation and recent cerebral ischemia. N Engl J Med 1995; 333(1): 5-10.

[http://dx.doi.org/10.1056/NEJM199507063330102] [PMID: 7776995]

[22]    Palareti G, Legnani C, Guazzaloca G, *et al.* Risks factors for highly unstable response to oral anticoagulation: a case-control study. Br J Haematol 2005; 129(1): 72-8.
[http://dx.doi.org/10.1111/j.1365-2141.2005.05417.x] [PMID: 15801958]

[23]    Connolly SJ, Pogue J, Eikelboom J, *et al.* Benefit of oral anticoagulant over antiplatelet therapy in atrial fibrillation depends on the quality of international normalized ratio control achieved by centers and countries as measured by time in therapeutic range. Circulation 2008; 118(20): 2029-37.
[http://dx.doi.org/10.1161/CIRCULATIONAHA.107.750000] [PMID: 18955670]

[24]    Witt DM, Delate T, Clark NP, *et al.* Outcomes and predictors of very stable INR control during chronic anticoagulation therapy. Blood 2009; 114(5): 952-6.
[http://dx.doi.org/10.1182/blood-2009-02-207928] [PMID: 19439733]

[25]    Fang MC, Chang Y, Hylek EM, *et al.* Advanced age, anticoagulation intensity, and risk for intracranial hemorrhage among patients taking warfarin for atrial fibrillation. Ann Intern Med 2004; 141(10): 745-52.
[http://dx.doi.org/10.7326/0003-4819-141-10-200411160-00005] [PMID: 15545674]

[26]    Steiner T, Rosand J, Diringer M. Intracerebral hemorrhage associated with oral anticoagulant therapy: current practices and unresolved questions. Stroke 2006; 37(1): 256-62.
[http://dx.doi.org/10.1161/01.STR.0000196989.09900.f8] [PMID: 16339459]

[27]    Ma M, Meretoja A, Churilov L, *et al.* Warfarin-associated intracerebral hemorrhage: volume, anticoagulation intensity and location. J Neurol Sci 2013; 332(1-2): 75-9.
[http://dx.doi.org/10.1016/j.jns.2013.06.020] [PMID: 23911098]

[28]    Dezee KJ, Shimeall WT, Douglas KM, Shumway NM, Omalley PG. Treatment of excessive anticoagulation with phytonadione (vitamin K): a meta-analysis. Arch Intern Med 2006; 166(4): 391-7.
[PMID: 16505257]

[29]    Watson HG, Baglin T, Laidlaw SL, Makris M, Preston FE. A comparison of the efficacy and rate of response to oral and intravenous Vitamin K in reversal of over-anticoagulation with warfarin. Br J Haematol 2001; 115(1): 145-9.
[http://dx.doi.org/10.1046/j.1365-2141.2001.03070.x] [PMID: 11722425]

[30]    Tazarourte K, Riou B, Tremey B, Samama C-M, Vicaut E, Vigué B. Guideline-concordant administration of prothrombin complex concentrate and vitamin K is associated with decreased mortality in patients with severe bleeding under vitamin K antagonist treatment (EPAHK study). Crit Care 2014; 18(2): R81.
[http://dx.doi.org/10.1186/cc13843] [PMID: 24762166]

[31]    Goldstein JN, Thomas SH, Frontiero V, *et al.* Timing of fresh frozen plasma administration and rapid correction of coagulopathy in warfarin-related intracerebral hemorrhage. Stroke 2006; 37(1): 151-5.
[http://dx.doi.org/10.1161/01.STR.0000195047.21562.23] [PMID: 16306465]

[32]    Bershad EM, Suarez JI. Prothrombin complex concentrates for oral anticoagulant therapy-related intracranial hemorrhage: a review of the literature. Neurocrit Care 2010; 12(3): 403-13.
[http://dx.doi.org/10.1007/s12028-009-9310-0] [PMID: 19967567]

[33] Keeling D, Baglin T, Tait C, *et al.* Guidelines on oral anticoagulation with warfarin - fourth edition. Br J Haematol 2011; 154(3): 311-24.
[http://dx.doi.org/10.1111/j.1365-2141.2011.08753.x] [PMID: 21671894]

[34] Tran HA, Chunilal SD, Harper PL, Tran H, Wood EM, Gallus AS. An update of consensus guidelines for warfarin reversal. Med J Aust 2013; 198(4): 198-9.
[http://dx.doi.org/10.5694/mja12.10614] [PMID: 23451962]

[35] Spahn DR, Bouillon B, Cerny V, *et al.* Management of bleeding and coagulopathy following major trauma: an updated European guideline. Crit Care 2013; 17(2): R76. [BioMed Central Ltd].
[http://dx.doi.org/10.1186/cc12685] [PMID: 23601765]

[36] Gong IY, Kim RB. Importance of pharmacokinetic profile and variability as determinants of dose and response to dabigatran, rivaroxaban, and apixaban. Can J Cardiol 2013; 29(7) (Suppl.): S24-33.
[http://dx.doi.org/10.1016/j.cjca.2013.04.002] [PMID: 23790595]

[37] Mueck W, Becka M, Kubitza D, Voith B, Zuehlsdorf M. Population model of the pharmacokinetics and pharmacodynamics of rivaroxaban oral, direct factor xa inhibitor healthy subjects. Int J Clin Pharmacol Ther 2007; 45(6): 335-44.
[http://dx.doi.org/10.5414/CPP45335] [PMID: 17595891]

[38] Jiang X, Crain EJ, Luettgen JM, Schumacher WA, Wong PC. Apixaban, an oral direct factor Xa inhibitor, inhibits human clot-bound factor Xa activity *in vitro*. Thromb Haemost 2009; 101(4): 780-2.
[PMID: 19350128]

[39] Ogata K, Mendell-Harary J, Tachibana M, *et al.* Clinical safety, tolerability, pharmacokinetics, and pharmacodynamics of the novel factor Xa inhibitor edoxaban in healthy volunteers. J Clin Pharmacol 2010; 50(7): 743-53.
[http://dx.doi.org/10.1177/0091270009351883] [PMID: 20081065]

[40] Ruff CT, Giugliano RP, Braunwald E, *et al.* Comparison of the efficacy and safety of new oral anticoagulants with warfarin in patients with atrial fibrillation: a meta-analysis of randomised trials. Lancet 2014; 383(9921): 955-62.
[http://dx.doi.org/10.1016/S0140-6736(13)62343-0] [PMID: 24315724]

[41] Sharma M, Cornelius VR, Patel JP, Davies JG, Molokhia M. Efficacy and harms od direct oral anticoagulants in the elderly for stroke prevention in atrial fibrillation and secondary prevention of venous thromboembolism. Circulation 2015; 132: 194-204.
[http://dx.doi.org/10.1161/CIRCULATIONAHA.114.013267] [PMID: 25995317]

[42] Jackson LR II, Becker RC. Novel oral anticoagulants: pharmacology, coagulation measures, and considerations for reversal. J Thromb Thrombolysis 2014; 37(3): 380-91.
[http://dx.doi.org/10.1007/s11239-013-0958-0] [PMID: 23928868]

[43] Heidbuchel H, Verhamme P, Alings M, *et al.* European Heart Rhythm Association Practical Guide on the use of new oral anticoagulants in patients with non-valvular atrial fibrillation. Europace 2013; 15(5): 625-51.
[http://dx.doi.org/10.1093/europace/eut083] [PMID: 23625942]

[44] Lippi G, Ardissino D, Quintavalla R, Cervellin G. Urgent monitoring of direct oral anticoagulants in patients with atrial fibrillation: a tentative approach based on routine laboratory tests. J Thromb

Thrombolysis 2014; 38(2): 269-74.
[http://dx.doi.org/10.1007/s11239-014-1082-5] [PMID: 24811247]

[45]    Douxfils J, Mullier F, Robert S, Chatelain C, Chatelain B, Dogné JM. Impact of dabigatran on a large panel of routine or specific coagulation assays. Laboratory recommendations for monitoring of dabigatran etexilate. Thromb Haemost 2012; 107(5): 985-97.
[http://dx.doi.org/10.1160/TH11-11-0804] [PMID: 22438031]

[46]    Stangier J, Feuring M. Using the HEMOCLOT direct thrombin inhibitor assay to determine plasma concentrations of dabigatran. Blood Coagul Fibrinolysis 2012; 23(2): 138-43.
[http://dx.doi.org/10.1097/MBC.0b013e32834f1b0c] [PMID: 22227958]

[47]    Mueck W, Lensing AW, Agnelli G, Decousus H, Prandoni P, Misselwitz F. Rivaroxaban: population pharmacokinetic analyses in patients treated for acute deep-vein thrombosis and exposure simulations in patients with atrial fibrillation treated for stroke prevention. Clin Pharmacokinet 2011; 50(10): 675-86.
[http://dx.doi.org/10.2165/11595320-000000000-00000] [PMID: 21895039]

[48]    Douxfils J, Mullier F, Loosen C, Chatelain C, Chatelain B, Dogné JM. Assessment of the impact of rivaroxaban on coagulation assays: laboratory recommendations for the monitoring of rivaroxaban and review of the literature. Thromb Res 2012; 130(6): 956-66.
[http://dx.doi.org/10.1016/j.thromres.2012.09.004] [PMID: 23006523]

[49]    Douxfils J, Chatelain C, Chatelain B, Dogné JM, Mullier F. Impact of apixaban on routine and specific coagulation assays: a practical laboratory guide. Thromb Haemost 2013; 110(2): 283-94.
[http://dx.doi.org/10.1160/TH12-12-0898] [PMID: 23765180]

[50]    Sarich TC, Seltzer JH, Berkowitz SD, *et al.* Novel oral anticoagulants and reversal agents: Considerations for clinical development. Am Heart J 2015; 169(6): 751-7.
[http://dx.doi.org/10.1016/j.ahj.2015.03.010] [PMID: 26027611]

[51]    Siegal DM, Garcia DA, Crowther MA. How I treat target-specific oral anticoagulant-associated bleeding. Blood 2014; 123(8): 1152-8.
[http://dx.doi.org/10.1182/blood-2013-09-529784] [PMID: 24385535]

[52]    Vanden Daelen S, Peetermans M, Vanassche T, Verhamme P, Vandermeulen E. Monitoring and reversal strategies for new oral anticoagulants. Expert Rev Cardiovasc Ther 2015; 13(1): 95-103.
[http://dx.doi.org/10.1586/14779072.2015.987126] [PMID: 25431993]

[53]    Zhou W, Schwarting S, Illanes S, *et al.* Hemostatic therapy in experimental intracerebral hemorrhage associated with the direct thrombin inhibitor dabigatran. Stroke 2011; 42(12): 3594-9.
[http://dx.doi.org/10.1161/STROKEAHA.111.624650] [PMID: 21998060]

[54]    Siegal DM, Crowther MA. Acute management of bleeding in patients on novel oral anticoagulants. Eur Heart J 2013; 34(7): 489-498b.
[http://dx.doi.org/10.1093/eurheartj/ehs408] [PMID: 23220847]

[55]    Eerenberg ES, Kamphuisen PW, Sijpkens MK, Meijers JC, Buller HR, Levi M. Reversal of rivaroxaban and dabigatran by prothrombin complex concentrate: a randomized, placebo-controlled, crossover study in healthy subjects. Circulation 2011; 124(14): 1573-9.
[http://dx.doi.org/10.1161/CIRCULATIONAHA.111.029017] [PMID: 21900088]

[56]   Levi M, Eerenberg E, Kamphuisen PW. Bleeding risk and reversal strategies for old and new anticoagulants and antiplatelet agents. J Thromb Haemost 2011; 9(9): 1705-12.
[http://dx.doi.org/10.1111/j.1538-7836.2011.04432.x] [PMID: 21729240]

[57]   Majeed A, Schulman S. Bleeding and antidotes in new oral anticoagulants. Best Pract Res Clin Haematol 2013; 26(2): 191-202.
[http://dx.doi.org/10.1016/j.beha.2013.07.001] [PMID: 23953907]

[58]   Stangier J, Rathgen K, Stähle H, Mazur D. Influence of renal impairment on the pharmacokinetics and pharmacodynamics of oral dabigatran etexilate: an open-label, parallel-group, single-centre study. Clin Pharmacokinet 2010; 49(4): 259-68.
[http://dx.doi.org/10.2165/11318170-000000000-00000] [PMID: 20214409]

[59]   Martin AC, Le Bonniec B, Fischer AM, *et al.* Evaluation of recombinant activated factor VII, prothrombin complex concentrate, and fibrinogen concentrate to reverse apixaban in a rabbit model of bleeding and thrombosis. Int J Cardiol 2013; 168(4): 4228-33.
[http://dx.doi.org/10.1016/j.ijcard.2013.07.152] [PMID: 23928345]

[60]   Perzborn E, Gruber A, Tinel H, *et al.* Reversal of rivaroxaban anticoagulation by haemostatic agents in rats and primates. Thromb Haemost 2013; 110(1): 162-72.
[http://dx.doi.org/10.1160/TH12-12-0907] [PMID: 23636219]

[61]   Steiner T, Böhm M, Dichgans M, *et al.* Recommendations for the emergency management of complications associated with the new direct oral anticoagulants (DOACs), apixaban, dabigatran and rivaroxaban. Clin Res Cardiol 2013; 102(6): 399-412.
[http://dx.doi.org/10.1007/s00392-013-0560-7] [PMID: 23669868]

[62]   Fukuda T, Honda Y, Kamisato C, Morishima Y, Shibano T. Reversal of anticoagulant effects of edoxaban, an oral, direct factor Xa inhibitor, with haemostatic agents. Thromb Haemost 2012; 107(2): 253-9.
[http://dx.doi.org/10.1160/TH11-09-0668] [PMID: 22186946]

[63]   Gonsalves WI, Patnaik MM. Management of bleeding complications in patients on new oral anticoagulants. J Hematol Transfus 2014; 2: 1015.

[64]   Dentali F, Marchesi C, Giorgi Pierfranceschi M, *et al.* Safety of prothrombin complex concentrates for rapid anticoagulation reversal of vitamin K antagonists. A meta-analysis. Thromb Haemost 2011; 106(3): 429-38.
[http://dx.doi.org/10.1160/TH11-01-0052] [PMID: 21800002]

[65]   Godier A, Miclot A, Le Bonniec B, *et al.* Evaluation of prothrombin complex concentrate and recombinant activated factor VII to reverse rivaroxaban in a rabbit model. Anesthesiology 2012; 116(1): 94-102.
[http://dx.doi.org/10.1097/ALN.0b013e318238c036] [PMID: 22042412]

[66]   Schiele F, van Ryn J, Canada K, *et al.* A specific antidote for dabigatran: functional and structural characterization. Blood 2013; 121(18): 3554-62.
[http://dx.doi.org/10.1182/blood-2012-11-468207] [PMID: 23476049]

[67]   Pollack CV Jr, Reilly PA, Eikelboom J, *et al.* Idarucizumab for dabigatran reversal. N Engl J Med 2015; 373(6): 511-20.

[http://dx.doi.org/10.1056/NEJMoa1502000] [PMID: 26095746]

[68]    Sarode R, Milling TJ Jr, Refaai MA, *et al.* Efficacy and safety of a 4-factor prothrombin complex concentrate in patients on vitamin K antagonists presenting with major bleeding: a randomized, plasma-controlled, phase IIIb study. Circulation 2013; 128(11): 1234-43.
[PMID: 23935011]

[69]    Lu G, DeGuzman FR, Hollenbach SJ, *et al.* A specific antidote for reversal of anticoagulation by direct and indirect inhibitors of coagulation factor Xa. Nat Med 2013; 19(4): 446-51.
[http://dx.doi.org/10.1038/nm.3102] [PMID: 23455714]

[70]    Crowther MM, Kitt M, Lu G, Conley PB, Hollenbach S, *et al.* A phase 2 randomized, double blind, placebo-controlled trial demonstrating reversal of rivaroxaban-induced anticoagulation in healthy subjects by Andexanet Alfa (PRT064445), an antidote for Fxa inhibitors. Blood 2013; 122(21): 3636.

[71]    Siegal DM, Curnutte JT, Connolly SJ, *et al.* Andexanet Alfa for the Reversal of Factor Xa Inhibitor Activity. N Engl J Med 2015; 373(25): 2413-24.
[http://dx.doi.org/10.1056/NEJMoa1510991] [PMID: 26559317]

# CHAPTER 5

# Cerebral Collateral Circulation in Acute Ischemic Stroke: Translational Evidence for Outcome Prediction and Modulation Strategies

Simone Beretta[*], Fausto De Angeli, Elisa Cuccione, Giada Padovano, Davide Carone, Alessandro Versace and Carlo Ferrarese

*Laboratory of Experimental Stroke Research, School of Medicine, University of Milano-Bicocca, Monza, Italy*

*Milan Center for Neuroscience (NeuroMi), Milan, Italy*

**Abstract:** Cerebral collateral circulation is a subsidiary vascular network, which is dynamically recruited after arterial occlusion, and represents a powerful determinant of ischemic stroke outcome. Although several methods may be used for assessing cerebral collaterals in the acute phase of ischemic stroke in humans and rodents, they are generally underutilized. The assessment of collateral status in acute stroke patients may improve patient selection and maximize benefit-to-risk ratio of acute recanalization therapies. The systematic assessment of collaterals in experimental stroke models may be used as a "stratification factor" in multiple regression analysis of neuroprotection studies, in order to control the within-group variability. Exploring the modulatory mechanisms of cerebral collaterals during acute ischemic stroke may promote the translational development of therapeutic strategies for increasing collateral flow and directly compare them in terms of efficacy, safety and feasibility. Collateral therapeutics may have a role in the hyperacute (even pre-hospital) phase of ischemic stroke, prior to recanalization therapies.

**Keywords:** Acute ischemic stroke, Cerebral collaterals, Collateral therapeutics, CT angiography, Experimental stroke models, Infarct size variability, Ischemic penumbra, MRI angiography, patient selection, Recanalization therapies.

[*] **Corresponding author Simone Beretta:** Laboratory of Experimental Stroke Research, School of Medicine, University of Milano-Bicocca, Via Cadore 48, 20900 Monza (MI) – Italy; Tel: +39-02.6448.8128; Fax: +39-02.6448.8108; E-mail: simone.beretta@unimib.it

Alberto Radaelli, Giuseppe Mancia, Carlo Ferrarese & Simone Beretta (Eds.)

## INTRODUCTION

Cerebral collateral circulation is an auxiliary vascular network that is dynamically recruited after arterial occlusion and has the potential to provide residual blood flow to ischemic tissue. During acute ischemic stroke, cerebral collateral flow is highly variable among different individuals and is emerging as a strong prognostic factor both in unselected stroke patients and in patients treated with intravenous rtPA or endovascular recanalization therapy [1]. Experimental stroke models may be fundamental for a better understanding of the adaptive and modulatory mechanisms that regulate cerebral collateral circulation. Researching this further may lead to the translational development of new stroke therapies centred on collateral flow modulation in the hyperacute stage of ischemic stroke, prior to recanalization therapies [2].

### Cerebral Collateral Circulation in Humans and Rodents

Many similarities can be found between humans and rodents cerebral collateral circulation. In both species the circle of Willis represents a compensatory system to rapidly redistribute blood flow in case of occlusion of cervical arteries. Moreover in both humans and rodents, each cerebral artery ramifies along the cortical surface to form a pial arteriolar network, creating anastomotic connections among different vascular territories, known as leptomeningeal anastomoses (LMAs). LMAs are mostly developed between cortical branches of middle cerebral artery (MCA) and ACA or posterior cerebral artery. When proximal occlusion of a cerebral artery occurs, dynamic blood flow diversion through these anastomoses might provide residual (retrograde) blood flow to the cortical surface of the occluded artery territory, distally from the occlusion (Fig. **1**). However there are also some notable differences in the cerebral collateral circulation anatomy in the two species. The circle of Willis in rodents does not include the anterior communicating artery and the proximal segments of anterior cerebral arteries (ACA) converge to form one single median artery called Azigos ACA. Another difference between the two species is that in rodents, the pterygopalatine artery originates from the proximal internal carotid artery (ICA) providing additional extracranial collateral connections between external carotid artery and ICA *via* many arterial branches to facial, orbital and meningeal districts.

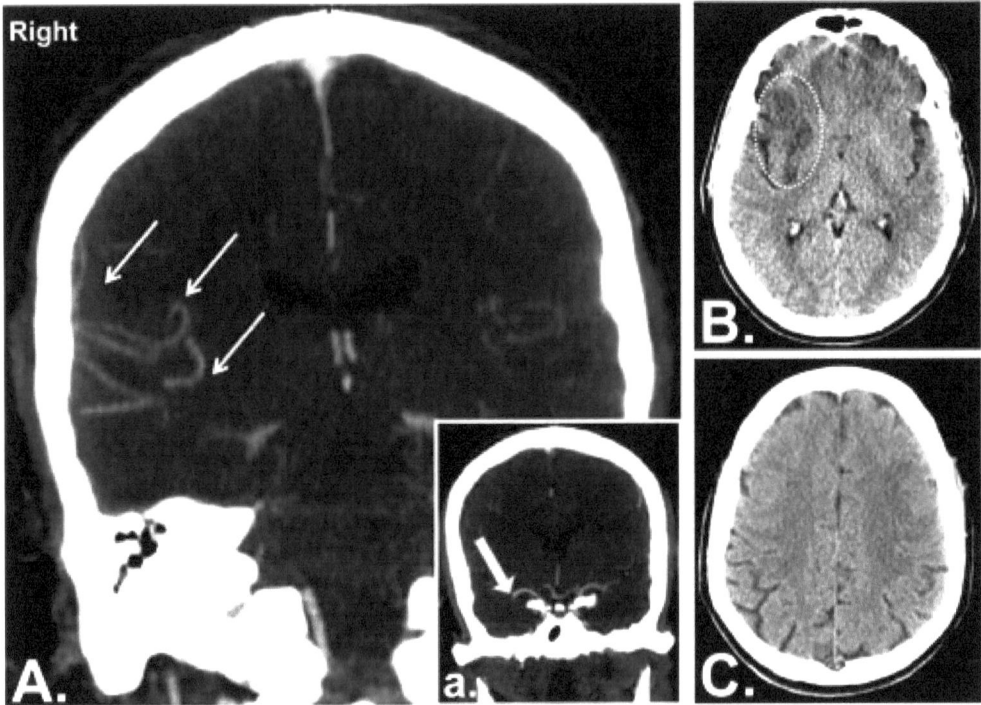

Fig. (1). Clinical imaging of cerebral collaterals during acute ischemic stroke using CT-angiography. Collateral vessels (**A**. small arrows) are visible in the right hemisphere. These vessels have been recruited after acute right MCA occlusion (**a**. large arrow). This patient was treated with intravenous thrombolysis and developed a small subcortical lesion (**B**), while the entire cortical territory was intact (**C**).

## Assessment of Cerebral Collateral Flow in Acute Stroke Patients

The anatomy of cerebral collaterals in acute stroke patients can be assessed using different diagnostic modalities (Table **1**) such as conventional digital subtraction angiography (DSA), CT angiography (CTA) or MR angiography (MRA). Functional performance can be studied through tissue perfusion evaluation *via* CT and MR perfusion techniques (PCT and PWI). At present, there is no agreement in clinical practice on which imaging should be performed, when after stroke and which patients would benefit most from cerebral collateral imaging. Recent studies have investigated the role of the circle of Willis in the development of collateral flow in ICA obstruction. [3, 4]. These studies were based on mathematical models and used transcranial Doppler ultrasound, digital contrast-enhanced angiography or magnetic resonance angiography. The relative importance of the separate components of the circle of Willis have thus been assessed, although no clear consensus is found among these reports [5].

**Table 1. Advantages, limitations, invasiveness and affordability of each technique for clinical assessment of cerebral collateral vessels in acute ischemic stroke.**

| Method | Advantages | Disadvantages | Risks | Cost |
|---|---|---|---|---|
| DSA | Evaluation of entire cerebrovascular system, plaque morphology and collateral circulation | Invasiveness Long duration Limited number of projections | Procedure-associated stroke, arterial dissections, allergic reactions to contrast agent, risk of renal function impairment | High |
| CTA | Direct visualization of collateral flow after arterial occlusion High spatial resolution | High radiation exposure Allergy risk Specific protocol needed | Allergic reactions to contrast agent Risk renal function impairment | Moderate |
| MRA | Multi-modal combination with other MRI sequences | Low spatial resolution Not feasible in agitated patients or in patients with non-MRI-conditional devices | Allergic reactions to contrast agent Non-MRI-conditional devices | High |
| PCT | Short duration | High radiation exposure Low amount of data Specific protocol needed | same as CTA | Moderate |
| PWI | Multi-modal combination with other MRI sequences | Low amount of data | same as MRA | High |

DSA is the gold standard for evaluating the recruitment of cerebral collaterals. The development of this technique reduces the dose of contrast, uses smaller catheters and shortens the length of the procedure [6]. Cerebral angiography permits an evaluation of the entire carotid artery system, providing information about tandem atherosclerotic disease, plaque morphology and collateral circulation which may affect management [7]. The disadvantages of angiography include its invasive nature, high cost, and risk of morbidity and mortality. The risk of morbidity is increased with cerebrovascular symptoms, advanced age, diabetes, hypertension, elevated serum creatinine and peripheral vascular disease. The size of the catheter, amount of contrast and procedure duration also affect complications rate. Although is considered the gold standard of carotid neurovascular imaging methods, conventional DSA has the disadvantage of a limited number of projections, typically two or three, representing the carotid artery. This limitation could lead to an underestimation of the degree of carotid stenosis in arteries that have asymmetrical rather than concentric stenotic lumen [8, 9].

CTA is able to provide direct visualization of collateral flow after arterial occlusion [10]. Patient presenting with proximal MCA occlusions showed a time dependent recruitment of flow to the symptomatic hemisphere through collateral vessels. Studying collateral vessels *via* CTA has given important advances in the current understanding of how collateral pathways influence outcome in acute stroke and the assessment of collaterals through CTA may provide a clinically useful method of selecting patients to benefit from intra-arterial therapies. CTA imaging can identify patients with diminished or absent collateral vessels in the symptomatic hemisphere. This group of patients experiences higher risk for further worsening. However, despite the abundance of emerging multimodal imaging techniques, there is a low amount of data demonstrating a strong correlation between an imaging finding and clinical outcome. Furthermore use of CTA reveals the extent of arterial collaterals by observing contrast filling of vessel lumens, but cannot account for any difference in volume of flow within collateral vessels that may be induced by occlusion [11].

MRA has been used to investigate collateral pathways, despite its lower spatial resolution compared to CTA [12] in view of the fact that is able to provide morphological and hemodynamic information concerning blood flow direction in individual vessels accurately. It is well known that the sensitivity of MRA decreases when blood flow velocity decreases. However, hemodynamic adaptations after ICA occlusion such as an increased flow through the collateral channels does result in improved sensitivity of MRA in detecting this vessels. A recent study has demonstrated how MRA can be used to investigate the anatomic variation of the collateral vessels in patients with severe carotid disease, to analyze how collateral vessels diameter changes in relation to varying grades of ICA obstruction and to analyze changes of LMAs diameter in relation to the presence or absence of collateral flow [13]. However, MRA is more expensive and time consuming than other techniques, and is less readily available. MRA may not be performed if the patient is critically ill, unable to stay supine, or has claustrophobia, a pacemaker or ferromagnetic implants [14]. Recent studies have shown a good correlation of MRA and conventional angiography in representing steno-occlusive lesions of the proximal intracranial arteries, but MRA alone has a potential for causing overestimation of stenosis [15, 16].

CT perfusion imaging can indicate the extent of irreversibly injured brain in the ischemic core and potentially salvageable but hypoperfused tissue in the ischemic penumbra. This technique allows to study the performance of collateral flow, which is indicated by preserved or increased cerebral blood volume (CBF) and augmented mean transit time [17]. Furthermore, CT perfusion imaging has evolved and fully automated, standardized volumetric processing can now be rapidly performed: brain tissue at risk for infarction (ischemic penumbra) can be distinguished from minimally hypoperfused tissue if the time to maximum delay is more than 6 seconds, while irreversibly injured brain (ischemic core) can be diagnosed if the relative cerebral blood flow is less than 30% of the normal tissue. In clinical practice, CT perfusion imaging could be used to exclude patients with large ischemic cores and without clinically significant salvageable tissue from endovascular therapy [18].

MR perfusion imaging offers the potential for measuring brain perfusion in acute stroke patients, at the time when treatment decisions based upon these measurements may affect outcomes dramatically. Because recanalization therapies offer both the potential of lifesaving rescue of underperfuse tissue and the risk of intracranial hemorrhage, the most active focus of research on MR perfusion imaging in acute stroke has been its potential application in refining the selection of patients for thrombolysis. However MR perfusion imaging has other potential roles such as establishing diagnosis, predicting prognosis and guiding other therapies designed to maintain cerebral perfusion FLAIR images on MR are able to show vascular hyper-intensities distal to an occluded cerebral artery, due to the presence of a slow, retrograde blood flow in collateral vessels [19]. PWI could assess the performance of collateral flow, showing cerebral tissue with relatively preserved CBF and prolonged blood transit time [20]. MR perfusion imaging has been used successfully to establish the diagnosis of cerebral ischemia in the absence of other objective evidence, and shows promise for selecting patients for thrombolytic therapy. Arterial spin-labelling MRI can detect brain regional hypoperfusion [21] and potentially identify the presence of leptomeningeal collateral routes [22]. However, this technique is rarely used in acute stroke imaging because of its relatively long imaging time and its difficulty in distinguishing between reduced blood flow and delayed transit times.

## Cerebral Collateral Flow as Stratification Factor in Pre-Clinical Neuroprotection Studies

More than 1000 putative neuroprotective agents have shown promising results in experimental stroke models [23, 24], however no successful translation has occurred in the phase-3 stroke clinical trials performed so far [25, 26].

One of the main reason behind this translational failure is thought to be the poor methodology that has characterized many preclinical studies, including study design, effective dose-finding, outcome assessment heterogeneity of stroke models and stroke severity, drug targeting and time window [27 - 29]. Outcome variability, and in particular infarct size, which is the most commonly used primary outcome, represents a well-recognized limitation of preclinical stroke models [30]. According to a recent meta-analysis, the average infarct size coefficient of variation of 502 control groups in preclinical stroke experiments was about 30% (ranging from 1.7% to 148%) [31]. The main consequence of dealing with high outcome variability is that a higher number of animals becomes necessary in order to have adequate statistical power, leading to an increase in the expenses and raising ethical issues. The reasons underlying infarct size variability in stroke models are not entirely understood. Although it has been demonstrated that surgical procedures, anaesthesia, rat strain, occluding filaments and physiological monitoring are associated with infarct size variability [32], factors related to inter-individual differences in cerebrovascular anatomy [33] and cerebral collateral circulation [34] have been reported. Interestingly, the National Centre for the Replacement, Refinement and Reduction of Animals in Research (NC3Rs) is currently funding a project (2014-2015) entitled "Determining the source of variability within experimental stroke models", which is mainly focused on vascular anatomy and reperfusion [35]. Cerebral hemodynamics variability during ischemia and the influence of drugs on CBF have both been largely neglected in preclinical research [36]. Monitoring CBF, including cerebral collateral flow, may help predicting outcome variability between treatment groups and detecting indirect neuroprotective effects in preclinical studies. Similarly to humans, the functional performance of collateral circulation during cerebral ischemia displays inter-individual variability in rodents [37]. Our work showed that the functional performance of the cerebral collaterals during MCAO in rats, assessed using multi-site LDF monitoring, predicted infarct size and functional outcome more accurately than conventional perfusion deficit in the ischemic core [34]. Additional experiments using the same method, in a series of 45 untreated animals, confirmed a highly significant correlation between stroke outcome and collateral flow during MCAO (Fig. **2**).

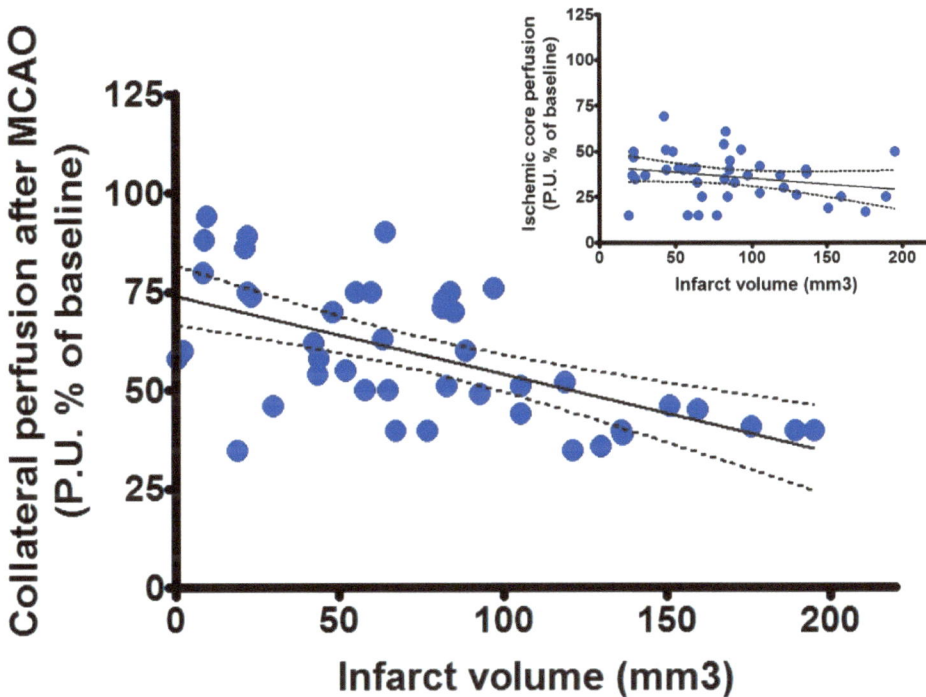

**Fig. (2).** Relationship between cerebral collateral flow during MCAO and stroke outcome in rats. Linear regression between infarct volume and perfusion deficit during MCAO in the territory of leptomeningeal collaterals, measured using multi-site laser Doppler, was calculated for 45 consecutive untreated rats (p < 0.0001; Pearson's r= -0.59). Notably, the correlation between infarct volume and perfusion deficit in the ischemic core (central MCA territory) was not significant (p = 0.14, smaller graph).

In experimental stroke studies, stratifying animals by collateral flow during MCAO represents a promising strategy to adjust for outcome variability. A simple method to stratify animals in term of pre-treatment perfusion deficit may be the use of cerebral collateral flow during MCAO as a covariate in multiple regression analysis, reducing the within group variability and improving efficacy analysis in preclinical neuroprotection studies. Further studies are required to determine more suitable methods, timing and statistical tool for collateral flow assessment in pre-clinical neuroprotection trials.

## Acute Therapeutic Modulation of Cerebral Collateral Flow

At present, intravenous thrombolysis with rtPA (Alteplase) performed within 4.5 hours from symptom onset and endovascular thrombectomy within 6 hours from symptom onset in presence of a large vessel occlusion represent the best therapeutic strategies available for acute ischemic stroke [38, 39]. However not only recanalization is not always achievable but when obtained it may be futile due to delayed reperfusion, vascular collapse downstream, re-occlusion, or hemorrhagic transformation [40, 41]. Vascular features beyond the occlusion are in fact often neglected [42]. Nonetheless, optimising ischemic penumbra perfusion thorough collateral blood flow modulation might represent a novel therapeutic strategy potentially implementable in the hyperacute (even pre-hospital) stage of ischemic stroke, prior to recanalization or neuroprotective therapies.

**Table 2. Potential strategies for modulation of cerebral collateral flow in acute ischemic stroke.**

| Strategies | | Risks | Cost | Results in Preclinical Stroke Models | Results and Feasibility in Human Stroke |
|---|---|---|---|---|---|
| Pressure Load | Induced hypertension | Haemorrhagic transformation, cardiac arrhythmias, myocardial ischemia | Low | Core and penumbra CBF augmentation through LMAs after distal MCAO in mice [43]. | Preliminary results indicate efficacy (small clinical studies) [44, 45]. High feasibility. |

*(Table 2) contd.....*

| Strategies | | Risks | Cost | Results in Preclinical Stroke Models | Results and Feasibility in Human Stroke |
|---|---|---|---|---|---|
| Intravascular Volume Load | Dextran and hydroxyethyl starch | Anaphylaxis, pulmonary edema, platelet dysfunction | Low | CBF augmentation and improved outcome in various stroke models [46]. | No benefit in early clinical trials (before the introduction of recanalization therapies) [47]. High feasibility. |
| | Albumin | Pulmonary edema, allergic reactions | Moderate | Cerebral perfusion enhancement through LMAs after distal MCAO in mice [48, 49]. | No benefit in a large RCT (administered after recanalization therapy) [50]. High feasibility. |
| Cerebral Vasodilation | Nitric Oxide Inhalation | Pulmonary irritation | Moderate | Selective arteriolar vasodilation in the penumbra and cortical CBF enhancement after MCAO in mice [52]. | No results available in human stroke. Moderate feasibility (inhalation delivery equipment needed). |
| | Sphenopalatine Ganglion Stimulation | Invasive (minor surgery) | High | Cortical arterioles vasodilation and CBF augmentation after photothrombosis [53] | Ongoing clinical trial [54]. Moderate feasibility (surgery needed). |
| | Sensory-induced Vasodilation | No risks known | Low | Gradual reperfusion through collaterals after MCAO in rats [56]. | No results available in human stroke. High feasibility. |
| | Acetazolamide | Paraesthesia, nausea, metabolic acidosis | Low | Negative effect on outcome if administered 48-54 hours after the onset of permanent MCAO [59]. | No results available in human acute stroke. Clinically used as diagnostic tool in chronic stroke. High feasibility. |

*(Table 2) contd.....*

| Strategies | | Risks | Cost | Results in Preclinical Stroke Models | Results and Feasibility in Human Stroke |
|---|---|---|---|---|---|
| Cerebral Flow Diversion | Head down tilt | Increase in intracranial venous pressure | Low | Cerebral perfusion augmentation after bilateral CCAO in mice [62]. | Increase in cerebral perfusion and blood flow velocity by flat head positioning (case series) [60, 61]. High feasibility. |
| | Partial aortic occlusion | Invasive (endovascular surgery) | High | Blood flow enhancement through LMAs after thromboembolic MCAO in rats [63]. | Clinical trial suggest efficacy in post-hoc subgroup analysis (further confirmation required) [64]. Moderate feasibility (endovascular procedure needed). |

A number of strategies (summarized in Table **2**) have the potential to modulate cerebral collateral flow during acute ischemic stroke, however extensive research is still required in both animal models and stroke patients to understand the optimal approach in term of benefit-to-risk ratio. A first strategy might be increasing systemic blood pressure. Phenylephrine is a selective α1-adrenergic receptor agonist able to induce systemic vasoconstriction with very limited effects on cerebral arteries. In rodents phenylephrine has been used to attain a 30% blood pressure increase after distal MCAO induction enhancing cortical CBF both in core and penumbra [43]. In small clinical studies, norepinephrine- o phenyle-phrine-induced hypertension was shown to improve the outcome in stroke patients [44, 45]; in these works however collateral circulation was not directly assessed, leaving its contribution unclear. Expanding the intravascular volume may constitute a second strategy. An increase in cerebral blood volume can be obtained by plasma expansion and haemodilution. This strategy was shown to improve cerebral perfusion in experimental stroke models [46]. However, in acute stroke trials performed in the 1990s, plasma expansion by dextran 40 and hydroxyethyl starch did not affect neurological outcome or mortality [47]. Notably, all these early clinical studies were performed in the pre-thrombolysis era and outside a meaningful therapeutic window (patients' enrolment was conducted many hours or even days after symptom onset) and cerebral collateral flow was not evaluated. Intravenous albumin administration has been reported to enhance cerebral perfusion and provide neuroprotection in preclinical works [48, 49]. However no benefit was found in a large randomized clinical trial that investigated the effects of intravenous albumin solution 25% in ischemic stroke patients compared to standard treatment [50]. Notably, 85% of these patients were treated with rtPA and intravenous albumin was administered on average 60 minutes after (not before) recanalization therapy. Inducing selective cerebral vasodilation may represent a third strategy. Nitric oxide (NO) is a strong endogenous vasodilator and has therapeutic potential for ischemic stroke [51]. In adult mice NO inhalation following MCAO induced a selective arteriolar vasodilation within the ischemic penumbra, likely through collateral arterioles, leading to decreased brain damage and improved functional outcome [52]. No data are available for inhaled nitric oxide in acute stroke patients. Sphenopalatine ganglion (SPG) electrostimulation activates parasympathetic fibers innervating intracranial vessels leading to their vasodilation. SPG-stimulation started after MCAO has been shown in preclinical studies to preserve DWI-PWI mismatch and reduce infarct size [53]. This technique has been demonstrated to be safe in ischemic stroke patients [54]. During ischemia collateral perfusion of affected regions could be non-invasively enhanced stimulating cerebral function through neurovascular coupling mechanisms (*i.e.* functional hyperaemia) [55]. Sensory cortical activation induced by whiskers stimulation in rats was shown to lead to a gradual reperfusion *via* MCA distal collaterals, when the treatment was initiated within a critical time window from MCAO onset [56]. No results are available for sensory stimulation in acute stroke patients. Acetazolamide, a carbonic anhydrase inhibitor, may also enable selective cerebral arteriolar vasodilation. By raising cerebral $CO_2$ levels acetazolamide was able to cause pial arteriolar vasodilation and increase cortical perfusion in piglets [57]. In clinical practice, acetazolamide is used to test hemispheric cerebrovascular reactivity in patients with chronic cerebrovascular occlusions [58]. Quite surprisingly, the only report of acetazolamide in experimental stroke dates back to 1971 [59], was performed in cats undergoing permanent MCAO (without reperfusion) and the drug was administered using a very late time window (48-54 hours after the onset ischemia). No results have been reported regarding the use of acetazolamide in acute stroke patients. Cerebral flow diversion represents a fourth strategy. Head positioning after acute vascular occlusion may affect through gravitational influences the pressure gradients in cerebral circulation, enhancing leptomeningeal recruitment. An increase in both cerebral perfusion and MCA blood flow velocity has been reported in stroke patients after flat head positioning [60, 61] and after 5° head-down tilt following bilateral CCAO in mice [62]. Flow diversion from the splanchnic circulation can be obtained through a temporary partial occlusion of the abdominal aorta. This procedure has been shown to increase blood flow through ACA-MCA leptomeningeal anastomoses after thromboembolic MCAO in rats, restoring it to baseline levels and maintaining stroke-induced vasodilation [63]. A randomized clinical trial in acute ischemic stroke patients has shown a tolerable safety profile and suggested efficacy in post-hoc subgroup analysis [64].

## CONCLUSION

A limited number of clinical and preclinical stroke studies focused on cerebral collateral circulation. Generally, neuroprotective effects are being sought, whereas the contribution of collateral blood flow is rarely considered or just inferred. Clinical and preclinical stroke research has the potential to directly study the adaptive capacity and modulatory mechanisms of cerebral collateral flow during focal cerebral ischemia, using different methods and in different conditions, with the ultimate goal of translating into clinical practice an effective strategy to enhance cerebral collateral flow in acute ischemic stroke.

## TAKE HOME MESSAGE

Cerebral collateral flow largely influences the temporal evolution of the ischemic lesion and the final stroke outcome. A significant inter-individual variability in the extent of collateral flow occurs after large vessel occlusion in acute stroke patients, which may be amenable to treatment with collateral therapeutics.

## CONFLICT OF INTEREST

The authors confirm that they have no conflict of interest to declare for this publication.

# DISCLOSURE

Part of this chapter has been previously published in Experimental & Translational Stroke Medicine20168:2 DOI: 10.1186/s13231-016-0015-0

# ACKNOWLEDGEMENTS

Declared none.

# REFERENCES

[1]    Campbell BC, Christensen S, Tress BM, *et al.* Failure of collateral blood flow is associated with infarct growth in ischemic stroke. J Cereb Blood Flow Metab 2013; 33(8): 1168-72.
[http://dx.doi.org/10.1038/jcbfm.2013.77] [PMID: 23652626]

[2]    Shuaib A, Butcher K, Mohammad AA, Saqqur M, Liebeskind DS. Collateral blood vessels in acute ischaemic stroke: a potential therapeutic target. Lancet Neurol 2011; 10(10): 909-21.
[http://dx.doi.org/10.1016/S1474-4422(11)70195-8] [PMID: 21939900]

[3]    Cassot F, Vergeur V, Bossuet P, Hillen B, Zagzoule M, Marc-Vergnes JP. Effects of anterior communicating artery diameter on cerebral hemodynamics in internal carotid artery disease. A model study. Circulation 1995; 92(10): 3122-31.
[http://dx.doi.org/10.1161/01.CIR.92.10.3122] [PMID: 7586284]

[4]    Hillen B, Drinkenburg BA, Hoogstraten HW, Post L. Analysis of flow and vascular resistance in a model of the circle of Willis. J Biomech 1988; 21(10): 807-14.
[http://dx.doi.org/10.1016/0021-9290(88)90013-9] [PMID: 3225267]

[5]    Hoksbergen AW, Fülesdi B, Legemate DA, Csiba L. Collateral configuration of the circle of Willis: transcranial color-coded duplex ultrasonography and comparison with postmortem anatomy. Stroke 2000; 31(6): 1346-51.
[http://dx.doi.org/10.1161/01.STR.31.6.1346] [PMID: 10835455]

[6]    Hankey GJ, Warlow CP, Sellar RJ. Cerebral angiographic risk in mild cerebrovascular disease. Stroke 1990; 21(2): 209-22.
[http://dx.doi.org/10.1161/01.STR.21.2.209] [PMID: 2406993]

[7]    Wolpert SM, Caplan LR. Current role of cerebral angiography in the diagnosis of cerebrovascular diseases. AJR Am J Roentgenol 1992; 159(1): 191-7.
[http://dx.doi.org/10.2214/ajr.159.1.1609697] [PMID: 1609697]

[8]    Edwards JH, Kricheff II, Riles T, Imparato A. Angiographically undetected ulceration of the carotid bifurcation as a cause of embolic stroke. Radiology 1979; 132(2): 369-73.
[http://dx.doi.org/10.1148/132.2.369] [PMID: 461794]

[9]    Bosanac Z, Miller RJ, Jain M. Rotational digital subtraction carotid angiography: technique and comparison with static digital subtraction angiography. Clin Radiol 1998; 53(9): 682-7.
[http://dx.doi.org/10.1016/S0009-9260(98)80295-X] [PMID: 9766722]

[10]   Maas MB, Lev MH, Ay H, *et al.* Collateral vessels on CT angiography predict outcome in acute

ischemic stroke. Stroke 2009; 40(9): 3001-5.
[http://dx.doi.org/10.1161/STROKEAHA.109.552513] [PMID: 19590055]

[11]   Maas MB, Lev MH, Ay H, *et al.* Collateral vessels on CT angiography predict outcome in acute
       ischemic stroke. Stroke 2009; 40(9): 3001-5.
       [http://dx.doi.org/10.1161/STROKEAHA.109.552513] [PMID: 19590055]

[12]   Kinoshita T, Ogawa T, Kado H, Sasaki N, Okudera T. CT angiography in the evaluation of intracranial
       occlusive disease with collateral circulation: comparison with MR angiography. Clin Imaging 2005;
       29(5): 303-6.
       [http://dx.doi.org/10.1016/j.clinimag.2005.01.030] [PMID: 16153534]

[13]   Hartkamp MJ, van Der Grond J, van Everdingen KJ, Hillen B, Mali WP. Circle of Willis collateral
       flow investigated by magnetic resonance angiography. Stroke 1999; 30(12): 2671-8.
       [http://dx.doi.org/10.1161/01.STR.30.12.2671] [PMID: 10582995]

[14]   Tsuruda JS, Saloner D, Anderson C. Noninvasive evaluation of cerebral ischemia. Trends for the
       1990s. Circulation 1991; 83(2) (Suppl.): I176-89.
       [PMID: 1991398]

[15]   Hirai T, Korogi Y, Ono K, *et al.* Prospective evaluation of suspected stenoocclusive disease of the
       intracranial artery: combined MR angiography and CT angiography compared with digital subtraction
       angiography. AJNR Am J Neuroradiol 2002; 23(1): 93-101.
       [PMID: 11827880]

[16]   Nederkoorn PJ, Elgersma OE, Mali WP, Eikelboom BC, Kappelle LJ, van der Graaf Y.
       Overestimation of carotid artery stenosis with magnetic resonance angiography compared with digital
       subtraction angiography. J Vasc Surg 2002; 36(4): 806-13.
       [http://dx.doi.org/10.1016/S0741-5214(02)00137-4] [PMID: 12368742]

[17]   Donahue J, Wintermark M. Perfusion CT and acute stroke imaging: foundations, applications, and
       literature review. J Neuroradiol 2015; 42(1): 21-9.
       [http://dx.doi.org/10.1016/j.neurad.2014.11.003] [PMID: 25636991]

[18]   Bruce CV, Campbell MD, Peter J, *et al.* for the EXTEND-IA Investigators* endovascular therapy for
       ischemic stroke with perfusion-imaging selection. N Engl J Med 2015; 372(1009): 1018.
       [http://dx.doi.org/10.1056/NEJMoa1414792] [PMID: 25671797]

[19]   Kim SJ, Ha YS, Ryoo S, *et al.* Sulcal effacement on fluid attenuation inversion recovery magnetic
       resonance imaging in hyperacute stroke: association with collateral flow and clinical outcomes. Stroke
       2012; 43(2): 386-92.
       [http://dx.doi.org/10.1161/STROKEAHA.111.638106] [PMID: 22096035]

[20]   Nicoli F, Lafaye de Micheaux P, Girard N. Perfusion-weighted imaging-derived collateral flow index
       is a predictor of MCA M1 recanalization after i.v. thrombolysis. AJNR Am J Neuroradiol 2013; 34(1):
       107-14.
       [http://dx.doi.org/10.3174/ajnr.A3174] [PMID: 22766675]

[21]   Hartkamp NS, van Osch MJ, Kappelle J, Bokkers RP. Arterial spin labeling magnetic resonance
       perfusion imaging in cerebral ischemia. Curr Opin Neurol 2014; 27(1): 42-53.
       [http://dx.doi.org/10.1097/WCO.0000000000000051] [PMID: 24300794]

[22]    Wu B, Wang X, Guo J, *et al.* Collateral circulation imaging: MR perfusion territory arterial spin-labeling at 3T. AJNR Am J Neuroradiol 2008; 29(10): 1855-60.
[http://dx.doi.org/10.3174/ajnr.A1259] [PMID: 18784211]

[23]    Lo EH, Ning M. Mechanisms and challenges in translational stroke research. J Investig Med 2016; pii: jim-2016-000104.

[24]    OCollins VE, Macleod MR, Donnan GA, Horky LL, van der Worp BH, Howells DW. 1,026 experimental treatments in acute stroke. Ann Neurol 2006; 59(3): 467-77.
[http://dx.doi.org/10.1002/ana.20741] [PMID: 16453316]

[25]    Stroke Trials Registry, Dallas: UT Southwestern Medical Center , 1997 [Accessed Aug 2015]; Available at: http://www.strokecenter.org/trials/. Accessed Aug 2015.

[26]    Llovera G, Liesz A. The next step in translational research: lessons learned from the first preclinical randomized controlled trial. J Neurochem 2016; 139 (Suppl. 2): 271-9.
[http://dx.doi.org/10.1111/jnc.13516] [PMID: 26968835]

[27]    Howells DW, Sena ES, Macleod MR. Bringing rigour to translational medicine. Nat Rev Neurol 2014; 10(1): 37-43.
[http://dx.doi.org/10.1038/nrneurol.2013.232] [PMID: 24247324]

[28]    Macleod MR, Fisher M, OCollins V, *et al.* Good laboratory practice: preventing introduction of bias at the bench. Stroke 2009; 40(3): e50-2.
[http://dx.doi.org/10.1161/STROKEAHA.108.525386] [PMID: 18703798]

[29]    Sutherland BA, Minnerup J, Balami JS, Arba F, Buchan AM, Kleinschnitz C. Neuroprotection for ischaemic stroke: translation from the bench to the bedside. Int J Stroke 2012; 7(5): 407-18.
[http://dx.doi.org/10.1111/j.1747-4949.2012.00770.x] [PMID: 22394615]

[30]    Howells DW, Porritt MJ, Rewell SS, *et al.* Different strokes for different folks: the rich diversity of animal models of focal cerebral ischemia. J Cereb Blood Flow Metab 2010; 30(8): 1412-31.
[http://dx.doi.org/10.1038/jcbfm.2010.66] [PMID: 20485296]

[31]    Ström JO, Ingberg E, Theodorsson A, Theodorsson E. Method parameters impact on mortality and variability in rat stroke experiments: a meta-analysis. BMC Neurosci 2013; 14: 41.
[http://dx.doi.org/10.1186/1471-2202-14-41] [PMID: 23548160]

[32]    Braeuninger S, Kleinschnitz C. Rodent models of focal cerebral ischemia: procedural pitfalls and translational problems. Exp Transl Stroke Med 2009; 1: 8.
[http://dx.doi.org/10.1186/2040-7378-1-8] [PMID: 20150986]

[33]    Barone FC, Knudsen DJ, Nelson AH, Feuerstein GZ, Willette RN. Mouse strain differences in susceptibility to cerebral ischemia are related to cerebral vascular anatomy. J Cereb Blood Flow Metab 1993; 13(4): 683-92.
[http://dx.doi.org/10.1038/jcbfm.1993.87] [PMID: 8314921]

[34]    Riva M, Pappadà GB, Papadakis M, *et al.* Hemodynamic monitoring of intracranial collateral flow predicts tissue and functional outcome in experimental ischemic stroke. Exp Neurol 2012; 233(2): 815-20.
[http://dx.doi.org/10.1016/j.expneurol.2011.12.006] [PMID: 22193110]

[35]  National Centre for Replacement, Refinement & Reduction of Animals in Research, London, UK. Determining the source of variability within experimental stroke models , 2015 [Accessed Aug 2015]; Available at: https://www.nc3rs.org.uk/determining-source- variability-within- experimental-stroke-models.

[36]  Sutherland BA, Papadakis M, Chen RL, Buchan AM. Cerebral blood flow alteration in neuroprotection following cerebral ischaemia. J Physiol 2011; 589(17): 4105-14.
[http://dx.doi.org/10.1113/jphysiol.2011.209601] [PMID: 21708904]

[37]  Oliff HS, Coyle P, Weber E. Rat strain and vendor differences in collateral anastomoses. J Cereb Blood Flow Metab 1997; 17(5): 571-6.
[http://dx.doi.org/10.1097/00004647-199705000-00012] [PMID: 9183296]

[38]  Jauch EC, Saver JL, Adams HP Jr, *et al.* Guidelines for the early management of patients with acute ischemic stroke: a guideline for healthcare professionals from the American Heart Association/American Stroke Association. Stroke 2013; 44(3): 870-947.
[http://dx.doi.org/10.1161/STR.0b013e318284056a] [PMID: 23370205]

[39]  Powers WJ, Derdeyn CP, Biller J, *et al.* American Heart Association Stroke Council. 2015 AHA/ASA Focused Update of the 2013 Guidelines for the Early Management of Patients With Acute Ischemic Stroke Regarding Endovascular Treatment: A Guideline for Healthcare Professionals From the American Heart Association/American Stroke Association. Stroke 2015; pii: STR.0000000000000074.
[http://dx.doi.org/10.1161/STR.000000000000007]

[40]  Espinosa de Rueda M, Parrilla G, Manzano-Fernández S, *et al.* Combined multimodal computed tomography score correlates with futile recanalization after thrombectomy in patients with acute stroke. Stroke 2015; 46(9): 2517-2.
[http://dx.doi.org/10.1161/STROKEAHA.114.008598]

[41]  Gomis M, Dávalos A. Recanalization and reperfusion therapies of acute ischemic stroke: what have we learned, what are the major research questions, and where are we headed? Front Neurol 2014; 5: 226.
[http://dx.doi.org/10.3389/fneur.2014.00226] [PMID: 25477857]

[42]  Liebeskind DS. Collaterals in acute stroke: beyond the clot. Neuroimaging Clin N Am 2005; 15(3): 553-573, x.
[http://dx.doi.org/10.1016/j.nic.2005.08.012] [PMID: 16360589]

[43]  Shin HK, Nishimura M, Jones PB, *et al.* Mild induced hypertension improves blood flow and oxygen metabolism in transient focal cerebral ischemia. Stroke 2008; 39(5): 1548-55.
[http://dx.doi.org/10.1161/STROKEAHA.107.499483] [PMID: 18340095]

[44]  Hillis AE, Ulatowski JA, Barker PB, *et al.* A pilot randomized trial of induced blood pressure elevation: effects on function and focal perfusion in acute and subacute stroke. Cerebrovasc Dis 2003; 16(3): 236-46.
[http://dx.doi.org/10.1159/000071122] [PMID: 12865611]

[45]  Marzan AS, Hungerbühler HJ, Studer A, Baumgartner RW, Georgiadis D. Feasibility and safety of norepinephrine-induced arterial hypertension in acute ischemic stroke. Neurology 2004; 62(7): 1193-5.
[http://dx.doi.org/10.1212/01.WNL.0000118303.45735.04] [PMID: 15079024]

[46]   Heros RC, Korosue K. Hemodilution for cerebral ischemia. Stroke 1989; 20(3): 423-7.
[http://dx.doi.org/10.1161/01.STR.20.3.423] [PMID: 2466352]

[47]   Chang TS, Jensen MB. Haemodilution for acute ischaemic stroke. Cochrane Database Syst Rev 2014;
8(8): CD000103.
[PMID: 25159027]

[48]   Belayev L, Zhao W, Pattany PM, *et al*. Diffusion-weighted magnetic resonance imaging confirms
marked neuroprotective efficacy of albumin therapy in focal cerebral ischemia. Stroke 1998; 29(12):
2587-99.
[http://dx.doi.org/10.1161/01.STR.29.12.2587] [PMID: 9836772]

[49]   Nimmagadda A, Park HP, Prado R, Ginsberg MD. Albumin therapy improves local vascular dynamics
in a rat model of primary microvascular thrombosis: a two-photon laser-scanning microscopy study.
Stroke 2008; 39(1): 198-204.
[http://dx.doi.org/10.1161/STROKEAHA.107.495598] [PMID: 18032741]

[50]   Ginsberg MD, Palesch YY, Hill MD, *et al*. High-dose albumin treatment for acute ischaemic stroke
(ALIAS) Part 2: a randomised, double-blind, phase 3, placebo-controlled trial. Lancet Neurol 2013;
12(11): 1049-58.
[http://dx.doi.org/10.1016/S1474-4422(13)70223-0] [PMID: 24076337]

[51]   Terpolilli NA, Moskowitz MA, Plesnila N. Nitric oxide: considerations for the treatment of ischemic
stroke. J Cereb Blood Flow Metab 2012; 32(7): 1332-46.
[http://dx.doi.org/10.1038/jcbfm.2012.12] [PMID: 22333622]

[52]   Terpolilli NA, Kim SW, Thal SC, *et al*. Inhalation of nitric oxide prevents ischemic brain damage in
experimental stroke by selective dilatation of collateral arterioles. Circ Res 2012; 110(5): 727-38.
[http://dx.doi.org/10.1161/CIRCRESAHA.111.253419] [PMID: 22207711]

[53]   Bar-Shir A, Shemesh N, Nossin-Manor R, Cohen Y. Late stimulation of the sphenopalatine-ganglion
in ischemic rats: improvement in N-acetyl-aspartate levels and diffusion weighted imaging
characteristics as seen by MR. J Magn Reson Imaging 2010; 31(6): 1355-63.
[http://dx.doi.org/10.1002/jmri.22110] [PMID: 20512887]

[54]   Khurana D, Kaul S, Bornstein NM. Implant for augmentation of cerebral blood flow trial 1: a pilot
study evaluating the safety and effectiveness of the Ischaemic Stroke System for treatment of acute
ischaemic stroke. Int J Stroke 2009; 4(6): 480-5.
[http://dx.doi.org/10.1111/j.1747-4949.2009.00385.x] [PMID: 19930060]

[55]   Attwell D, Buchan AM, Charpak S, Lauritzen M, Macvicar BA, Newman EA. Glial and neuronal
control of brain blood flow. Nature 2010; 468(7321): 232-43.
[http://dx.doi.org/10.1038/nature09613] [PMID: 21068832]

[56]   Lay CC, Davis MF, Chen-Bee CH, Frostig RD. Mild sensory stimulation reestablishes cortical
function during the acute phase of ischemia. J Neurosci 2011; 31(32): 11495-504.
[http://dx.doi.org/10.1523/JNEUROSCI.1741-11.2011] [PMID: 21832179]

[57]   Domoki F, Zimmermann A, Tóth-Szuki V, Busija DW, Bari F. Acetazolamide induces indomethacin
and ischaemia-sensitive pial arteriolar vasodilation in the piglet. Acta Paediatr 2008; 97(3): 280-4.
[http://dx.doi.org/10.1111/j.1651-2227.2007.00615.x] [PMID: 18298774]

[58] Ogasawara K, Ogawa A, Yoshimoto T. Cerebrovascular reactivity to acetazolamide and outcome in patients with symptomatic internal carotid or middle cerebral artery occlusion: a xenon-133 single-photon emission computed tomography study. Stroke 2002; 33(7): 1857-62.
[http://dx.doi.org/10.1161/01.STR.0000019511.81583.A8] [PMID: 12105366]

[59] Regli F, Yamaguchi T, Waltz AG. Effects of acetazolamide on cerebral ischemia and infarction after experimental occlusion of middle cerebral artery. Stroke 1971; 2(5): 456-60.
[http://dx.doi.org/10.1161/01.STR.2.5.456] [PMID: 5000028]

[60] Schwarz S, Georgiadis D, Aschoff A, Schwab S. Effects of body position on intracranial pressure and cerebral perfusion in patients with large hemispheric stroke. Stroke 2002; 33(2): 497-501.
[http://dx.doi.org/10.1161/hs0202.102376] [PMID: 11823659]

[61] Wojner-Alexander AW, Garami Z, Chernyshev OY, Alexandrov AV. Heads down: flat positioning improves blood flow velocity in acute ischemic stroke. Neurology 2005; 64(8): 1354-7.
[http://dx.doi.org/10.1212/01.WNL.0000158284.41705.A5] [PMID: 15851722]

[62] Nagatani K, Nawashiro H, Takeuchi S, Otani N, Wada K, Shima K. Effects of a head-down tilt on cerebral blood flow in mice during bilateral common carotid artery occlusion. Asian J Neurosurg 2012; 7(4): 171-3.
[http://dx.doi.org/10.4103/1793-5482.106648] [PMID: 23559983]

[63] Winship IR, Armitage GA, Ramakrishnan G, Dong B, Todd KG, Shuaib A. Augmenting collateral blood flow during ischemic stroke *via* transient aortic occlusion. J Cereb Blood Flow Metab 2014; 34(1): 61-71.
[http://dx.doi.org/10.1038/jcbfm.2013.162] [PMID: 24045399]

[64] Shuaib A, Bornstein NM, Diener HC, *et al.* Partial aortic occlusion for cerebral perfusion augmentation: safety and efficacy of NeuroFlo in Acute Ischemic Stroke trial. Stroke 2011; 42(6): 1680-90.
[http://dx.doi.org/10.1161/STROKEAHA.110.609933] [PMID: 21566232]

# CHAPTER 6

# Life in the Penumbra with the BRODERICK PROBE®

P.A. Broderick[1,2,3,*], L. Wenning[1,4] and Y-S. Li[1,4]

[1] Department of Physiology, Pharmacology and Neuroscience, The City University of New York School of Medicine, The Sophie Davis Program in Biomedical Education, The City College of New York, New York, NY USA

[2] Department of Biology, CUNY Grad. Ctr., New York, NY USA

[3] Department of Neurology, NYU Langone Medical Center and Comprehensive Epilepsy Center, New York, NY USA

[4] Department of Anesthesiology, NYU Langone Medical Center, New York, NY USA

**Abstract:** The penumbra is an area of living brain tissue immediately surrounding the necrotic core of an ischemic or thrombolytic stroke. The penumbra may remain viable several hours post-stroke due to blood flow from collateral arteries. Thus, this area of peri-infarct tissue is a therapeutic target for post- stroke and neuroprotective treatment modalities. Due to the fact that the ratio of viable to non-viable tissue decreases with time, Factor Xa and Factor II inhibitors such as enoxaparin and thrombolytics such as recombinant tissue plasminogen activator (r-tPA) must be administered immediately for optimal, synergistic treatment outcomes. The Broderick Lab is the first to study penumbral brain neurochemistry after causal acute ischemic stroke (AIS) by middle cerebral artery occlusion (MCAO) *in vivo*, as well as to comprehend the effects of enoxaparin (Lovenox®) and reperfusion *via in vivo* biochip nanotheranostics actually imaging the penumbra and its surrounding tissue intravascularly. Indeed, using Neuromolecular Imaging (NMI) with BRODERICK PROBE® nanobiosensors, animals were studied as their own control and each side of the brain was imaged *in vivo*, online, and in real time. NMI is a technology that uniquely images the baseline state of subjects before a disease state occurs, thereby establishing an intra-subject control

* **Corresponding author P.A. Broderick:** Department of Physiology, Pharmacology and Neuroscience, The City University of New York School of Medicine, The Sophie Davis Program in Biomedical Education, The City College of New York, New York, NY USA; Tel: (212)650-5479, (212)650-7764; Emails: broderick@med.cuny.edu, Patricia.Broderick@nyumc.org

Alberto Radaelli, Giuseppe Mancia, Carlo Ferrarese & Simone Beretta (Eds.)

model. In the same subject, with no gliosis, both the infarcted and peri-infarcted regions were imaged before, during, and after enoxaparin administration. Such imaging is available only with NMI nanobiosensor technology. In fact, with this new NMI nanobiosensor technology, the specificity of comparing baselines during drug and disease states is high because of the ability of NMI to compare baselines in thousands of previous studies of prescient and non-prescient mammals *in vivo*. Concurrently, Dual Laser Doppler Flowmetry (DLDF) was used to monitor cerebral blood perfusion. The results of this study demonstrate that, using intra-subject studies online (a) NMI profiles for dorsal striatum in basal ganglia are baseline values, ipsilaterally and contralaterally. (b) Diminished cerebral blood perfusion from AIS produces a significant increase of DA and 5-HT neurotransmitter concentrations, as well as associated metabolites and precursors, in motor neurons. (c) Enoxaparin alleviates oxygen deficiency by enhancing blood perfusion and reduces DA-induced brain trauma, enabling brain repair and regeneration. (d) Enoxaparin increases 5-HT release from motor neurons within the ipsilateral, lesioned hemisphere, as well as in the contralateral, non-lesioned hemisphere, particularly during the reperfusion stage. This serotonergic effect demonstrates the potential use of enoxaparin as an antidepressant, which would be clinically relevant for treating the depression that oftentimes is co-morbid with AIS. (e) The area of post-stroke infarcts is significantly reduced upon reperfusion; and (f) Cerebral blood perfusion is augmented in a compensatory manner by both enoxaparin therapy and reperfusion within both hemispheres, particularly the contralateral hemisphere. Thus, this research demonstrates the efficacy of enoxaparin in preserving the viability of the penumbra in stroke victims and supports consideration of the combined use of enoxaparin with r-TPA in standard stroke treatment protocols in order to harness the brain's intrinsic repair system. Moreover, these studies demonstrate the power of NMI nanotechnology in conjunction with BRODERICK PROBE® theranostic nanobiosensors to reliably study the intricacies of stroke in order to develop further neuroprotective treatments and allow personalized medicine to be realized.

**Keywords:** Anti-platelet, Brain attack, Brain repair, Cerebral blood perfusion, Enoxaparin, Imaging, Infarct, Intravascular, Ischemia, Lovenox®, Micro-circulation, Nanobiosensors, Nanodiagnostics, Nanotheranostics, Nano-therapeutics, Neuromolecular Imaging, Occlusion, Peri-infarct, Personalized medicine, Point of care, Reperfusion, Sensors, Stroke, Surgery, Theranostics, thrombolytic, Tissue imaging.

# INTRODUCTION

"Umbra," "penumbra," and "antumbra" are Latin terms used to describe different eclipse relationships between the earth and the moon. "Umbra" is Latin for shadow and can either describe a total or partial planetary eclipse caused by the inner core of Earth's shadow blocking all sunlight from reaching the moon. An umbra generates a dramatic effect with a total lunar umbra creating a blood moon and a partial umbra casting a bite-like lunar shadow on the moon's surface. Similarly, an "antumbra" creates a striking appearance as the total circumference of the earth is encompassed by the luminous body of the moon, thereby creating a glistening, ring-like lunar eclipse. In contrast, a "penumbra" describes the moon falling into the outer, annular shadow of the earth, which results in a subtle darkening of the moon's exterior that is often missed by the naked eye. [1]

In medicine, penumbra refers to the living neural tissue encircling an infarcted core secondary to ischemic stroke. This viable peri-infarct region is visually analogous to the circular shadow left by a penumbral eclipse. The penumbra is literally a region of brain suffering from a dimming of its former vitality as a result of arterial occlusion. In this shadow zone, components of the ischemic lesion tentatively remain alive. However, the viability of penumbral tissue decreases with time if it remains in a prolonged ischemic state. In contrast, the necrotic core encompassed by the tenuously living penumbra is analogous to the umbra. Indeed, the necrotic core has already been muted by total cell death. Thus, the penumbra is an effective therapeutic target for the prevention of additional neuronal cell death after stroke. Due to the fact that the ratio of viable to non-viable penumbral tissue decreases with time, clotting factor inhibitors such as enoxaparin and thrombolytics such as recombinant tissue plasminogen activator (r-tPA) must be administered immediately for optimal treatment outcomes. Fig. (**1**) shows an image of a thrombus occluding an artery that can result in ischemia with viable penumbral tissue.

Indeed, enoxaparin (Lovenox®) is a first-line anti-platelet and anti-thrombotic agent that inhibits Factor Xa and Factor II in the clotting cascade. Enoxaparin is a low molecular weight heparin that impedes the formation of clots, reduces brain edema [2], reduces cerebral infarcts [3], restores both cognitive and motor impairments post-Traumatic Brain Injury in the murine model [3], and may be a neuroprotectant [4]. Moreover, enoxaparin curbs infarct size during reperfusion, which further reduces brain edema by limiting the release of cytotoxic, inflammatory necrotic substances by atherosclerotic plaques [5]. Compared to heparin, enoxaparin is associated with less platelet reactivity during hemodialysis, is safer to use in individuals with end stage renal disease [6], and is associated with a lower bleeding risk [7]. Similarly, research has demonstrated that enoxaparin is preferred over heparin treatment for both post- stroke thromboembolism [8] and AIS [9, 10]. Enoxaparin targets the etiology of AIS by inhibiting monocytic adhesion to endothelial cells [11]. For all of these reasons, the current research focuses on the use of enoxaparin to preserve the penumbra post-stroke.

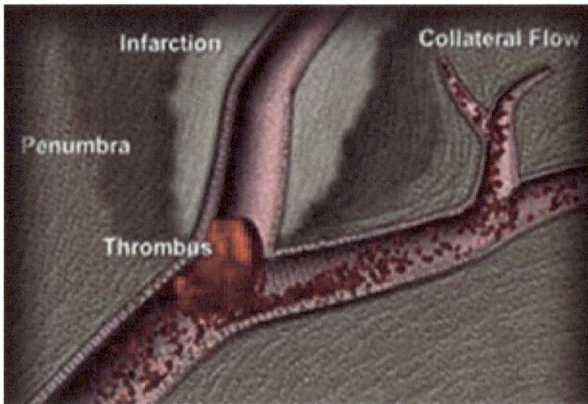

**Fig. (1).** Image of a thrombus occluding an artery with resultant ischemic core surrounded by a viable penumbra in brain tissue. (The Internet Stroke Center; retrieved May 21, 2016 from http://www.strokecenter.org/professionals/brain-anatomy/cellular-injury-during-ischemia/the-ischemic-penu mbra/)

Stroke is a cerebrovascular incident that is typically caused by a diminished or absolute lack of oxygen-containing blood flow to neural tissue, which initiates the ischemic cascade of tissue factor release and blood clotting. The etiology of this cerebrovascular accident may be due to a clot blocking blood flow through a vessel or a broken vessel wall leading to blood loss directly into brain tissue. If deprived of oxygen for more than three hours, irreversible neuronal cell death occurs. The typical etiology of stroke is arteriosclerosis. As atherosclerotic plaques grow in size and take up 75% of the arterial lumen, the resultant decrease in blood flow initiates the clotting cascade. Platelets are deposited on lumen walls by Platelet Endothelial Cell Adhesion Molecules (PECAM), and tissue factors generate thrombin in order to cleave fibrinogen to the active form fibrin. As fibrin, platelets, and tissue factor conglomerate as blood clots upon endothelial linings in response to vessel wall injury, showers of small emboli are released as plaques disintegrate. Unfortunately, these emboli may travel to the brain to cause stroke. Similarly, in patients with atrial fibrillation, irregularly irregular atrial contractions prevent the atrium from releasing its full end diastolic volume to the ventricles. In this manner, atrial fibrillation promotes blood stasis, clot formation, and resultant emboli traveling from the heart to the brain *via* the internal carotid artery. The end result of either peripheral emboli from arteriosclerosis or cardiac emboli from atrial fibrillation to the brain is arterial occlusion and consequent acute ischemic stroke (AIS). Stroke occurs every minute worldwide [12], and is, consequently, a crucial medical issue that demands further elucidation.

Despite the fact that necrotic, post-stroke brain tissue, may not always perform the function of regeneration, a non-damaged part of the brain may compensate by taking over the function of the damaged part of the brain. This typically involves long-distance, interhemispheric axonal sprouting contralateral to the location of stroke. However, optimal recovery occurs when function returns to undamaged regions on the ipsilateral hemisphere *via* intrahemispheric axonal sprouting where the stroke occurred [13]. This mechanism of recovery describes neuroplasticity, a phenomenon that is most dramatically apparent in young children who rapidly strengthen neural connections as they interact with their environment and briskly prune away neural connections that they do not use [14]. The former example of strengthening neural circuits through functional use *via* engagement with the environment is the basis of stroke rehabilitation. Indeed, this is the concept behind encouraging stroke patients to use disabled limbs. As demonstrated by Forrester *et al.* (2008), post-stroke gait function may be improved by mediating CNS plasticity through long-term treadmill exercise [15]. Similarly, the non-prescient mammalian model of stroke has demonstrated that an enriched environment providing extensive opportunities for physical engagement and sensory stimulation encourages the proliferation and neurogenesis of subventricular neural stem cells in adult rats with stroke lesions [16]. Moreover, the Bennett group studied hind limb movement of a hemisected spinal cord and observed a virtual "stepping response", which demonstrated serotonergic temporal synchrony. Previous experimental, *in vivo* NMI data from the Broderick Lab [17] supports the Bennett Group (2010) paper [18] and exhibits temporal synchrony between 5-HT and movement in the exact same motor neuroanatomical region of the basal ganglia. Indeed, Broderick (2013) was the first to demonstrate that temporal synchrony between 5-HT and movement occurs during natural behavior and is made dysfunctional during brain and spinal cord injury due to the fact that 5-HT and rhythmic movement are inextricable. Fig. (**2**) shows schematic images of blood vessel endothelial lining undergoing clot formation.

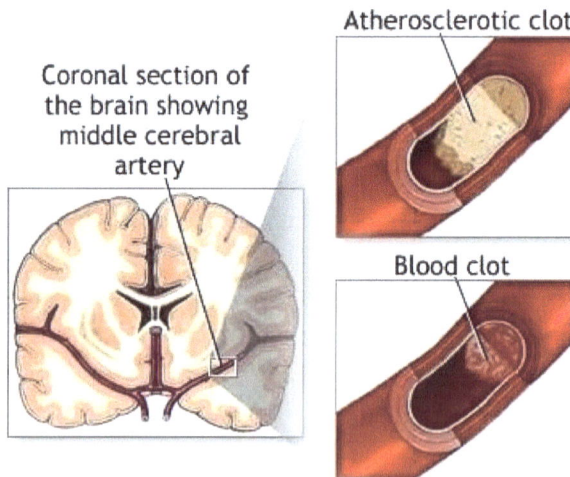

**Fig. (2).** (Left): Coronal section demonstrating the location of the middle cerebral artery relative to the basal ganglia. (Right): Upper and lower schematic images of blood vessel endothelial lining creating a blood clot. Adapted from: http://stroke.about.com/od/causesofstroke/a/lacunar_strokes.htm.

In the present paper, AIS is artificially induced by MCAO in the animal brain. MCAO was pioneered by Hayakawa and Waltz in 1975 using the craniotomy method. In our experiment, we executed the Zea Longa *et al.* (1989) midline neck incision method involving a nylon monofilament suture of the external carotid artery stump [19, 20 - 28]. Using Neuromolecular Imaging (NMI) with BRODERICK PROBE® nanobiosensors, animals were studied as their own control and each side of the brain was imaged *in vivo*, online, and in real time [29 - 31]. With this technology, the Broderick lab assessed 5-HT and DA with corresponding metabolites and precursors in the penumbra, throughout the development, occurrence, and resolution of stroke in the dorsal striatum. Indeed, NMI uses an analyzer/detector with a semiderivative/semidifferential circuit above a linear circuit, modified with a reduction electrical circuit [32] to sharpen signaling that takes place with electron transfer kinetics. This circuit selectively and separately images several neurochemicals within seconds. Moreover, unlike spectroscopy and chromatography, NMI studies may be performed *in vivo* over months without glial formation using nanobiosensors comprised of fatty acid constituents of the normal animal and human brain that are resistant to bacterial growth. [32 - 40] In particular, these NMI laurate nanobiosensors enhance electron transfer kinetics *via* the lauric acid hydrophobic head and hydrophilic tail that reduce surface tension and augment both signal resolution and speed [32 - 34, 37-39].

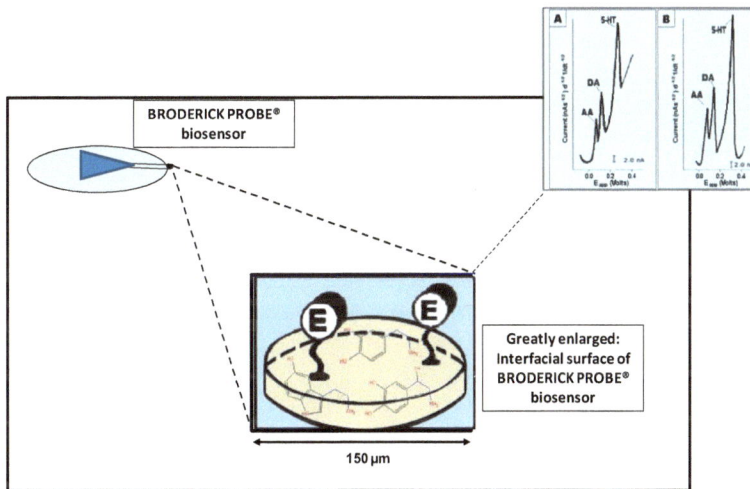

**Fig. (3).** Diagram demonstrating the mechanism of electron transfer involved in NMI. Biosensor insertion causes the selective transfer of electrons from neurotransmitters (NTs) in corresponding areas of the brain. Each biosensor formulation and NT demonstrates fluctuating hydrophilicity, hydrophobicity and polarity that affects the cationic or anionic properties of carbon conduction, which promotes the electron transfer mechanism. This picture was drawn by the corresponding author. The data are original raw data from the Broderick Laboratory.

In addition to determining the neuronal mechanism of action for stroke, these nanobiosensors were used to research enoxaparin. Indeed, in the same subject, with no gliosis, both the infarcted and peri-infarcted regions were imaged before, during, and after enoxaparin administration with concurrent monitoring of cerebral blood flow perfusion using Dual Laser Doppler Flowmetry. A schematic of the nanobiosensors is shown in Fig. (**3**).

Fig. (**4**) shows how the BRODERICK PROBE® works in concert with related nanobiotechnologies involved in the process of NMI.

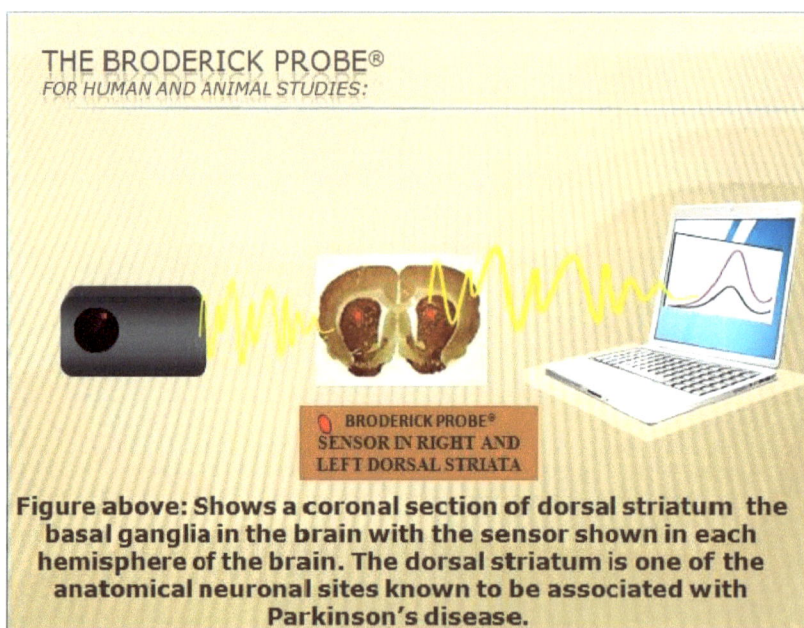

THE BRODERICK PROBE®
FOR HUMAN AND ANIMAL STUDIES:

BRODERICK PROBE®
SENSOR IN RIGHT AND
LEFT DORSAL STRIATA

Figure above: Shows a coronal section of dorsal striatum the basal ganglia in the brain with the sensor shown in each hemisphere of the brain. The dorsal striatum is one of the anatomical neuronal sites known to be associated with Parkinson's disease.

**Fig. (4).** This diagram depicts how the BRODERICK PROBE® works in concert with the NMI-related nanobiotechnologies. Simply apply a voltage potential to the BRODERICK PROBE® nanobiosensor, voltage is converted to current, and a software application will show NMI signals on a suitable monitor such as a laptop or cell phone. NMI studies are performed in the dorsal striata in the mammalian brain of the live subject. Note: The terms, nanobiosensor and biosensor, are used interchangeably. Abbreviations: AA is ascorbic acid; DA is dopamine; 5-HT is serotonin. This diagram was drawn by the corresponding author.

## METHODS

Using NMI with BRODERICK PROBE® nanobiosensors, DA and 5-HT were imaged during baseline, experimental, AIS, enoxaparin, and reperfusion stages on line and *in vivo* in 16 animals using an intra-animal control model. Indeed, all animals (N = 16) were used as their own baseline by separately imaging the non-lesioned brain hemisphere to obtain data for the control study group (N = 16)

(Group A). Ipsilateral (lesioned) and contralateral hemispheres of dorsal striatum were imaged independently, and Dual Laser Doppler Flowmetry (DLDF) was used concurrently to monitor Cerebral Blood Flow (Oxy Flo, Oxford Optronics, Oxford UK).

In the experimental study group (N = 16) (Group B), middle cerebral artery occlusion using the nylon intraluminal suture method was performed for quantitative histopathologies *via* midline neck incision [19] in order to delineate areas of infarction both before and after enoxaparin administration and subsequent reperfusion.

Using pentobarbital Na (100 mg/kg, intraperitoneal (ip)), animals were humanely sacrificed to prepare coronal brain sections to be viewed on a microscope slide. Coronal mounts were soaked in 2,3,5-triphenyltetrazolium chloride (TTC) for fifteen minutes, preserved with 10% formalin, and processed by the Image J program (National Institute of Health) to record the infarction percentage before and after both enoxaparin treatment and reperfusion. Please refer to the results section to view quantitative histopathology pictures.

Experimental Design for Neuromolecular Imaging (NMI) and Dual Laser Doppler Flow (DLDF):

NMI and DLDF experimental design is presented below. Studies were independently conducted in each hemisphere for Group A (intra-control, non-lesioned hemisphere) and Group B (experimental, lesioned hemisphere).

a. Control (non-lesioned) NMI and DLDF were conducted for 0.5 hours on the dorsal striatum of each hemisphere.
b. Using the Zea Longa *et al.* 1989 middle cerebral artery occlusion (MCAO) nylon intraluminal suture method [19], focal transient cerebral ischemia was generated in one hemisphere.
c. NMI and DLDF were maintained for one-half hour on each MCAO ipsilateral (lesioned) and contralateral (non- lesioned) hemispheres of DStr.
d. During MCAO, enoxaparin was administered (10 mg/kg subcutaneously (sc)) while LDF and NMI were continued for 0.5 hours on each hemisphere of dorsal striatum.

e. Reperfusion co-occurred with enoxaparin administration until the third hour. In separate studies, reperfusion co-occurred with enoxaparin treatment to 4.5 hours while DLDF and NMI were continued on each hemisphere.

f. On the same day, animals were sacrificed.

g. In two separate groups, infarct size (lesion) was also studied; one group was sacrificed at 1.5 hours reperfusion time, whereas the other group was sacrificed at 3 hours reperfusion time.

## *In vitro* Calibration Procedures

BRODERICK PROBE® biosensors are manufactured on site. Details of the nanobiosensor construction and design are published [32 - 34, 37 - 40]. *In vitro*, nanobiosensors are pre-calibrated using freshly prepared, deoxygenated physiological saline-phosphate buffer solution (0.01 M, pH = 7.4 consisting of nmol aliquots of DA, 5-HT, HVA, L-TP, ascorbic acid, somatostatin, dynorphin A (1-17) and uric acid (99% purity, Sigma-Aldrich, St. Louis, MO) [32 - 34, 37 - 40]. Saline-phosphate buffer calibration curves are published [41].

## *In vivo* Surgical Procedures

These studies are in accordance with the Institutional Animal Care and Use Committee (IACUC) of The City College of New York, The City University of New York with approval from the National Institutes of Health (NIH). Charles River Laboratories in Kingston, NY provided male, Sprague Dawley, Caesarean-derived, virus-free, laboratory rats *(Rattus norvegicus)*. Upon arrival, animals are housed for approximately one week in the Marshak Vivarium in order to promote environmental acclimation before surgery. Non-prescient mammals are given Purina Rat Chow and water *ad libitum*. A twelve hour dark-light cycle is maintained in the Vivarium and in the Broderick Lab where studies are performed in order to maintain each animal's circadian rhythm. Surgery commences with an i.p. injection of Na pentobarbital (50 mg/kg in a dilute 6% solution). BRODERICK PROBE® laurate biosensors are inserted (Kopf Stereotaxic, Tujunga, CA) within the dorsal striatum using stereotaxic coordinates (AP = +2.5; ML = +2.6; DV = −4.0) [42]; an Ag/AgCl microreference and stainless steel micro auxiliary are put in contact with dura mater. Indicator laurate biosensors are secured with Splintline Acrylic (Lang Dental, Il.). Using a thermometer and rectal probe (Fisher Sci., Fadem, NJ), temperature is monitored continuously and sustained at 37.5 ± 0.5 °C with an aquamatic K module heating pad (Amer. Hosp. Supply, Edison, NJ).

For the duration of surgery, corneal, pinnal, and leg flexion responses are examined and additional doses of Na pentobarbital are provided to sustain adequate depth and pharmacokinetic induction of anesthesia. Additional doses of Na pentobarbital are administered as needed to complete the study under anesthesia. Physiologic saline equaling the non-prescient mammal's body weight in cc's is administered *via* intraperitoneal injection to preserve adequate electrolyte and volumetric status. The surgery takes a total of three to four hours.

### Image Scanning Procedures

Potentials are applied at a scan rate of 10 mV/s with time constants of 5 and 1 second tau from −0.2 V to +0.9 V with respect to an Ag/AgCl (1 M NaCl) electrode. After neurochemical charging and reduction in the circumferential tissues, the indicator nanobiosensors reveal returning oxidative current from NTs. Each scan, which includes several discriminately oxidized NTs, is finished in 60 seconds. In the first 25 seconds, non-faradaic charging current is eliminated. In these *in vitro* laurate studies, 5-HT and DA are sequentially detected in two waveforms with a characteristic signature based on its specific oxidative potential (voltage). *In vivo*, oxidation (half wave) potentials for these laureate nanobiosensors are detected from lowest to highest with DA at 0.14 V and 5-HT at 0.31 V. Other neurochemical signatures are demonstrated in the present paper with each specified oxidation potential falling within a range of +/−0.015 V. In nano- and pico-amperes, current is plotted as a function of potential.

### Interpretation and Analysis of Data *via* Electrochemical Methods

The current produced by a particular redox reaction is proportional to the neurochemical concentration according to the Cottrell equation, which enabled the calculation of each neurochemical concentration by direct proportionality to its current [43].

In order to reduce between-animal variations such that each subject may serve as its own control, data was interpreted using the Cottrell Equation and fluctuations in DA, 5-HT, HVA and L-TP concentration are presented as percent changes. Images were submitted for statistical analysis using 95% Confidence Limits. P-values < 0.05 are considered to be statistically significant compared to baseline, control values.

## Middle Cerebral Artery Occlusion  According to the  Method of Zea Longa *et al.*, 1989

The middle cerebral artery occlusion was conducted according to the method of Zea Longa *et al.*, 1989 [19]. The common carotid artery was visualized through a midline neck incision using a Nikon SMZ 800 microscope (Diagnostic Instruments) with High Intensity Nova 2000 Illuminator (Morrell, Instr., LI, NY).

The nylon monofilament is withdrawn from the external carotid artery stump branching off of the internal carotid artery in order to achieve reperfusion. Animal weight is used to calibrate a small animal ventilator (Model 685) (Harvard Apparatus, MA) that is kept within reach should it be needed.

### Preparation of the Monofilament Nylon Suture

The nylon monofilament tip is blunted with a soldering apparatus, and the diameter of this suture tip remains 0.2 mm.

Of note, several researchers in the field of MCAO tested different laboratory rodent species and found that the occlusion procedure outcome is limited in the spontaneously hypertensive laboratory rodent [44].

It is also significant that MCAO investigators have searched for several types of suture modification involving silicone coating and heat-treated poly-L-lysine to perform this surgery (for review, see [45]). Our method of manufacturing thread is somewhat similar to that of Belayev *et al.* [28].

Most importantly, it must be emphasized that the new focal point for stroke treatment is the penumbra, and NMI with BRODERICK PROBE® nanobiosensors are providing a valuable tool for reaching this salvageable area of the brain to treat victims of stroke [46 - 48].

## Dual Laser Doppler Flowmetry (DLDF)

DLDF separately measures erythrocyte perfusion in both ipsilateral and contralateral dorsal striatum hemispheres as directly related to microvascular blood flow (Oxyflo, OXFORDTM Ltd., UK). The DLDF stereotaxic coordinates for the placement of optic sensors are: AP = −1.2 mm, ML = +2.6, DV = −1.0 mm posterior to bregma [42]. Measurements are recorded in the relative scale of blood perfusion units. NMI utilizes electron transfer, and DLDF harnesses the Brownian motion of a suspension of latex spheres; interestingly, common motility standards routinely utilized in the public domain are used to control this random movement. DLDF is used to illuminate the dorsal striatum with optical light fiber sensors that emit low power laser light. Part of this laser light is scattered within the dorsal striatum, while other portions of this light are dispersed back to the laser light sensor. Moreover, a separate optical fiber collects the backscattered light from the dorsal striatum and eventually returns the backscattered light to the perfusion monitor. The majority of the light is dispersed by neuronal tissue within the immobile dorsal striatum. However, some light is dispersed back to mobile erythrocytes. Therefore, when the light is scattered back to the monitor, signal processing is actually taking the light from moving red blood cells, and the blood perfusion output signal is proportional to erythrocyte perfusion. The following equation defines the transport of blood cells through microvasculature: MP = NE x VE, *i.e.*, Microvascular perfusion = number of mobile erythrocytes multiplied by erythrocyte velocity.

Hence, Blood Perfusion Units (BPUs) are equivalent to the product of mean blood cell perfusion and mean blood cell velocity in the minute portion of dorsal striatum that is posterior to bregma and is illuminated by optical light sensors. The perfusion parameter is defined by the optical spectrum of light emitted from the small portion of dorsal striatum with a +/- 5V output to the analogue recording signal.

As previously mentioned, NMI harnesses electron transfer in a minute portion of dorsal striatum to create images of neurotransmitter molecules as they are read by the carbon-based BRODERICK PROBE® nanobiosensor according to millivolts of potential transformed by potentiostat operational amplifiers into nanoamperes of current. The specific diameter of the BRODERICK PROBE® nanobiosensor defines the neuroimaging parameter; patents for NMI include diameters of nano-micro-millimeters [33, 34]. Output to the analogue recording signal is +/−15 V [32].

## RESULTS AND DISCUSSION

### NMI Data, Quantitative Histopathologic, and DLDF Data

Fig. (**5**) shows on line, *in vivo* data taken from the ipsilateral, pre-lesioned hemisphere of Group A animals *via* NMI nanobiotechnology and the BRODERICK PROBE® laurate nanobiosensors. Pre-lesioned, on line, *in vivo* studies show data taken from the hemisphere that is not yet lesioned.

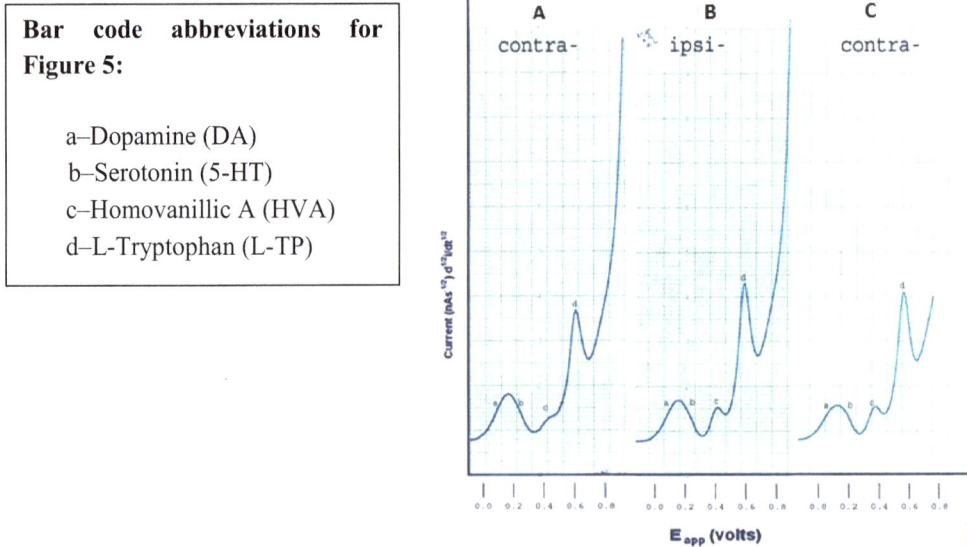

**Bar code abbreviations for Figure 5:**

    a–Dopamine (DA)
    b–Serotonin (5-HT)
    c–Homovanillic A (HVA)
    d–L-Tryptophan (L-TP)

**Fig. (5).** NMI baseline scans of neurotransmitters of contralateral (A & C-contra) and ipsilateral (B-ipsi) hemispheres before infarction on the ipsilateral side are produced. NMI scans of two pre-infarction, contralateral (A & C-contra) hemispheres are provided to demonstrate the reliability of this control group; the neurotransmitter levels between groups A and C differ within standard error. X-axis is applied potential (MilliVolts), and y-axis is current (NanoAmperes). E app means applied potential. Potential is represented with the letter, "E".

Results demonstrate that each brain hemisphere exhibits different neurochemical properties even in its baseline state, thus emphasizing the importance of NMI in its ability to compare same subject data and in doing so, promote personalized medicine. Note that the rationale for delineation of the term, ipsi, means that this is the hemisphere that will undergo the lesion made in the middle cerebral artery in that said hemisphere. The hemisphere chosen is completely arbitrary. The take home message is that one hemisphere exhibits higher synaptic release of neurotransmitters, precursors and metabolites than does the other hemisphere. Moreover, note that these data clearly demonstrate baseline differences between hemispheres in the baseline state before any drug or disease has occurred or is in progress. Therefore, the data represent the baseline neurotransmitter synaptic imaging performance for each of the ensuing stroke, treatment, and recovery stages. The nanotheranostics of disease and treatment is shown as studied by NMI and these novel nanobiosensors. Importantly, these nanobiosensor nanotheranostics with NMI go beyond current nanotheranostics because baseline control neurotransmitter environment/environtome is enabled.

In Fig. (**6**) below, on line, *in vivo* MCAO injury data followed by stroke treatment data are shown. The injury was produced by blocking blood flow through the middle cerebral artery *via* entrance through the carotid artery. The treatment studied is enoxaparin (Lovenox®). The data are taken from the ipsilateral, post-lesioned hemisphere of Group A animals using the unique NMI nanobiotechnology and the BRODERICK PROBE® laurate nanobiosensors. The data demonstrate that MCAO injury significantly increased the release of DA, HVA, 5-HT, and L-TP while on line and *in vivo*, whereas the stroke treatment, enoxaparin, significantly reduced the increase of DA, HVA, 5-HT, and L-TP that occurred in response to MCAO injury.

Thus, NMI shows that the hallmarks of TBI are significantly enhanced biogenic release of both DA and 5-HT in selective electroactive, electrochemical signals, as well as characteristic metabolite and precursor responses ($p < 0.05$). The BRODERICK PROBE® shows significantly enhanced 5-HT, HVA and L-TP with a ten-fold increase in the electroactive signal denoting DA response during MCAO (Slide A). The DA-ergic profile of TBI is significantly reduced while 5-HT and its precursor, L-TP, are significantly increased by enoxaparin. Due to the electrical properties of the semiderivative circuit, the increase in 5-HT occurs below the x axis in slides B and C. DA exhibits its maximum decrease at 25 minutes post-enoxaparin administration. Concurrently, 5-HT, HVA and L-TP begin to show downward signal processing in dorsal striatum.

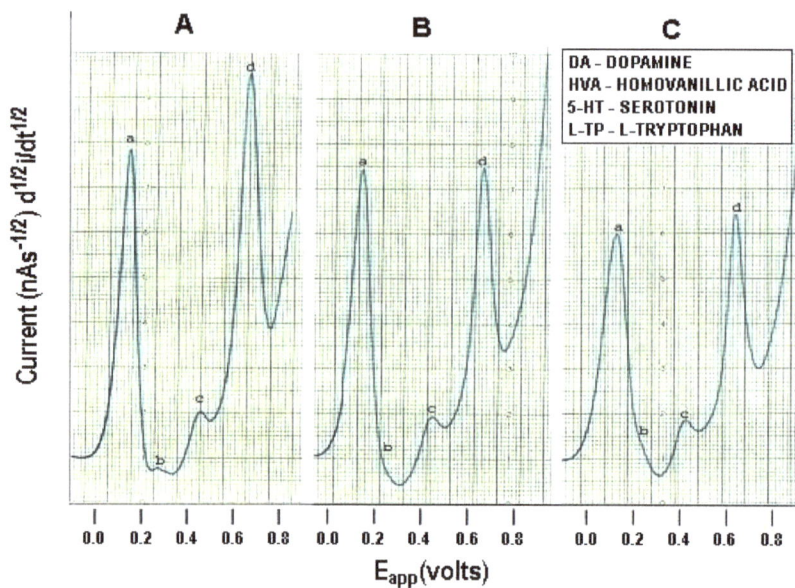

NMI: IPSILATERAL (LESIONED) HEMISPHERE

A. EFFECT OF MCAO ON NEUROTRANSMITTERS
B. EFFECT OF ENOXAPARIN ON MCAO, ADMINISTERED AT 5 MINUTES
C. EFFECT OF ENOXAPARIN ON MCAO, ADMINISTERED AT 25 MINUTES

a) dopamine (b) serotonin (c) homovanillic acid (d) L-tryptophan.

**Fig. (6).** These are original N M I data from ipsilateral hemisphere after MCAO injury followed by enoxaparin therapy. Scale: 10 mm = 2 na current; sensitivity setting is 5 na/volt. Data are derived from ipsilateral hemisphere. See Fig. (**5**) for baseline/control values, which were obtained using our NMI technology that provided intra-subject controls. Oxidation potential for HVA is 0.46 V = +/− 0.015 V; oxidation potential for L-TP is 0.68 V +/−0.015 V.

Unfortunately, there is little research interpreting neurotransmitter response in the context of stroke and MCAO. Nonetheless, one group of researchers detected a transient decrease in the DA metabolite, 3,4- dihydroxyphenylacetic acid (DOPAC), during stroke and attribute this *in vitro* finding to cortical degeneration [49]. These findings are confirmed by the present *in vivo* results. Furthermore, a dramatic elevation in DA with a transient reduction in DOPAC metabolite is consistent with the slower turnover likely resulting from the dramatic, *in vivo* increase in DA that is induced by stroke. Furthermore, aside from NMI, there is more DA imaging research using modalities such as magnetic resonance [50 - 52]. However, there is only one study using positron emission tomography (PET) that focuses on DA imaging, but not release [51]. The authors of this PET study state that the results concerning 5-HT release are limited and vague.

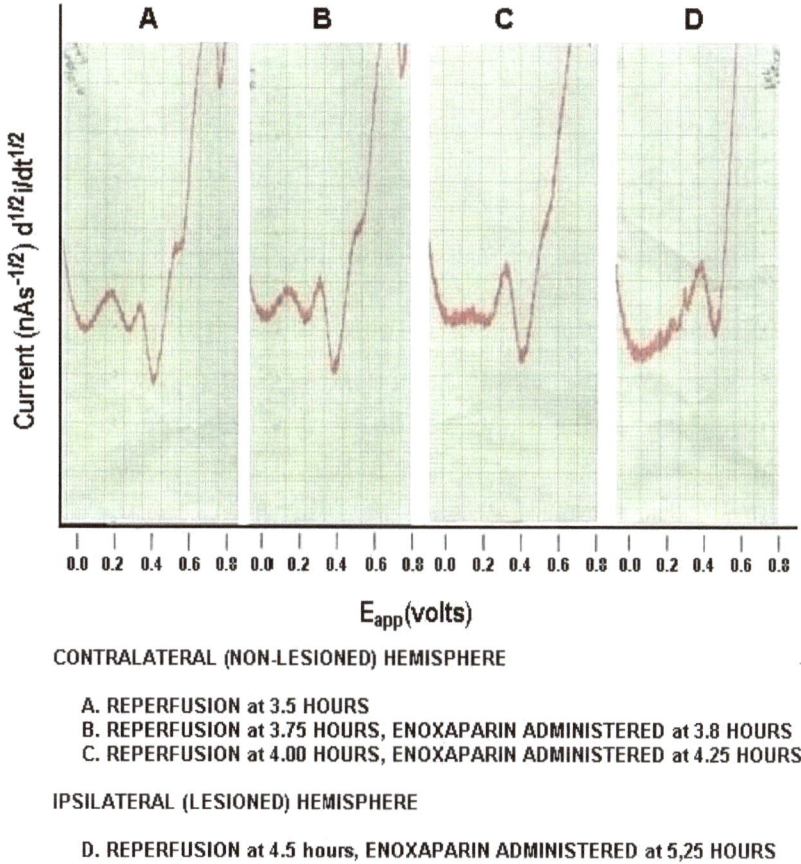

**Fig. (7).** Original data of NMI after MCAO, enoxaparin and reperfusion; NMI from contralateral and ipsilateral hemispheres.

Moreover, Fig. (7) further demonstrates on line, *in vivo* representative data (Group A) derived from NMI biotechnology and the BRODERICK PROBE® laurate biosensors. An experimentally different reperfusion time was used for these studies. Interestingly, DA and both 5-HT metabolite and precursor are able to reduce TBI-associated DA systems while augmenting 5-HT systems. The enhancement of 5-HT suggests that enoxaparin may alleviate mood disorders that are typically co-morbid with stroke. Indeed, DA is decreased to baseline and 5-HT release is increased ten-fold over baseline control values. In fact, post-stroke depression has been assuaged by atypical antipsychotic medications and 5-HT reuptake inhibitors [53, 54].

A review of 5-HT literature reveals a conflicted relationship between 5-HT and stroke. Indeed, although 5-HT release can lessen the depression co-morbid with stroke, serotonergic compounds may also induce stroke in patients who have a predisposition to cardiovascular events such as stroke. Moreover, 5-HT may cause adverse gastrointestinal responses especially when there is a profusion of 5-HT in gastrointestinal tract platelets such as that observed in both autistic children and patients predisposed to stroke [55 - 66]. Nonetheless, the data here do suggest that enoxaparin may alleviate stroke-induced depression. Future studies are needed to elucidate the triple role of enoxaparin as an anti-depressant, anti-platelet, and anti-thrombotic in stroke patients.

Moreover, our research highlights the efficacy of enoxaparin in preventing re-occlusion after reperfusion, as well as to treat stroke-induced depression. Thus, we propose that this versatile drug has the potential to be used with r-tPA in the treatment of AIS. According to 2008 European Cooperative Acute Stroke Study (ECASS) III guidelines that are currently considered the gold standard for AIS treatment, FDA-approved IV r-tPA should be given to patients who are not suffering from other medical issues such as brain hemorrhage or major infarction within 3 to 4.5 hours of stroke onset for optimal neurological outcomes [67]. In the present paper, we would like to encourage further scientific investigation regarding the concurrent administration of enoxaparin with IV r-tPA as part of standard stroke protocol. Indeed, researchers at NYU Langone School of Medicine suggested that enoxaparin may be a neuroprotectant after identifying a reduction in intracellular $Ca^{2+}$ release by Purkinje fibers [4]. This work was furthered by French scientists who studied the neuroprotective effects of enoxaparin and found that it acts synergistically with the naturally occurring tissue plasminogen activator (tPA) found on endothelial cells, thereby widening the therapeutic window for enoxaparin in the murine model. Other research based on the previous animal model suggests that enoxaparin may be an effective prophylactic agent for stroke [68, 69]. Moreover, in the Second Trial of Heparin and Aspirin Reperfusion Therapy (HART II), enoxaparin was an effective adjunct to r-tPA thrombolysis with aspirin in acute myocardial infarction [70]. Thus, based on this cumulative research, we suggest that enoxaparin be studied as a potential adjunct to r-tPA in AIS treatment protocol.

Our DLDF infarction data verify the results of other studies. Bederson *et al.*, 1986 published a coronal section showing the same percentage of infarct tissue in basal ganglia as the Broderick Lab found [25]. At both 1.5 and 3 hours, infarct reduction *via* enoxaparin and reperfusion are clearly significant at the $p < 0.05$ level. Indeed, the infarcts are virtually undetectable confirming previous data that demonstrate the effectiveness of enoxaparin in reducing both infarcts and edema [2 - 11, 68, 69, 71 - 86]. Fig. (**8a**) below shows the results derived from DLDF on the ipsilateral hemisphere. Most studies have investigated only ipsilateral DLDF, and our work confirms previous results [2 - 11, 68, 69, 71 - 86].

To our knowledge, the present studies are the first to present contralateral findings on line with concurrent DLDF data. Notably, in response to the occlusion of the ipsilateral middle cerebral artery, the contralateral hemisphere shows a significant compensatory effect. The aforementioned contralateral compensation observed in our research illustrates the phenomenon of neuroplasticity described in the Introduction of this paper. Indeed, further understanding of the mechanism of neuroplasticity is paramount to the development of effective therapeutic strategies for augmenting brain repair. Fortunately, improved stroke therapies are currently being developed based on novel insights into intrinsic brain repair. Functional magnetic resonance imaging (fMRI) has already demonstrated that a temporal relationship between task-related motor system activation is associated with recovery after stroke [87]. Thus, further research is currently devoted to understanding the mechanism of post-stroke recovery. In particular, Genetically Encoded Voltage Indicators (GEVI), a project funded by the Obama administration's Brain Research through Advancing Innovative Neurotechnologies (BRAIN) initiative, may convert the simultaneous, electrical firing of large populations of neurons into minute flashes of light with enhanced resolution [88], which may allow investigators to better understand the cellular re-wiring of the brain after stroke.

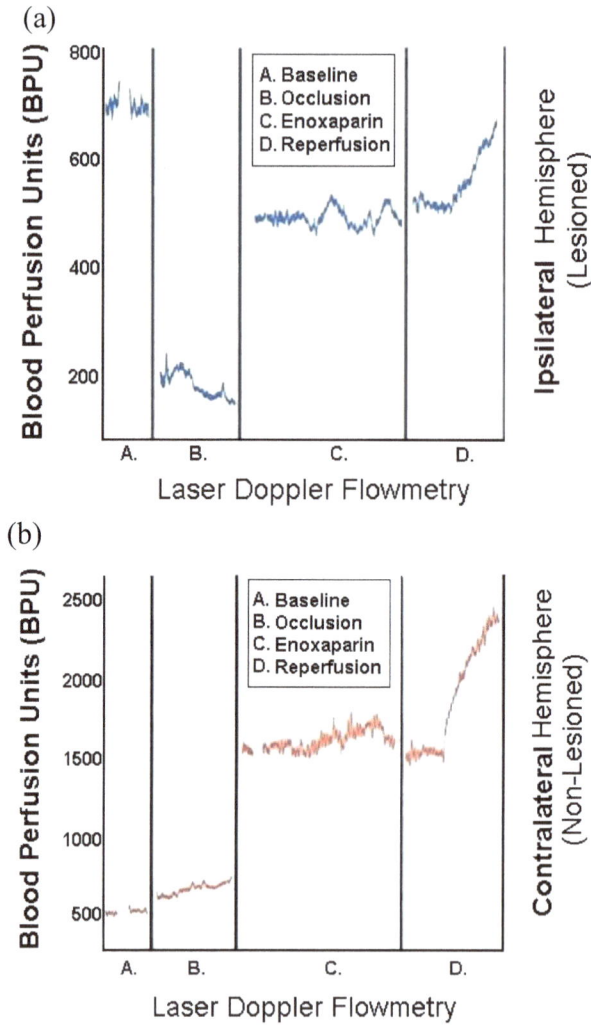

**Fig. (8). (a)** Original data: results derived from DLDF from ipsilateral hemisphere; **(b)** Original data: results derived from DLDF from contralateral hemisphere.

Similarly, new, ongoing research is demonstrating that the stroke-damaged brain may respond to intense physical therapy even after the typical stroke recovery period of 6 months. Indeed, in a randomized, controlled trial conducted by the Locomotor Experience Applied Post-Stroke (LEAPS) study, intense physical therapy involving in-home exercises and specially outfitted treadmills was more physically challenging than standard rehabilitation exercises and produced a greater improvement in walking six months post-stroke compared to the standard of care [89].

Stroke patients may use non-invasive, electroencephalogram (EEG)-based brain-computer interface (BCI) technologies to exert control over their environment by manipulating a computer cursor or limb orthosis. Indeed, in a 2012 study [90], a woman left paralyzed by stroke used a brain-machine interface *via* implanted electrodes to generate neuronal signals to drink from a bottle of coffee using a robotic arm. Moreover, BCI technology may aid in brain repair by guiding activity-dependent brain plasticity *via* EEG signals. In this manner, the user of EEG-BCI technology may view the current activity of their motor cortex in order to lower abnormal activity by following rehabilitation protocols, thereby improving muscle control [91]. Similarly, therapeutic exoskeletons in the form of motor-powered mechanical braces supporting limbs may be used to aid in walking or lifting, while simultaneously allowing post-stroke patients to interact with the environment or environtome in a manner that activates neural intrinsic repair mechanisms [92, 93]. Moreover, NMI with the BRODERICK PROBE® may be used in concert with these and other novel therapies for stroke to dramatically broaden the horizon for stroke therapies.

Fig. (**9**) displays characteristic infarcts at the 1.5 hour and 3.0 hour studies of enoxaparin and reperfusion. Reperfusion is achieved by withdrawal of the nylon monofilament suture from the internal carotid artery *via* the external carotid artery stump. Reperfusion may prevent ischemic necrosis by restoring blood flow to hypoxic tissues. However, reperfusion itself may cause microvascular tissue injury. Indeed, after endothelial cell walls have been deprived of oxygen, they have increased membrane permeability, which promotes extravasation of fluids across vessel tissues. This extravasation causes endothelial cells to release more reactive oxygen species and less nitric oxide, thereby inducing an inflammatory response that promotes apoptosis. Moreover, white blood cells that come into contact with extravasated sites release interleukins and free radicals that further exacerbate this inflammatory response [94, 95]. Thus, in order to minimize inflammatory microvascular injury, reperfusion of the middle cerebral artery was actually started during ongoing enoxaparin treatment. Very interestingly, enoxaparin significantly reduces dorsal striatum infarcts post-MCAO, and reperfusion produces the additional positive effect of infarct reduction in the context of enoxaparin administration. This is clearly observed in the enoxaparin, reperfusion 3 hour time period.

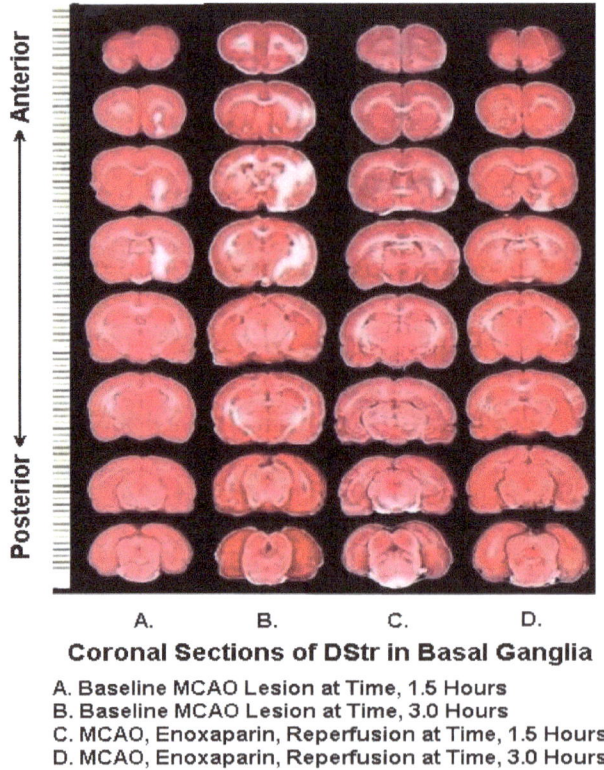

**Coronal Sections of DStr in Basal Ganglia**

A. Baseline MCAO Lesion at Time, 1.5 Hours
B. Baseline MCAO Lesion at Time, 3.0 Hours
C. MCAO, Enoxaparin, Reperfusion at Time, 1.5 Hours
D. MCAO, Enoxaparin, Reperfusion at Time, 3.0 Hours

**Fig. (9).** Original data of quantitative histopathologies at reperfusion, time 1.5 and 3 hours.

Figs. (**7** to **9**) are reprinted from Sensors, Broderick and Kolodny, print, 2010; on line, 2011 with permission from MDPI in Basel, Switzerland and Beijing, China. The citation is listed under Nanotheranostics in the Appendix.

## SUMMARY AND CONCLUSION

In summary, results show that, (a) intra-subject data of dorsal striatal neuronal circuitry in basal ganglia obtained online *via* the BRODERICK PROBE® is at baseline values. (b) AIS produces a significant increase in neurotransmitters DA and 5-HT, precursors and metabolites, in motor neurons; this effect occurred simultaneously with diminished cerebral blood perfusion. (c) Enoxaparin decreases DA-induced brain trauma in motor neurons while assuaging oxygen deficiency by increasing blood perfusion. (d) Enoxaparin enhances 5-HT release from motor neurons within the ipsilateral hemisphere (site of lesioned hemisphere) as well as in the opposite hemisphere (contralateral) relative to the acute ischemic lesion, particularly in the reperfusion stage as detected by novel nanobiotechnology for stroke therapy known as NMI. Due to the fact that AIS is often co-morbid with clinical depression, the serotonergic, possibly antidepressant effect of enoxaparin, is critical. (e) Reperfusion (removal of the arterial occlusion) significantly decreases AIS infarct size; and (f) cerebral blood perfusion is increased in a compensatory manner by both enoxaparin therapy and reperfusion; interestingly, this compensatory response occurs in both hemispheres but more extensively within the contralateral hemisphere.

Therefore, in conclusion, enoxaparin is an effective anti-platelet and anti-thrombotic agent with multifaceted applications. As demonstrated by our research, enoxaparin minimizes reperfusion injury upon reversal of MCAO in the murine model; and it may also be used to treat post-stroke depression due to its ability to increase 5-HT levels. Moreover, due to its synergy with r-tPA, research regarding the use of enoxaparin as an adjuvant to r-tPA therapy for acute ischemic stroke is warranted. On behalf of stroke victims, this important work incorporates the clinical aspects of neurodegenerative brain disease while presenting applications of other brain technologies. Indeed, this scientific undertaking demonstrates the reliability, reproducibility, and versatility of the NMI biotechnology and the BRODERICK PROBE® microelectrodes/biosensors. More importantly, this technology adds a much-needed tool to the existing but limited *in vivo* nanotheranostic literature. Not only has the BRODERICK PROBE® *in vivo* nanotheranostic technology been implemented in the diagnosis and treatment of human epilepsy patients, but it is the only *in vivo* biochip nanotheranostic to implement an intra-subject control in animal models of intravascular and tissue imaging.

In the Appendix, we provide commentaries on two selected published articles that shed light on the topic of stroke therapies. The first paper was selected for its interesting slant on harnessing the mechanic force of blood flow in the treatment of stroke.

Table **1** is published within the context of the second paper, which was selected for its contribution to epigenetics and stroke.

**Table 1.** This table describes epigenetic regulatory mechanisms that are relevant to stroke [97].

| Epigenetic Mechanism | DNA Methylation | Histone Code Modifications, Remodeling, and Higher-Order Chromatin Formation |
|---|---|---|
| **Description** | Refers to the transfer of methyl groups from SAM to cytosine residues in various genomic regions | Refer to highly integrated epigenetic mechanisms that modulate chromatin structure and function at single nucleotides (histone code modification), specific gene loci (nucleosome remodeling), and more extensive genomic regions (higher-order chromatin formation) |
| | Mediated by DNA methyltransferase enzymes | Mediated by histone-, nucleosome-, and chromatin-modifying enzymes that are often components of large, multifunctional epigenetic macromolecular complexes |
| | Regulates gene expression as well as diverse cellular processes, including maintenance of genomic stability, XCI, and genomic imprinting | Play vital roles in executing genomic programs such as gene activation and silencing |
| **Relevance to stroke** | Levels are increased in the ischemic brain and may be responsible for promoting neural cell death | Histone acetylation levels are perturbed in the ischemic brain and may be associated with mediating neural cell death and protective responses, including excitotoxicity, oxidative stress, inflammation, cell cycle regulation, DNA repair, and apoptosis |
| | Deficiency of methylenetetrahydrofolate reductase, which is involved in the formation of SAM, causes hyperhomocysteinemia and an increased risk of stroke | Abnormal chromatin is a key feature of necrotic cell death and apoptotic cell death, which are both associated with neural injury in stroke |
| | Extent of XCI in female heterozygotes with Fabry disease determines clinical involvement, including risk | Schimke immune-osseous dysplasia is a disease characterized by increased risk of stroke, which is caused by mutation of a nucleosome remodeling enzyme (*i.e.,* SMARCAL1) |
| | Imprinted GNAS genomic locus is important for glucose and lipid metabolism and platelet function | Antichromatin and antihistone antibodies are found in systemic lupus erythematosus, which is associated with an increased risk of stroke due to multiple factors |
| | Abnormal DNA methylation is associated with atherosclerosis, obesity, insulin resistance, kidney disease, cancer, and autoimmunity | Chromatin dynamics are important for modulating cholesterol synthesis, transport, and metabolic pathways |

Abbreviations: SAM, S-adenosylmethionine; SMARCAL1, SWI/SNF-related, matrix-associated, actin-dependent regulator of chromatin, subfamily A-like 1; XCI, X chromosome inactivation.

Table **2** originates from the Broderick Laboratory and for the first time organizes stroke nanotechnologies available since 2001 by implementation in Diagnosis, Therapy, or a combination of both. This detailed table entitled "Nanotechnology in Stroke: An Overview of Human and Animal Models" systematically lists Nanodiagnostics, Nanotheranostics and Nanotherapeutics in separate columns. References corresponding to Table **2** citations are listed directly under Table **2** for ease of access to the original research.

**Table 2. Nanotechnology in Stroke - An Overview of Human and Animal Models.**

| Nanodiagnostics: Nanotechnology for Imaging | Nanotheranostics: Nanotechnology for Diagnosis/Imaging and Treatment | Nanotherapeutics: Nanotechnology for Treatment |
|---|---|---|
| **Animated dextran iron oxide particle** for MRI *via* P-selectin - targeted contrast agent [1] | **Anticholinergic-HSP72 vectorized stealth immunoliposomes** that carry citicoline and are traceable by MRI & fluorescence [18] | **Amine-modified single-walled carbon nanotubes** for stem cell nanoscaffold transplantation [27] |
| **Carbon nanotubes** for extracellular glutamate monitoring in real-time [2] | **Aptamer Based Circuit** monitors serum thrombin level and activity and delivers appropriate amount of inhibitory anti-coagulant [19] | **Buckminsterfullerene** to deliver neuroprotective, water-soluble hexasulfonated C(60) (FC(4)S) intraperitoneal pre-treatment for permanent MCAO [28] |
| **Fibrin-targeting peptide (GPR, Gly-Pro-Arg)** [3,4] | **Fluorescent Polystyrene Nanospheres** for drug delivery and on-site diagnosis [20] | **Carbon nanofibers** [5] |
| **Functionalized nanoshells** for Photoacoustic Tomography Imaging with Contrast Agents [5] | **Liposomes** for delivery of (18)F-labeled Liposome-encapsulated hemoglobin (LEH) for PET scan and oxygen delivery [21] | **Carbon nanotube** with monoclonal antibody or to promote neural growth [5] |
| **Lipid-encapsulated perfluorocarbon nanoparticles** containing gadolinium-chelate for *in vivo* MRI detecting thrombus formation [6] | **Magnetofluorescent crosslinked dextran-coated iron oxide nanoparticles** conjugated to tPA with FXIIIa-targeted fibrinolytic nanoagent for thrombolysis [22] | **Carboxyfullerene** intracerebroventricular infusion for neuroprotection [29] |

*(Table 2) contd.....*

| Nanodiagnostics: Nanotechnology for Imaging | Nanotheranostics: Nanotechnology for Diagnosis/Imaging and Treatment | Nanotherapeutics: Nanotechnology for Treatment |
|---|---|---|
| **Lipopeptide nanoparticles carrying fluorescently-labeled pentapeptide Cys-Arg-G-u-Lys-Ala (CREKA)** to visualize clotted serum plasma proteins such as fibrin to target atherosclerosis [7] *via* MRI [8] | **Neuromolecular Imaging (NMI)** with *in vivo* **BRODERICK PROBE®** **nanobiosensors** to check validity of murine stroke model and efficacy of enoxaparin post-stroke and during reperfusion [23]; to diagnose human epilepsy during surgery with future studies dedicated to prolonged use of biosensors in humans undergoing intracranial EEG studies, as well as novel surgical and pharmacological strategies to treat seizures [24]; to test validity of murine Parkinson's model and biphasic properties of bromocriptine therapy [25] | **Cerium oxide nanoparticles (nanoceria)** for neuroprotection and reactive oxygen species reduction [30] |
| **Perfluorocarbon nanoemulsion** for $^{19}$FMRI markers [9] to visualize inflammatory processes *in vivo* [10] | **Shear-Activated Nanotherapeutic** to target thrombolysis or imaging agent to stenotic site [26] | **Dendrimer drug conjugate** [5] |
| **pH-responsive polymeric micelles** triggered by acidic environment of ischemia to visualize on MRI [11] | | **Echogenic liposomes (ELIP)** for xenon gas delivery [31] |
| **Polysaccharide fucoidan nanosystem for** *in vivo* **P-selectin detection** *via* single-photon emission CT imaging [12] | | **Electrospun nanofibers** as scaffolds for neural tissue engineering [32] |
| **Quantum dots** conjugated with fluorescent particles [5] for labeling and imaging of bone marrow stromal cells [13] | | **e-PAM-R**, a biodegradable arginine ester of PAMAM dendrimer for siRNA delivery [33] |
| **Single-walled carbon nanotubes (SWNTs)** for online glucose and lactate monitoring in the ischemic brain [14] | | **Gelatin and zinc acetate tPA delivery nanosystem** for I.V. thrombolysis [34] |

(Table 2) contd.....

| Nanodiagnostics: Nanotechnology for Imaging | Nanotheranostics: Nanotechnology for Diagnosis/Imaging and Treatment | Nanotherapeutics: Nanotechnology for Treatment |
|---|---|---|
| **Single-walled carbon nanotube (SWNT)-modified glassy carbon electrode** for integration with *in vivo* microdialysis ascorbate depletion monitoring [15] | | **Liposome** functionalized with monoclonal antibodies [5] |
| **Ultrasmall superparamagnetic iron oxide (USPIO) nanoparticles** for MRI visualization of macrophage recruitment in ischemic brain [16] | | **Magnetically powered rotating nanomotors** to accelerate tPA-mediated thrombolysis [35] |
| **Urinary nanomarker assay** using iron oxide nanoworms with thrombin-cleavable peptides to detect urine thrombin activity *via* synthetic reporter system to estimate thrombosis level *in vivo* [17] | | **Nanocapsules** containing indomethacin [36] |
| | | **Nanocrystals** for PX-18 drug delivery [37] |
| | | **Perfluorocarbon Nanoparticles** for thrombolysis [38] |
| | | **pH-sensitive nitroxyl radical-containing nanoparticles (NPs)** for prolonged drug circulation with NPs disintegrating at low pH [39] |
| | | **Polyactide nanocapsules** containing quercetin [40] |
| | | **Poly(D,L-lactose co-glycolide) nanoparticles** for drug delivery [41] |
| | | **Polyethylene glycol (PEG)-coated chitosan nanospheres** conjugated to an anti-mouse transferrin receptor monoclonal antibody [42] |
| | | **Polymeric micelles** with entrapped drug [5] |
| | | **Polymeric poly (n-butyl cyanoacrylate) PBCA nanoparticles** for tacrine drug delivery [43] |

*(Table 2) contd.....*

| Nanodiagnostics: Nanotechnology for Imaging | Nanotheranostics: Nanotechnology for Diagnosis/Imaging and Treatment | Nanotherapeutics: Nanotechnology for Treatment |
|---|---|---|
| | | **Puerarin-loaded poly (butylcyanoacrylate) nanoparticles (PBCN)** for neuroprotection in ischemia [44] |
| | | **Quantum dots** for siRNA delivery [45] |
| | | **Self-assembling peptide nanofibers** for neuroregeneration *via in vivo* injection [46] |
| | | **Silicon wafers** with nanoscale surface topograph [5] |
| | | **Solid lipid nanoparticles (SLNs)** for increased circulation time of daidzein [47] and drug-delivery of puerarin [48] |
| | | **Superoxide dismutase enzyme and targeted anti-NMDA (N-methyl-D-aspartate) receptor 1 (NR1) antibody nanoparticles** to limit reperfusion injury [49] |
| | | **Superparamagnetic Iron-Oxide (SPIO) nanoparticles** to monitor human stem cell transplantation [50] *via* contrast agents visible by MRI [51] such as chitosan [52] or ferumoxide [53] |
| | | **tPA-bound magnetite nanoparticles** for targeted local thrombolysis [54] |
| | | **Urokinase-type plasminogen activator (uPA)-coated, self-assembled chitosan and tripolyphosphate nanoparticles** for clot lysis [55] |

This table organizes a literature review of nanotechnology in stroke from 2001 to the present. The nanotechnology is organized by function into 3 categories: nanotechnology for diagnosis (Nanodiagnostics); nanotechnology for both therapy and diagnostics (Nanotheranostics); and nanotechnology for therapy (Nanotherapeutics). As demonstrated, there is a relative lack of Nanotheranostics compared to both Nanodiagnostics and Nanotherapeutics.

# NOTES FOR TABLE 2

[1]    Jin AY, Tuor UI, Rushforth D, *et al.* Magnetic resonance molecular imaging of post-stroke neuroinflammation with a P-selectin targeted iron oxide nanoparticle. Contrast Media Mol Imaging 2009; 4(6): 305-11.

[http://dx.doi.org/10.1002/cmmi.292] [PMID: 19941323]

[2]     Lee HJ, Park J, Yoon OJ, *et al.* Amine-modified single-walled carbon nanotubes protect neurons from injury in a rat stroke model. Nat Nanotechnol 2011; 6(2): 121-5.
[http://dx.doi.org/10.1038/nnano.2010.281] [PMID: 21278749]

[3]     McCarthy JR, Patel P, Botnaru I, Haghayeghi P, Weissleder R, Jaffer FA. Multimodal nanoagents for the detection of intravascular thrombi. Bioconjug Chem 2009; 20(6): 1251-5.
[http://dx.doi.org/10.1021/bc9001163] [PMID: 19456115]

[4]     Obermeyer AC, Capehart SL, Jarman JB, Francis MB. Multivalent viral capsids with internal cargo for fibrin imaging. PLoS One 2014; 9(6): e100678.
[http://dx.doi.org/10.1371/journal.pone.0100678] [PMID: 24960118]

[5]     Nair SB, Dileep A, Rajanikant GK. Nanotechnology based diagnostic and therapeutic strategies for neuroscience with special emphasis on ischemic stroke. Current Medicinal Chemistry 2012; 19: 0001-13.
[http://dx.doi.org/10.2174/092986712798992138]

[6]     Flacke S, Fischer S, Scott MJ, *et al.* Novel MRI contrast agent for molecular imaging of fibrin: implications for detecting vulnerable plaques. Circulation 2001; 104(11): 1280-5.
[http://dx.doi.org/10.1161/hc3601.094303] [PMID: 11551880]

[7]     Peters D, Kastantin M, Kotamraju VR, *et al.* Targeting atherosclerosis by using modular, multifunctional micelles. Proc Natl Acad Sci USA 2009; 106(24): 9815-9.
[http://dx.doi.org/10.1073/pnas.0903369106] [PMID: 19487682]

[8]     Makowski MR, Forbes SC, Blume U, *et al. In vivo* assessment of intraplaque and endothelial fibrin in ApoE(-/-) mice by molecular MRI. Atherosclerosis 2012; 222(1): 43-9.
[http://dx.doi.org/10.1016/j.atherosclerosis.2012.01.008] [PMID: 22284956]

[9]     Grapentin C, Barnert S, Schubert R. Monitoring the stability of Perfluorocarbon Nanoemulsions by Cryo-TEM image analysis and dynamic light scattering. PLoS One 2015; 10(6): e0130674.
[http://dx.doi.org/10.1371/journal.pone.0130674] [PMID: 26098661]

[10]    Flögel U, Ding Z, Hardung H, *et al. In vivo* monitoring of inflammation after cardiac and cerebral ischemia by fluorine magnetic resonance imaging. Circulation 2008; 118(2): 140-8.
[http://dx.doi.org/10.1161/CIRCULATIONAHA.107.737890] [PMID: 18574049]

[11]    Gao GH, Lee JW, Nguyen MK, *et al.* pH-responsive polymeric micelle based on PEG-poly(-amino ester)/(amido amine) as intelligent vehicle for magnetic resonance imaging in detection of cerebral ischemic area. J Control Release 2011; 155(1): 11-7.
[http://dx.doi.org/10.1016/j.jconrel.2010.09.012] [PMID: 20854855]

[12]    Rouzet F, Bachelet-Violette L, Alsac JM, *et al.* Radiolabeled fucoidan as a p-selectin targeting agent for *in vivo* imaging of platelet-rich thrombus and endothelial activation. J Nucl Med 2011; 52(9): 1433-40.
[http://dx.doi.org/10.2967/jnumed.110.085852] [PMID: 21849401]

[13]    Kawabori M, Kuroda S, Sugiyama T, *et al.* Intracerebral, but not intravenous, transplantation of bone marrow stromal cells enhances functional recovery in rat cerebral infarct: An optical imaging study. Neuropathology 2012; 32(3): 217-6.

[http://dx.doi.org/10.1111/j.1440-1789.2011.01260.x] [PMID: 22007875]

[14]  Lin Y, Zhu N, Yu P, Su L, Mao L. Physiologically relevant online electrochemical method for continuous and simultaneous monitoring of striatum glucose and lactate following global cerebral ischemia/reperfusion. Anal Chem 2009; 81(6): 2067-74.
[http://dx.doi.org/10.1021/ac801946s] [PMID: 19281258]

[15]  Zhang M, Liu K, Gong K, Su L, Chen Y, Mao L. Continuous on-line monitoring of extracellular ascorbate depletion in the rat striatum induced by global ischemia with carbon nanotube-modified glassy carbon electrode integrated into a thin-layer radial flow cell. Anal Chem 2005; 77(19): 6234-42.
[http://dx.doi.org/10.1021/ac051188d] [PMID: 16194084]

[16]  Saleh A, Schroeter M, Ringelstein A, *et al.* Iron oxide particle-enhanced MRI suggests variability of brain inflammation at early stages after ischemic stroke. Stroke 2007; 38(10): 2733-7.
[http://dx.doi.org/10.1161/STROKEAHA.107.481788] [PMID: 17717318]

[17]  Lin KY, Kwong GA, Warren AD, Wood DK, Bhatia SN. Nanoparticles that sense thrombin activity as synthetic urinary biomarkers of thrombosis. ACS Nano 2013; 7(10): 9001-9.
[http://dx.doi.org/10.1021/nn403550c] [PMID: 24015809]

[18]  Agulla J, Brea D, Campos F, *et al. In vivo* theranostics at the peri-infarct region in cerebral ischemia. Theranostics 2013; 4(1): 90-105.
[http://dx.doi.org/10.7150/thno.7088] [PMID: 24396517]

[19]  Han D, Zhu Z, Wu C, *et al.* A logical molecular circuit for programmable and autonomous regulation of protein activity using DNA aptamer-protein interactions. J Am Chem Soc 2012; 134(51): 20797-804.
[http://dx.doi.org/10.1021/ja310428s] [PMID: 23194304]

[20]  Yang CS, Chang CH, Tsai PJ, Chen WY, Tseng FG, Lo LW. Nanoparticle-based *in vivo* investigation on blood-brain barrier permeability following ischemia and reperfusion. Anal Chem 2004; 76(15): 4465-71.
[http://dx.doi.org/10.1021/ac035491v] [PMID: 15283589]

[21]  Urakami T, Kawaguchi AT, Akai S, *et al. In vivo* distribution of liposome-encapsulated hemoglobin determined by positron emission tomography. Artif Organs 2009; 33(2): 164-8.
[http://dx.doi.org/10.1111/j.1525-1594.2008.00702.x] [PMID: 19178462]

[22]  McCarthy JR, Sazonova IY, Erdem SS, *et al.* Multifunctional nanoagent for thrombus-targeted fibrinolytic therapy. Nanomedicine (Lond) 2012; 7(7): 1017-28.
[http://dx.doi.org/10.2217/nnm.11.179] [PMID: 22348271]

[23]  Broderick PA, Wenning L, Li Y-S. Life in the Penumbra with the BRODERICK PROBE®. In: Radaelli A, Mancia G, Ferrarese C, Beretta S, Eds. Current Development in Stroke: Chapter 6 - New Concepts in Stroke Diagnosis and Therapy [e-book]. Available from: Bentham Science electronic collection: Bentham Science Publishers 2017; pp. 131-75.

[24]  Broderick PA, Doyle WK, Pacia SV, Kuzniecky RI, Devinsky O, Kolodny EH. A clinical trial of an advanced diagnostic biomedical device for epilepsy patients. J Long Term Eff Med Implants 2008; 18: 50.
[http://dx.doi.org/10.1615/JLongTermEffMedImplants.v18.i1.480]

[25]  Broderick PA, Kolodny EH. Real-time imaging of biomarkers in the Parkinsons brain: Pharmaceutical therapy with bromocriptine. Pharmaceuticals 2009; 2(3): 236-49.
[http://dx.doi.org/10.3390/ph2030236] [PMID: 27713237]

[26]  Korin N, Gounis MJ, Wakhloo AK, Ingber DE. Targeted drug delivery to flow-obstructed blood vessels using mechanically activated nanotherapeutics. JAMA Neurol 2015; 72(1): 119-22.
[http://dx.doi.org/10.1001/jamaneurol.2014.2886] [PMID: 25365638]

[27]  Lee GJ, Choi SK, Choi S, Park JH, Park HK. Enzyme-immobilized CNT network probe for *in vivo* neurotransmitter detection. Methods Mol Biol 2011; 743: 65-75.
[http://dx.doi.org/10.1007/978-1-61779-132-1_6] [PMID: 21553183]

[28]  Yang DY, Wang MF, Chen IL, Chan YC, Lee MS, Cheng FC. Systemic administration of a water-soluble hexasulfonated C(60) (FC(4)S) reduces cerebral ischemia-induced infarct volume in gerbils. Neurosci Lett 2001; 311(2): 121-4.
[http://dx.doi.org/10.1016/S0304-3940(01)02153-X] [PMID: 11567793]

[29]  Lin AM, Fang SF, Lin SZ, Chou CK, Luh TY, Ho LT. Local carboxyfullerene protects cortical infarction in rat brain. Neurosci Res 2002; 43(4): 317-21.
[http://dx.doi.org/10.1016/S0168-0102(02)00056-1] [PMID: 12135775]

[30]  Estevez AY, Pritchard S, Harper K, *et al.* Neuroprotective mechanisms of cerium oxide nanoparticles in a mouse hippocampal brain slice model of ischemia. Free Radic Biol Med 2011; 51(6): 1155-63.
[http://dx.doi.org/10.1016/j.freeradbiomed.2011.06.006] [PMID: 21704154]

[31]  Britton GL, Kim H, Kee PH, *et al. In vivo* therapeutic gas delivery for neuroprotection with echogenic liposomes. Circulation 2010; 122(16): 1578-87.
[http://dx.doi.org/10.1161/CIRCULATIONAHA.109.879338] [PMID: 20921443]

[32]  Lee JY, Bashur CA, Goldstein AS, Schmidt CE. Polypyrrole-coated electrospun PLGA nanofibers for neural tissue applications. Biomaterials 2009; 30(26): 4325-35.
[http://dx.doi.org/10.1016/j.biomaterials.2009.04.042] [PMID: 19501901]

[33]  Kim ID, Lim CM, Kim JB, *et al.* Neuroprotection by biodegradable PAMAM ester (e-PAM--)-mediated HMGB1 siRNA delivery in primary cortical cultures and in the postischemic brain. J Control Release 2010; 142(3): 422-30.
[http://dx.doi.org/10.1016/j.jconrel.2009.11.011] [PMID: 19944723]

[34]  Kawata H, Uesugi Y, Soeda T, *et al.* A new drug delivery system for intravenous coronary thrombolysis with thrombus targeting and stealth activity recoverable by ultrasound. J Am Coll Cardiol 2012; 60(24): 2550-7.
[http://dx.doi.org/10.1016/j.jacc.2012.08.1008] [PMID: 23158532]

[35]  Cheng R, Huang W, Huang L, *et al.* Acceleration of tissue plasminogen activator-mediated thrombolysis by magnetically powered nanomotors. ACS Nano 2014; 8(8): 7746-54.
[http://dx.doi.org/10.1021/nn5029955] [PMID: 25006696]

[36]  Bernardi A, Frozza RL, Horn AP, *et al.* Protective effects of indomethacin-loaded nanocapsules against oxygen-glucose deprivation in organotypic hippocampal slice cultures: involvement of neuroinflammation. Neurochem Int 2010; 57(6): 629-36.
[http://dx.doi.org/10.1016/j.neuint.2010.07.012] [PMID: 20691236]

[37] Wang Q, Sun AY, Pardeike J, Müller RH, Simonyi A, Sun GY. Neuroprotective effects of a nanocrystal formulation of sPLA(2) inhibitor PX-18 in cerebral ischemia/reperfusion in gerbils. Brain Res 2009; 1285: 188-95.
[http://dx.doi.org/10.1016/j.brainres.2009.06.022] [PMID: 19527696]

[38] Marsh JN, Hu G, Scott MJ, *et al.* A fibrin-specific thrombolytic nanomedicine approach to acute ischemic stroke. Nanomedicine (Lond) 2011; 6(4): 605-15.
[http://dx.doi.org/10.2217/nnm.11.21] [PMID: 21506686]

[39] Yoshitomi T, Nagasaki Y. Nitroxyl radical-containing nanoparticles for novel nanomedicine against oxidative stress injury. Nanomedicine (Lond) 2011; 6(3): 509-18.
[http://dx.doi.org/10.2217/nnm.11.13] [PMID: 21542688]

[40] Das S, Mandal AK, Ghosh A, Panda S, Das N, Sarkar S. Nanoparticulated quercetin in combating age related cerebral oxidative injury. Curr Aging Sci 2008; 1(3): 169-74.
[http://dx.doi.org/10.2174/1874609810801030169] [PMID: 20021389]

[41] Reddy MK, Labhasetwar V. Nanoparticle-mediated delivery of superoxide dismutase to the brain: an effective strategy to reduce ischemia-reperfusion injury. FASEB J 2009; 23(5): 1384-95.
[http://dx.doi.org/10.1096/fj.08-116947] [PMID: 19124559]

[42] Karatas H, Aktas Y, Gursoy-Ozdemir Y, *et al.* A nanomedicine transports a peptide caspase-3 inhibitor across the blood-brain barrier and provides neuroprotection. J Neurosci 2009; 29(44): 13761-9.
[http://dx.doi.org/10.1523/JNEUROSCI.4246-09.2009] [PMID: 19889988]

[43] Wilson B, Samanta MK, Santhi K, Kumar KP, Paramakrishnan N, Suresh B. Targeted delivery of tacrine into the brain with polysorbate 80-coated poly(n-butylcyanoacrylate) nanoparticles. Eur J Pharm Biopharm 2008; 70(1): 75-84.
[http://dx.doi.org/10.1016/j.ejpb.2008.03.009] [PMID: 18472255]

[44] Zhao LX, Liu AC, Yu SW, *et al.* The permeability of puerarin loaded poly(butylcyanoacrylate) nanoparticles coated with polysorbate 80 on the blood-brain barrier and its protective effect against cerebral ischemia/reperfusion injury. Biol Pharm Bull 2013; 36(8): 1263-70.
[http://dx.doi.org/10.1248/bpb.b12-00769] [PMID: 23902970]

[45] Bonoiu A, Mahajan SD, Ye L, *et al.* MMP-9 gene silencing by a quantum dot-siRNA nanoplex delivery to maintain the integrity of the blood brain barrier. Brain Res 2009; 1282: 142-55.
[http://dx.doi.org/10.1016/j.brainres.2009.05.047] [PMID: 19477169]

[46] Tysseling-Mattiace VM, Sahni V, Niece KL, *et al.* Self-assembling nanofibers inhibit glial scar formation and promote axon elongation after spinal cord injury. J Neurosci 2008; 28(14): 3814-23.
[http://dx.doi.org/10.1523/JNEUROSCI.0143-08.2008] [PMID: 18385339]

[47] Gao Y, Gu W, Chen L, Xu Z, Li Y. The role of daidzein-loaded sterically stabilized solid lipid nanoparticles in therapy for cardio-cerebrovascular diseases. Biomaterials 2008; 29(30): 4129-36.
[http://dx.doi.org/10.1016/j.biomaterials.2008.07.008] [PMID: 18667234]

[48] Zhu L, Luo CF, Yuan M, Chen MS, Ji H. Molecular mechanism of protective effect of puerarin solid lipid nanoparticle on cerebral ischemia-reperfusion injury in gerbils. Zhong Yao Cai 2010; 33(12): 1900-4.

[PMID: 21548369]

[49]   Yun X, Maximov VD, Yu J, Zhu H, Vertegel AA, Kindy MS. Nanoparticles for targeted delivery of antioxidant enzymes to the brain after cerebral ischemia and reperfusion injury. J Cereb Blood Flow Metab 2013; 33(4): 583-92.
[http://dx.doi.org/10.1038/jcbfm.2012.209] [PMID: 23385198]

[50]   Jendelová P, Herynek V, Urdzíková L, *et al.* Magnetic resonance tracking of transplanted bone marrow and embryonic stem cells labeled by iron oxide nanoparticles in rat brain and spinal cord. J Neurosci Res 2004; 76(2): 232-43.
[http://dx.doi.org/10.1002/jnr.20041] [PMID: 15048921]

[51]   Liu CH, Huang S, Cui J, *et al.* MR contrast probes that trace gene transcripts for cerebral ischemia in live animals. FASEB J 2007; 21(11): 3004-15.
[http://dx.doi.org/10.1096/fj.07-8203com] [PMID: 17478745]

[52]   Reddy AM, Kwak BK, Shim HJ, *et al. In vivo* tracking of mesenchymal stem cells labeled with a novel chitosan-coated superparamagnetic iron oxide nanoparticles using 3.0T MRI. J Korean Med Sci 2010; 25(2): 211-9.
[http://dx.doi.org/10.3346/jkms.2010.25.2.211] [PMID: 20119572]

[53]   Song M, Kim Y, Kim Y, *et al.* MRI tracking of intravenously transplanted human neural stem cells in rat focal ischemia model. Neurosci Res 2009; 64(2): 235-9.
[http://dx.doi.org/10.1016/j.neures.2009.03.006] [PMID: 19428705]

[54]   Ma YH, Wu SY, Wu T, Chang YJ, Hua MY, Chen JP. Magnetically targeted thrombolysis with recombinant tissue plasminogen activator bound to polyacrylic acid-coated nanoparticles. Biomaterials 2009; 30(19): 3343-51.
[http://dx.doi.org/10.1016/j.biomaterials.2009.02.034] [PMID: 19299010]

[55]   Jin HJ, Zhang H, Sun ML, Zhang BG, Zhang JW. Urokinase-coated chitosan nanoparticles for thrombolytic therapy: preparation and pharmacodynamics *in vivo*. J Thromb Thrombolysis 2013; 36(4): 458-68.
[http://dx.doi.org/10.1007/s11239-013-0951-7] [PMID: 23728739]

## Appendix: Overview of Nanotechnology Platforms for Stroke Diagnosis and Treatment

We have selected two papers for detailed commentary. The first selected paper is, *Targeted Drug Delivery to Flow-Obstructed Blood Vessels Using Mechanically Activated Nanotherapeutics by Korin N, Gounis MJ, Wakhloo AK, and Ingber DE. JAMA Neurol 2015; 72(1): 119-122* [96].

Shear stress, shear force and shearing mechanisms are concepts from physics that have been effectively translated to medical treatment. For example, shearing effects applied tangentially differentially affect those applied vertically. Thus, applying these concepts to the physiology of both central and peripheral blood flow demonstrated that narrowed blood vessels exert greater shear stress because this aspect of force is concomitant with reduced surface area. Therefore, the physiologic term for these shearing dynamics is "hemodynamics" and the units for hemodynamics are called dynes/cm$^2$.

In physiologic circulatory and microcirculating systems, shear stresses in functionally intact blood vessels remain within tight limits (1-70 dynes/cm$^2$) depending on the location within the vascular tree. However, in arterial vascular diseases, hemodynamic conditions can stray from these normal values significantly, so much so that an arterial constriction of 95% can produce shear stresses greater than 1000 dynes/cm$^2$. As a result of greater dyne values, the molecular medley of platelets, red blood cells, white blood cells and other constituents including cytokines, sense significantly high shear stresses, enabling clumping of these molecules to form "clots". These clots coagulate along the wall of the narrowed blood vessel lumen. In essence, the clots are comprised of an amalgamation of solid blood components, as well as any molecules that travel in serum. The final response is plaque formation whether atherosclerotic derived or not.

As depicted in Fig. (**10**), the purpose of mechanically injecting nanoparticles to be "clot busters" is to "fight" the "shear stress" in the narrowed lumen with the shear stress created by a mechanical vehicle carrying nanoparticles. Once the mechanically inserted r-tPA nanoparticles or other examples of such, are deployed within the narrowed lumen, the dyne units for each nanoparticle is only about 100 to 200 nm. Voilà! The shear stress of each nanoparticle can and will be the "clot buster", in fact, reducing the chances of very debilitating and life-changing strokes. Nanotechnology with nanoparticles dramatically advances the nanotherapeutics for unfortunate stroke victims.

The second selected paper is, *The Emerging Role of Epigenetics in Stroke: III. Neural Stem Cell Biology and Regenerative Medicine by Qureshi IA and Mehler MF. Arch Neurol 2011; 68(3): 294-302* [97].

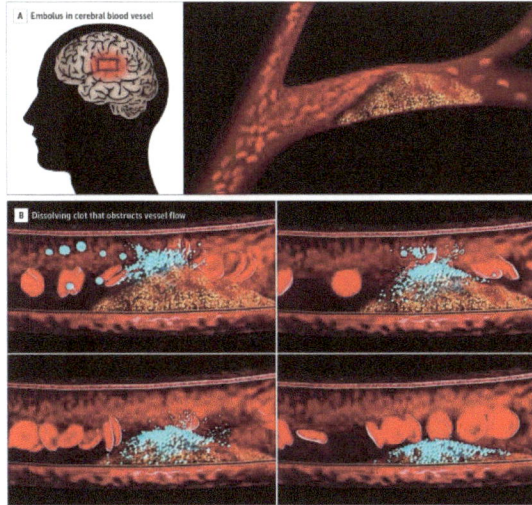

**Fig. (10).** Shear-activated nanotherapeutics for thrombolytic therapies are depicted in the image below. A, Ischemic stroke is produced by an embolus that lodges in cerebral blood vessels and obstructs blood flow. B, Local elevated shear stress in the narrowed lumen results from partial obstruction of vessel flow by the embolus. After these elevated shear stresses break apart the tissue plasminogen activator–coated, shear-activated nanotherapeutics, they are deployed locally to progressively dissolve the clot [96]. The figure was created by Kristin Johnson (Boston Children's Hospital, Boston, Massachusetts).

The adage that reads, "Never judge a book by its cover" is entirely appropriate in the case of the burgeoning and exciting field of epigenetics. It is amazing that each cell in the living being has the same genome but it is the "inside" that is different. The "inside" is comprised of cell- and tissue-specific profiles of gene transcription and posttranscriptional-RNA-processing. Indeed, here on the "inside" is where we will find the pathophysiology of stroke, as well as the subsequent treatments for stroke. The authors from the Albert Einstein College of Medicine go on to describe examples of these transcription processes as quality control, RNA modifications, translation, and transport are discriminately controlled by multiple layers of interlaced epigenetic mechanisms. The epigenetic interactions include DNA methylation; histone code modifications, nucleosome remodeling, and higher-order chromatin formation; noncoding RNA; and RNA editing. Also, it is important to remember that dynamic changes occur in the epigenome throughout life. Thus, normal development, adult homeostasis and aging are manipulated by the epigenome, and these revisions in the genome are further affected by the environment *via* the environtome. Therefore, targeting the epigenome for diagnosis and treatment of stroke is a critical new path to pursue if, in fact, we are serious about taking care of the stroke patient as well as the patient susceptible to stroke. Fortunately, there are some drugs that are already approved by the US Food and Drug Administration, and these medications have direct or indirect effects on epigenetic mechanisms. In this excellent piece of literature, these pharmacotherapeutic agents are described.

Indeed, a book should never be judged by its cover. It is amazing that the genome inside each cell of the living organism is comprised of the same genome, yet diverse outcomes may be generated by the interior mechanisms of these uniform genomes. Thus, we discuss breakthrough work on exogenous and endogenous transplantation mechanisms. Promising treatments for stroke include the transplantation of exogenous stem cells and the activation of endogenous neural stem and progenitor cells (NSPCs). These cells can regulate intrinsic responses to ischemic insult and may even directly integrate into injured neural networks. Epigenetic reprogramming denotes an innovative strategy for augmenting the intrinsic potential of the brain to protect and repair itself by regulating pathologic neural gene expression and stimulating the restatement of fundamental neural developmental processes.

Interestingly, there is another often said adage that comes to mind here as well. It is The Theory of Recapitulation, also called the biogenetic law or embryological parallelism. Ernst Haeckel phrased this theory as "ontogeny recapitulates phylogeny". Since embryos also evolve in different ways, within the field of developmental biology, the theory of recapitulation may be seen as an aside and not dogma, even discredited. Yet, since ontogeny is the development and growth of an individual (*e.g.* the development from an embryo during gestation) and phylogeny is the evolutionary history of a species, the idea may be weaker but is still accurate. A rationale for this thinking is the knowledge that embryonic stages develop to a fully formed offspring, and these stages repeat ("recapitulate") the stages of evolution. Perhaps "ontogeny recapitulates phylogeny" is not completely out of the question in the futuristic realm of stem cell epigenetics.

## CONFLICT OF INTEREST

The authors confirm that the authors have no conflict of interest to declare for this publication.

## ACKNOWLEDGEMENTS

The author wishes to thank the Broderick Brain Foundation, the F.M. Kirby Foundation, the Center for Advanced Technology, CUNY, and the MacKenzie Foundation for partial support of our laboratory and students during these studies. It is important to note that since this body of work, the development and pioneering of Neuromolecular Imaging (NMI) and the BRODERICK PROBE® (named in honor of the father of the corresponding author) has taken place diligently for many years. Other grants including the National Institute of Health, National Institute on Drug Abuse, The Lowenstein Foundation, the FACES and PACE Foundations for Epilepsy, and The Upjohn Pharmacia Company in Michigan deserve honorable mention.

## REFERENCES

[1]     Mobberley M. Total solar eclipses and how to observe them. New York: Springer 2007.
        [http://dx.doi.org/10.1007/978-0-387-69828-1]

[2]     Pratt J, Boudeau P, Uzan A, Imperato A, Stutzmann J. Enoxaparin reduces cerebral edemaafter photothrombotic injury in the rat. Haemostasis 1998; 28(2): 78-85.
        [PMID: 10087432]

[3]     Wahl F, Grosjean-Piot O, Bareyre F, Uzan A, Stutzmann JM. Enoxaparin reduces brain edema, cerebral lesions, and improves motor and cognitive impairments induced by a traumatic brain injury in rats. J Neurotrauma 2000; 17(11): 1055-65.
        [http://dx.doi.org/10.1089/neu.2000.17.1055] [PMID: 11101208]

[4]     Jonas S, Sugimori M, Llinás R. Is low molecular weight heparin a neuroprotectant? Ann N Y Acad Sci 1997; 825: 389-93.
        [http://dx.doi.org/10.1111/j.1749-6632.1997.tb48449.x] [PMID: 9370003]

[5]     Libersan D, Khalil A, Dagenais P, *et al.* The low molecular weight heparin, enoxaparin, limits infarct size at reperfusion in the dog. Cardiovasc Res 1998; 37(3): 656-66.
        [http://dx.doi.org/10.1016/S0008-6363(97)00292-7] [PMID: 9659449]

[6]     Aggarwal A, Whitaker DA, Rimmer JM, *et al.* Attenuation of platelet reactivity by enoxaparin compared with unfractionated heparin in patients undergoing haemodialysis. Nephrol Dial Transplant 2004; 19(6): 1559-63.
        [http://dx.doi.org/10.1093/ndt/gfh209] [PMID: 15034156]

[7]     Uzan A. [Thrombosis and ischemia: experimental data]. Arch Mal Coeur Vaiss 2002; 95(Spec No 7): 31-5.
        [PMID: 12500602]

[8]     Groch J. Enoxaparin outdoes heparin for post-stroke venous thromboembolism [Internet] , 2010 [[cited 9 December 2010].]; Available from: http://www.medpagetoday.com/Neurology/Strokes/5473.

[9]     Walling AD. Enoxaparin preferred following acute ischemic stroke. Am Fam Physician 2007; 76: 1859-64.

[10]    Sherman DG, Albers GW, Bladin C, *et al.* PREVAIL Investigators. The efficacy and safety of enoxaparin *versus* unfractionated heparin for the prevention of venous thromboembolism after acute ischemic stroke: an open-label randomized comparison. Lancet 2007; 369: 1347-55.
        [http://dx.doi.org/10.1016/S0140-6736(07)60633-3] [PMID: 17448820]

[11]    Manduteanu I, Voinea M, Capraru M, Dragomir E, Simionescu M. A novel attribute of enoxaparin: inhibition of monocyte adhesion to endothelial cells by a mechanism involving cell adhesion molecules. Pharmacology 2002; 65(1): 32-7.
        [http://dx.doi.org/10.1159/000056183] [PMID: 11901299]

[12]    Barnhart R. The Barnhart Concise Dictionary of Etymology. New York: Collins Reference 1995.

[13]    Carmichael ST. Plasticity of cortical projections after stroke. Neuroscientist 2003; 9(1): 64-75.
        [http://dx.doi.org/10.1177/1073858402239592] [PMID: 12580341]

[14]    Kolb B, Gibb R. Brain plasticity and behaviour in the developing brain. J Can Acad Child Adolesc Psychiatry 2011; 20(4): 265-76.
        [PMID: 22114608]

[15]    Forrester LW, Wheaton LA, Luft AR. Exercise-mediated locomotor recovery and lower-limb neuroplasticity after stroke. J Rehabil Res Dev 2008; 45(2): 205-20.
        [http://dx.doi.org/10.1682/JRRD.2007.02.0034] [PMID: 18566939]

[16]    Komitova M, Mattsson B, Johansson BB, Eriksson PS. Enriched environment increases neural stem/progenitor cell proliferation and neurogenesis in the subventricular zone of stroke-lesioned adult rats. Stroke 2005; 36(6): 1278-82.
        [http://dx.doi.org/10.1161/01.STR.0000166197.94147.59] [PMID: 15879324]

[17]    Broderick PA. Neuromolecular imaging shows temporal synchrony patterns between serotonin and movement within neuronal motor circuits in the brain. Brain Sci 2013; 3(2): 992-1012.
        [http://dx.doi.org/10.3390/brainsci3020992] [PMID: 24961434]

[18]    Fouad K, Rank MM, Vavrek R, Murray KC, Sanelli L, Bennett DJ. Locomotion after spinal cord injury depends on constitutive activity in serotonin receptors. J Neurophysiol 2010; 104(6): 2975-84.
        [http://dx.doi.org/10.1152/jn.00499.2010] [PMID: 20861436]

[19]    Longa EZ, Weinstein PR, Carlson S, Cummins R. Reversible middle cerebral artery occlusion without craniectomy in rats. Stroke 1989; 20(1): 84-91.
        [http://dx.doi.org/10.1161/01.STR.20.1.84] [PMID: 2643202]

[20]    Howells DW, Porritt MJ, Rewell SS, *et al.* Different strokes for different folks: the rich diversity of animal models of focal cerebral ischemia. J Cereb Blood Flow Metab 2010; 30(8): 1412-31.
        [http://dx.doi.org/10.1038/jcbfm.2010.66] [PMID: 20485296]

[21]   Bacigaluppi M, Comi G, Hermann DM. Animal models of ischemic stroke. Part two: modeling cerebral ischemia. Open Neurol J 2010; 4: 34-8.
[PMID: 20721320]

[22]   Hayakawa T, Waltz AG. Immediate effects of cerebral ischemia: evolution and resolution of neurological deficits after experimental occlusion of one middle cerebral artery in conscious cats. Stroke 1975; 6(3): 321-7.
[http://dx.doi.org/10.1161/01.STR.6.3.321] [PMID: 1154469]

[23]   Aspey BS, Taylor FL, Terruli M, Harrison MJ. Temporary middle cerebral artery occlusion in the rat: consistent protocol for a model of stroke and reperfusion. Neuropathol Appl Neurobiol 2000; 26(3): 232-42.
[http://dx.doi.org/10.1046/j.1365-2990.2000.00221.x] [PMID: 10886681]

[24]   Coyle P. Middle cerebral artery occlusion in the young rat. Stroke 1982; 13(6): 855-9.
[http://dx.doi.org/10.1161/01.STR.13.6.855] [PMID: 7147305]

[25]   Bederson JB, Pitts LH, Tsuji M, Nishimura MC, Davis RL, Bartkowski H. Rat middle cerebral artery occlusion: evaluation of the model and development of a neurologic examination. Stroke 1986; 17(3): 472-6.
[http://dx.doi.org/10.1161/01.STR.17.3.472] [PMID: 3715945]

[26]   Zhao W, Ginsberg MD, Prado R, Belayer MD. Depiction of infarct frequency distribution by Computer-Assisted Image Mapping in rat brain with middle cerebral artery occlusion. Stroke 1996; 27: 1112-7.
[http://dx.doi.org/10.1161/01.STR.27.6.1112] [PMID: 8650723]

[27]   Masada T, Hua Y, Xi G, Ennis SR, Keep RF. Attenuation of ischemic brain edema and cerebrovascular injury after ischemic preconditioning in the rat. J Cereb Blood Flow Metab 2001; 21(1): 22-33.
[http://dx.doi.org/10.1097/00004647-200101000-00004] [PMID: 11149665]

[28]   Belayev L, Alanso BS, Busto R, Zhao W, Ginsberg MD. Middle cerebral artery in the rat by intraluminal suture. Stroke 1996; 27: 166-1623.
[http://dx.doi.org/10.1161/01.STR.27.9.1616] [PMID: 8784138]

[29]   Broderick PA, Pacia SV. Identification, diagnosis, and treatment of neuropathologies, neurotoxicities, tumors and brain and spinal cord injuries using microelectrodes with microvoltammetry. USPTO_US 7,112,319, 2006.

[30]   Broderick PA, Pacia SV. Identification, diagnosis, and treatment of neuropathologies, neurotoxicities, tumors, and brain and spinal cord injuries using microelectrodes with microvoltammetry USPTO USSN Patent #2011/13/083,810. Pending 2011.

[31]   Broderick PA. Noninvasive Photonic Sensor with Polymer Memory Transduction using Organic and Inorganic Elements as Platforms. USPTO Provisional Patent 2015.

[32]   Broderick PA. Cathodic Electrochemical Current Arrangement with Telemetric Application. US Patent 4,883,057, 1989.

[33]   Broderick PA. Microelectrodes and their use in cathodic electrochemical current arrangement with telemetric application. US Patent 5,433,710, 1995.

[34]   Broderick PA. Microelectrodes and their use in an electrochemical arrangement with telemetric application. US Patent 5,938,903, 1999.

[35]   Broderick PA, Doyle WK, Pacia SV, Kuzniecky RI, Devinsky O, Kolodny EH, Eds. Intraoperative Neuromolecular Imaging (NMI) in neocortex of epilepsy patients: Comparison with resected neocortical epileptogenic tissue. Annual Meeting of the American Epilepsy Society. 2009 Dec 4-8; Boston, MA. 2009.

[36]   Broderick PA, Doyle WK, Pacia SV, Kuzniecky RI, Devinsky O, Kolodny EH. A clinical trial of an advanced diagnostic biomedical device for epilepsy patients. J Long Term Eff Med Implants 2008; 18: 50.
[http://dx.doi.org/10.1615/JLongTermEffMedImplants.v18.i1.480]

[37]   Broderick PA, Pacia SV. Identification, diagnosis, and treatment of neuropathologies, neurotoxicities, tumors and brain and spinal cord injuries using microelectrodes with microvoltammetry. US Patent 7,112,319, 2006.

[38]   Broderick PA. Distinguishing *in vitro* electrochemical signatures for norepinephrine and dopamine. Neurosci Lett 1988; 95(1-3): 275-80.
[http://dx.doi.org/10.1016/0304-3940(88)90670-2] [PMID: 3226613]

[39]   Broderick PA. Characterizing stearate probes *in vitro* for the electrochemical detection of dopamine and serotonin. Brain Res 1989; 495(1): 115-21.
[http://dx.doi.org/10.1016/0006-8993(89)91224-9] [PMID: 2776030]

[40]   Broderick PA. Studies of oxidative stress mechanisms using a morphine / ascorbate animal model and novel N-stearoyl cerebroside and laurate sensors. J Neural Transm (Vienna) 2008; 115(1): 7-17.
[http://dx.doi.org/10.1007/s00702-007-0809-2] [PMID: 17896074]

[41]   Broderick PA, Pacia SV, Doyle WK, Devinsky O. Monoamine neurotransmitters in resected hippocampal subparcellations from neocortical and mesial temporal lobe epilepsy patients: *in situ* microvoltammetric studies. Brain Res 2000; 878(1-2): 48-63.
[http://dx.doi.org/10.1016/S0006-8993(00)02678-0] [PMID: 10996135]

[42]   Pelligrino LJ, Pelligrino AS, Cushman AJ. A Stereotaxic Atlas of the Rat Brain. New York: Plenum Press 1979.

[43]   Broderick PA, Kolodny EH. Biosensors for brain trauma and dual laser doppler flowmetry: enoxaparin simultaneously reduces stroke-induced dopamine and blood flow while enhancing serotonin and blood flow in motor neurons of brain, *in vivo*. Sensors (Basel) 2011; 11(1): 138-61.
[http://dx.doi.org/10.3390/s11010013] [PMID: 22346571]

[44]   Coyle P, Jokelainen PT. Differential outcome to middle cerebral artery occlusion in spontaneously hypertensive stroke-prone rats (SHRSP) and Wistar Kyoto (WKY) rats. Stroke 1983; 14(4): 605-11.
[http://dx.doi.org/10.1161/01.STR.14.4.605] [PMID: 6658939]

[45]   Spratt NJ, Fernandez J, Chen M, *et al.* Modification of the method of thread manufacture improves stroke induction rate and reduces mortality after thread-occlusion of the middle cerebral artery in young or aged rats. J Neurosci Methods 2006; 155(2): 285-90.
[http://dx.doi.org/10.1016/j.jneumeth.2006.01.020] [PMID: 16513179]

[46]   Phan TG, Wright PM, Markus R, Howells DW, Davis SM, Donnan GA. Salvaging the ischaemic

penumbra: more than just reperfusion? Clin Exp Pharmacol Physiol 2002; 29(1-2): 1-10.
[http://dx.doi.org/10.1046/j.1440-1681.2002.03609.x] [PMID: 11917903]

[47]    Memezawa H, Minamisawa H, Smith ML, Siesjö BK. Ischemic penumbra in a model of reversible middle cerebral artery occlusion in the rat. Exp Brain Res 1992; 89(1): 67-78.
[http://dx.doi.org/10.1007/BF00229002] [PMID: 1601103]

[48]    Saita K, Chen M, Spratt NJ, *et al.* Imaging the ischemic penumbra with 18F-fluoromisonidazole in a rat model of ischemic stroke. Stroke 2004; 35(4): 975-80.
[http://dx.doi.org/10.1161/01.STR.0000121647.01941.ba] [PMID: 15017016]

[49]    Materossi C, Maoret T, Rozzini R, Spano PF, Trabucchi M. Effect of right middle cerebral artery occlusion on striatal dopaminergic function. J Neural Transm 1982; 53(4): 257-64.
[http://dx.doi.org/10.1007/BF01252037] [PMID: 7108507]

[50]    Koizumi H, Fujisawa H, Kurokawa T, *et al.* Recovered neuronal viability revealed by Iodine-12--iomazenil SPECT following traumatic brain injury. J Cereb Blood Flow Metab 2010; 30(10): 1673-81.
[http://dx.doi.org/10.1038/jcbfm.2010.75] [PMID: 20683454]

[51]    Paterson LM, Tyacke RJ, Nutt DJ, Knudsen GM. Measuring endogenous 5-HT release by emission tomography: promises and pitfalls. J Cereb Blood Flow Metab 2010; 30(10): 1682-706.
[http://dx.doi.org/10.1038/jcbfm.2010.104] [PMID: 20664611]

[52]    van Meer MP, van der Marel K, Otte WM, Berkelbach van der Sprenkel JW, Dijkhuizen RM. Correspondence between altered functional and structural connectivity in the contralesional sensorimotor cortex after unilateral stroke in rats: a combined resting-state functional MRI and manganese-enhanced MRI study. J Cereb Blood Flow Metab 2010; 30(10): 1707-11.
[http://dx.doi.org/10.1038/jcbfm.2010.124] [PMID: 20664609]

[53]    Nunes JV, Broderick PA. Novel research translates to clinical cases of schizophrenic and cocaine psychosis. Neuropsychiatr Dis Treat 2007; 3(4): 475-85.
[PMID: 19300576]

[54]    Yulug B. Neuroprotective treatment strategies for poststroke mood disorders: A minireview on atypical neuroleptic drugs and selective serotonin re-uptake inhibitors. Brain Res Bull 2009; 80(3): 95-9.
[http://dx.doi.org/10.1016/j.brainresbull.2009.06.013] [PMID: 19576272]

[55]    Miedema I, Horvath KM, Uyttenboogaart M, *et al.* Effect of selective serotonin re-uptake inhibitors (SSRIs) on functional outcome in patients with acute ischemic stroke treated with tPA. J Neurol Sci 2010; 293(1-2): 65-7.
[http://dx.doi.org/10.1016/j.jns.2010.03.004] [PMID: 20381072]

[56]    Berends HI, Nijlant J, van Putten M, Movig KL, IJzerman MJ. Single dose of fluoxetine increases muscle activation in chronic stroke patients. Clin Neuropharmacol 2009; 32(1): 1-5.
[PMID: 19536922]

[57]    (No authors listed, Article in Russian). Interaction effect of serotonin transporter gene and brain-derived neurotrophic factor on the platelet serotonin content in stroke patients. Zh Nevrol Psikhiatr Im S S Korsakova 2010; 110: 42-5.

[58]   Berends HI, Nijlant JM, Movig KL, Van Putten MJ, Jannink MJ, Ijzerman MJ. The clinical use of drugs influencing neurotransmitters in the brain to promote motor recovery after stroke; a Cochrane systematic review. Eur J Phys Rehabil Med 2009; 45(4): 621-30.
       [PMID: 20032921]

[59]   Ptak K, Yamanishi T, Aungst J, *et al.* Raphé neurons stimulate respiratory circuit activity by multiple mechanisms *via* endogenously released serotonin and substance P. J Neurosci 2009; 29(12): 3720-37.
       [http://dx.doi.org/10.1523/JNEUROSCI.5271-08.2009] [PMID: 19321769]

[60]   Ried LD, Jia H, Cameon R, Feng H, Wang X, Tueth M. Does prestroke depression impact poststroke depression and treatment? Am J Geriatr Psychiatry 2010; 18(7): 624-33.
       [http://dx.doi.org/10.1097/JGP.0b013e3181ca822b] [PMID: 20220578]

[61]   Trifirò G, Dieleman J, Sen EF, Gambassi G, Sturkenboom MC. Risk of ischemic stroke associated with antidepressant drug use in elderly persons. J Clin Psychopharmacol 2010; 30(3): 252-8.
       [http://dx.doi.org/10.1097/JCP.0b013e3181dca10a] [PMID: 20473059]

[62]   Wang SH, Zhang ZJ, Guo YJ, Sui YX, Sun Y. Involvement of serotonin neurotransmission in hippocampal neurogenesis and behavioral responses in a rat model of post-stroke depression. Pharmacol Biochem Behav 2010; 95(1): 129-37.
       [http://dx.doi.org/10.1016/j.pbb.2009.12.017] [PMID: 20045434]

[63]   Wessinger S, Kaplan M, Choi L, *et al.* Increased use of selective serotonin reuptake inhibitors in patients admitted with gastrointestinal haemorrhage: a multicentre retrospective analysis. Aliment Pharmacol Ther 2006; 23(7): 937-44.
       [http://dx.doi.org/10.1111/j.1365-2036.2006.02859.x] [PMID: 16573796]

[64]   Carneiro AM, Cook EH, Murphy DL, Blakely RD. Interactions between integrin alphaIIbbeta3 and the serotonin transporter regulate serotonin transport and platelet aggregation in mice and humans. J Clin Invest 2008; 118(4): 1544-52.
       [http://dx.doi.org/10.1172/JCI33374] [PMID: 18317590]

[65]   Macleod MR, OCollins T, Horky LL, Howells DW, Donnan GA. Systematic review and meta-analysis of the efficacy of melatonin in experimental stroke. J Pineal Res 2005; 38(1): 35-41.
       [http://dx.doi.org/10.1111/j.1600-079X.2004.00172.x] [PMID: 15617535]

[66]   Nakayama H, Ginsberg MD, Dietrich WD. (S)-emopamil, a novel calcium channel blocker and serotonin S2 antagonist, markedly reduces infarct size following middle cerebral artery occlusion in the rat. Neurology 1988; 38(11): 1667-73.
       [http://dx.doi.org/10.1212/WNL.38.11.1667] [PMID: 3185899]

[67]   Hacke W, Kaste M, Bluhmki E, *et al.* Thrombolysis with alteplase 3 to 4.5 hours after acute ischemic stroke. N Engl J Med 2008; 359(13): 1317-29.
       [http://dx.doi.org/10.1056/NEJMoa0804656] [PMID: 18815396]

[68]   Quartermain D, Li YS, Jonas S. The low molecular weight heparin enoxaparin reduces infarct size in a rat model of temporary focal ischemia. Cerebrovasc Dis 2003; 16(4): 346-55.
       [http://dx.doi.org/10.1159/000072556] [PMID: 13130175]

[69]   Quartermain D, Li YS, Jonas S. Acute enoxaparin treatment widens the therapeutic window for tPA in a mouse model of embolic stroke. Neurol Res 2007; 29(5): 469-75.

[http://dx.doi.org/10.1179/016164107X164102] [PMID: 17535591]

[70]    Ross AM, Molhoek P, Lundergan C, *et al.* Randomized comparison of enoxaparin, a low-molecula-
        -weight heparin, with unfractionated heparin adjunctive to recombinant tissue plasminogen activator
        thrombolysis and aspirin HART II. Circulation 2001; 104: 648-52.
        [http://dx.doi.org/10.1161/hc3101.093866] [PMID: 11489769]

[71]    Ay H, Furie KL, Singhal A, Smith WS, Sorensen AG, Koroshetz WJ. An evidence-based causative
        classification system for acute ischemic stroke. Ann Neurol 2005; 58(5): 688-97.
        [http://dx.doi.org/10.1002/ana.20617] [PMID: 16240340]

[72]    Deb P, Sharma S, Hassan KM. Pathophysiologic mechanisms of acute ischemic stroke: An overview
        with emphasis on therapeutic significance beyond thrombolysis. Pathophysiology 2010; 17(3): 197-
        218.
        [http://dx.doi.org/10.1016/j.pathophys.2009.12.001] [PMID: 20074922]

[73]    Stroke: Hope Through Research [Internet] , 1999 [cited 9 December 2010]; Available from:
        http://www.ninds.nih.gov/disorders/stroke/detail_stroke.htm.

[74]    Paciaroni M, Caso V, Agnelli G. The concept of ischemic penumbra in acute stroke and therapeutic
        opportunities. Eur Neurol 2009; 61(6): 321-30.
        [http://dx.doi.org/10.1159/000210544] [PMID: 19365124]

[75]    Furie B, Furie BC. Mechanisms of thrombus formation. N Engl J Med 2008; 359(9): 938-49.
        [http://dx.doi.org/10.1056/NEJMra0801082] [PMID: 18753650]

[76]    Donnan GA, Fisher M, Macleod M, Davis SM. Stroke. Lancet 2008; 371(9624): 1612-23.
        [http://dx.doi.org/10.1016/S0140-6736(08)60694-7] [PMID: 18468545]

[77]    Rothwell PM, Eliasziw M, Gutnikov SA, *et al.* Analysis of pooled data from the randomised
        controlled trials of endarterectomy for symptomatic carotid stenosis. Lancet 2003; 361(9352): 107-16.
        [http://dx.doi.org/10.1016/S0140-6736(03)12228-3] [PMID: 12531577]

[78]    Ederle J, Brown MM. The evidence for medicine *versus* surgery for carotid stenosis. Eur J Radiol
        2006; 60(1): 3-7.
        [http://dx.doi.org/10.1016/j.ejrad.2006.05.021] [PMID: 16920313]

[79]    Yanaka K, Spellman SR, McCarthy JB, Oegema TR Jr, Low WC, Camarata PJ. Reduction of brain
        injury using heparin to inhibit leukocyte accumulation in a rat model of transient focal cerebral
        ischemia. I. Protective mechanism. J Neurosurg 1996; 85(6): 1102-7.
        [http://dx.doi.org/10.3171/jns.1996.85.6.1102] [PMID: 8929502]

[80]    Fareed J, Iqbal O, Cunanan J, *et al.* Changing trends in anti-coagulant therapies. Are heparins and oral
        anti-coagulants challenged? Int Angiol 2008; 27(3): 176-92.
        [PMID: 18506123]

[81]    Furman MI, Krueger LA, Frelinger AL III, *et al.* GPIIb-IIIa antagonist-induced reduction in platelet
        surface factor V/Va binding and phosphatidylserine expression in whole blood. Thromb Haemost
        2000; 84(3): 492-8.
        [PMID: 11019977]

[82]    Rebello SS, Kasiewski CJ, Bentley RG, *et al.* Superiority of enoxaparin over heparin in combination
        with a GPIIb/IIIa receptor antagonist during coronary thrombolysis in dogs. Thromb Res 2001; 102(3):

261-71.
[http://dx.doi.org/10.1016/S0049-3848(01)00242-0] [PMID: 11369420]

[83]   Wahl F, Obrenovitch TP, Hardy AM, Plotkine M, Boulu R, Symon L. Extracellular glutamate during focal cerebral ischaemia in rats: time course and calcium dependency. J Neurochem 1994; 63(3): 1003-11.
[http://dx.doi.org/10.1046/j.1471-4159.1994.63031003.x] [PMID: 7914220]

[84]   Mary V, Wahl F, Uzan A, Stutzmann JM. Enoxaparin in experimental stroke: neuroprotection and therapeutic window of opportunity. Stroke 2001; 32(4): 993-9.
[http://dx.doi.org/10.1161/01.STR.32.4.993] [PMID: 11283402]

[85]   Stutzmann JM, Mary V, Wahl F, Grosjean-Piot O, Uzan A, Pratt J. Neuroprotective profile of enoxaparin, a low molecular weight heparin, in *in vivo* models of cerebral ischemia or traumatic brain injury in rats: a review. CNS Drug Rev 2002; 8(1): 1-30.
[http://dx.doi.org/10.1111/j.1527-3458.2002.tb00213.x] [PMID: 12070524]

[86]   Tanne D, Katzav A, Beilin O, *et al.* Interaction of inflammation, thrombosis, aspirin and enoxaparin in CNS experimental antiphospholipid syndrome. Neurobiol Dis 2008; 30(1): 56-64.
[http://dx.doi.org/10.1016/j.nbd.2007.12.004] [PMID: 18308578]

[87]   Ward NS, Brown MM, Thompson AJ, Frackowiak RS. Neural correlates of motor recovery after stroke: a longitudinal fMRI study. Brain 2003; 126(Pt 11): 2476-96.
[http://dx.doi.org/10.1093/brain/awg245] [PMID: 12937084]

[88]   Antic SD, Knopfel T. Sparse, strong, and large area targeting of genetically encoded indicators [Internet]. Pending project funded by the Obama Administration Brain Research through Advancing Innovative Neurotechnologies® (BRAIN) initiative and NIH. , 2015 [[cited 26 May 2016]]; Available from: https://projectreporter.nih.gov/project_info_description.cfm?icde=0&aid=9037189.

[89]   Duncan PW, Sullivan KJ, Behrman AL, *et al.* Protocol for the Locomotor Experience Applied Post-stroke (LEAPS) trial: a randomized controlled trial. BMC Neurol 2007; 7: 39.
[http://dx.doi.org/10.1186/1471-2377-7-39] [PMID: 17996052]

[90]   Hochberg LR, Bacher D, Jarosiewicz B, *et al.* Reach and grasp by people with tetraplegia using a neurally controlled robotic arm. Nature 2012; 485(7398): 372-5.
[http://dx.doi.org/10.1038/nature11076] [PMID: 22596161]

[91]   Daly JJ, Wolpaw JR. Brain-computer interfaces in neurological rehabilitation. Lancet Neurol 2008; 7(11): 1032-43.
[http://dx.doi.org/10.1016/S1474-4422(08)70223-0] [PMID: 18835541]

[92]   Perry JC, Rosen J. *Member, IEEE*, Burns S. Upper-Limb Powered Exoskeleton Design. IEEE/ASME Trans Mechatron 2007; 12(4): 408-17.
[http://dx.doi.org/10.1109/TMECH.2007.901934]

[93]   Bortole M, Pons JL. Converging Clinical and Engineering Research on Neurorehabilitation, Volume 1 of the series Biosystems & Biorobotics. Development of a Exoskeleton for Lower Limb Rehabilitation. New York: Springer 2013; pp. 85-90.

[94]   Carden DL, Granger DN. Pathophysiology of ischaemia-reperfusion injury. J Pathol 2000; 190(3): 255-66.

[http://dx.doi.org/10.1002/(SICI)1096-9896(200002)190:3<255::AID-PATH526>3.0.CO;2-6] [PMID: 10685060]

[95]   Crippen D. ACS Surgery: Principles and Practice Online. Brain failure and brain death [Internet] 2005. WebMD,       Inc.       [cited       26       May       2016].       Available       from: http://www.academia.edu/20547702/27_BRAIN_FAILURE_AND_BRAIN_DEATH.

[96]   Korin N, Gounis MJ, Wakhloo AK, Ingber DE. Targeted drug delivery to flow-obstructed blood vessels using mechanically activated nanotherapeutics. JAMA Neurol 2015; 72(1): 119-22. [http://dx.doi.org/10.1001/jamaneurol.2014.2886] [PMID: 25365638]

[97]   Qureshi IA, Mehler MF. The emerging role of epigenetics in stroke: III. Neural stem cell biology and regenerative medicine. Arch Neurol 2011; 68(3): 294-302. [http://dx.doi.org/10.1001/archneurol.2011.6] [PMID: 21403016]

**CHAPTER 7**

# On the Influence of Normalization Strategies for Perfusion MRI in Acute Stroke

**Mathilde Giacalone, Carole Frindel, Robin Zagala, Tae-Hee Cho, Yves Berthezène, Norbert Nighoghossian** and **David Rousseau**[*]

*Université de Lyon, CREATIS, CNRS UMR5220, Inserm U1206, INSA-Lyon, Université Claude Bernard Lyon 1, France*

**Abstract:** Normalization of magnetic resonance images with a given reference is a common preprocessing task which is rarely discussed. We review and address this question for a specific neuro-imaging problem of practical huge interest. We investigate the influence of the location of region of interest used for normalization of perfusion maps obtained with perfusion magnetic resonance imaging in the framework of the study of acute stroke. We demonstrate that a slice by slice normalization based on the whole hemisphere strategy optimally reduces the variability of the predictive value of the different perfusion maps. Interestingly, this is obtained for all the tested perfusion maps both from numerical simulation of perfusion MRI and from perfusion maps of real patients through a Neyman-Pearson detection strategy. These are important results to ease the quantitative assessment of stroke lesion from perfusion MRI on cohorts of patients. The proposed methodology could easily be transposed to other medical imaging problems where normalization of images is necessary.

**Keywords:** Acute stroke, Image processing, Ischemic penumbra, Ischemic stroke, Medical Imaging, MRI, Neuroimaging, Normalization, Perfusion maps, Perfusion MRI.

## INTRODUCTION

Perfusion-weighted imaging (PWI) is a magnetic resonance sequence increasingly

[*] **Corresponding author David Rousseau:** Université de Lyon, CREATIS, CNRS UMR5220, Inserm U1206, INSA-Lyon, Université Claude Bernard Lyon 1, France; Tel/Fax: ??????????; Email: david.rousseau@univ-lyon1.fr

used in the acute stroke setting. In its quantitative version, as pioneered in [1], maps of Cerebral Blood Flow (CBF), Cerebral Blood Volume (CBV), Mean Time Transit (MTT) and Time To Peak (TTP) can be derived noninvasively by dynamic imaging of a bolus injection of gadolinium contrast agent and subsequent data analysis from the time course of the tracer in both tissue and middle cerebral artery and deconvolution as shown in Fig. (**1**) for two human patients. Although used in clinics, there are still unsolved open questions on the determination of the optimal processing for the quantitative extraction of hemodynamic parameters. This is highlighted when PWI is compared to positron emission tomography (PET) imaging [2 - 5]. As stressed in [6], this is especially true for acute stroke because the images are of rather low quality due to emergency of the clinical context and the risk of possible movement of the patient. Because the method is inherently sensitive to vascular delays and dispersion effects, these maps have to be normalized to facilitate inter-individual quantitative evaluation [7 - 9]. Normalization can be considered in this context at two levels. Temporal normalization by deconvolution of the arterial input function [10, 11] and spatial normalization by division with hemodynamic values taken in a reference area. Please note that spatio-temporal normalization has also recently been introduced in [12]. In this chapter, we deal with spatial normalization. This normalization is usually done in the contralateral hemisphere unaffected by the stroke lesion. However, there are multiple ways of performing this normalization [13 - 20]. Spatial normalization by division of hemodynamic parameters from the contralateral hemisphere has been done for stroke with mirror ROI of the same slice [13, 14], with contralateral white matter of the whole hemisphere [15, 16], with mean white matter of a single slice [17] with contralateral voxel [18, 19] or with average in grey matter [20]. To the best of our knowledge, however, no comparison of various possible methods for this spatial normalization has been undertaken so far. In this work, we compared nine different normalization strategies in four different perfusion hemodynamic parameters (TTP, MTT, CBF, and CBV). This includes three normalization levels: to a reference slice (RS), to a volume (V) or slice by slice (SS) as shown in Fig. (**2**).

In addition, the region of interest for normalization can be chosen in the white matter (WM), can be taken as the whole contralateral hemisphere (WH), or can be defined as the contralateral "mirror" volume of the diffusion mask lesion (DIFF) as illustrated in Fig. (**3**).

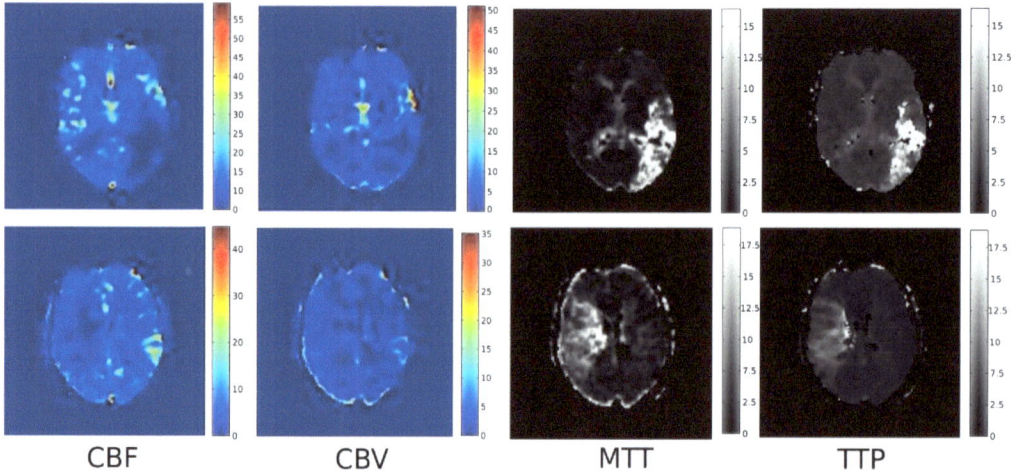

**Fig. (1).** Examples of perfusion parametric maps for two patients (one patient per line) with ischemic stroke. CBF and CBV are expressed in arbitrary units and, MTT and TTP in seconds. One can observe that the value ranges are not the same between the two patients.

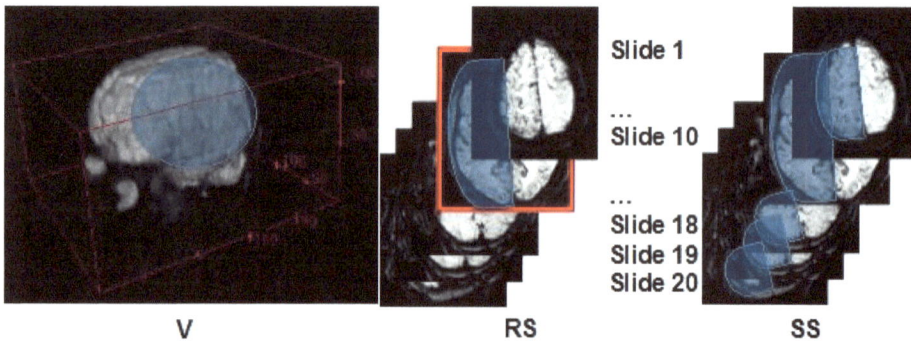

**Fig. (2).** Various levels tested for the normalization of perfusion parametric maps. The normalization is made using a unique reference slice just under the ventricle (RS), the entire contralateral volume (V) or slice by slice (SS).

To confront the performance of these nine combinations of normalization levels and normalization ROI, the comparison endpoint was the variability of the prediction of the final lesion after thresholding the parametric perfusion hemodynamic maps. Several studies have performed comparisons of various PWI post-processing methods using a variety of perfusion maps, normalization methods and comparison schemes. However, none have been done so far on the normalization strategies in terms of prediction of the final infarct lesion and none to our knowledge on the normalization strategies in terms of inter-individual variability.

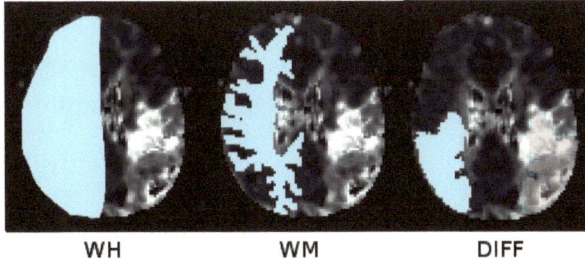

**Fig. (3).** Various ROI tested for normalization of perfusion maps with WH in the whole hemisphere, WM white matter in the contralateral hemisphere and DIFF in the diffusion mask.

## SUBJECTS AND METHODS

We analyzed patients from the European cohort I-KNOW which included patients with acute anterior circulation ischemic stroke that were studied by MRI with PWI and T1 at admission and follow-up T2 Flair imaging one month later. A subset of these patients had a subacute MRI 2-3h after the first scan allowing for assessment of tissue reperfusion based on MR angiography and PWI. Inclusion criteria were: patients presenting (thrombolysis) and presenting acute ischemic stroke, with or without treatment. Exclusion criteria were: patients with tissue reperfusion or with a too small final infarct lesion on T2 Flair imaging. 13 patients were finally included in this study.

MRI was performed with a 1.5-T clinical imager (Siemens Avanto) at admission (H0) and 2–3 h after the first scan (H2). The follow-up scan was achieved one month later for final infarct lesion assessment on T2 FLAIR sequences. Imaging protocol included the following sequences: (1) echoplanar PWI, using bolus passage-of-contrast with 0.1 mmol/kg of gadopentetate dimeglumine (2) axial T1 and (3) time-of-flight angiography were performed on H0 and H2 scans, and (4) axial FLAIR was performed on follow-up. The echoplanar PWI were 2D sequences with rather thick slices of 6 mm.

PWI images were transferred to a dedicated workstation and analyzed using in-house algorithms developed in Matlab 2012 (Mathworks Inc.). Perfusion maps of time-to-peak (TTP), mean transit time (MTT), cerebral blood volume (CBV), and cerebral blood flow (CBF) maps were generated on a pixel-by-pixel basis by standard singular value decomposition of $\Delta$R2* time curves. Perfusion-weighted imaging within 3 hours of symptom onset and 90-day T2-weighted imaging were coregistered.

The white matter mask were generated from T1-weighted images as shown in Fig. (**4**). We used BET (Brain Extraction Tool) and FAST (FMRIB's Automated Segmentation Tool) within the FSL (FMRIB Software Library) suite of tools to delete non-brain tissues from the T1-weighted image and segment the resulting image of the brain into different tissue types (Grey Matter, White Matter and CSF). Concerning the contralateral "mirror" volume of the diffusion mask lesion (DIFF) and the contralateral hemisphere, they are created after manual positioning of the axis of symmetry of the brain.

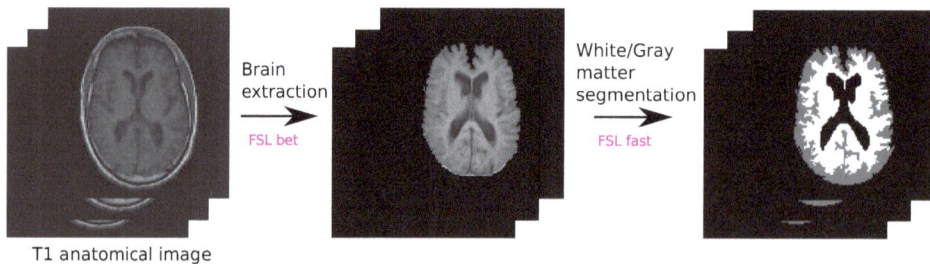

**Fig. (4).** White/grey matter segmentation flow chart.

We used Receiver Operating Characteristic (ROC) analysis to assess the performance of the nine normalization strategies on inter-individual comparisons when thresholding a PWI parametric map in order to retrieve the final lesion. ROC analysis is a well-established and comprehensive method, where the probability of good detection is plotted as a function of the probability of false alarm, to evaluate the efficacy of a continuous parameter in predicting a binary outcome and can be viewed as an analysis testing the predictive performance of a PWI map across all possible thresholds.

To assess the inter-individual variability of the prediction resulting from the choice of the normalization strategy, we developed four ROC descriptors. The first descriptor, called *all ROC*, computes the average standard deviation along the ROC curves for the N patients. The second descriptor, called *min*, corresponds to the standard deviation along the ROC curves at a specific point, *i.e.* the closest point to upper left corner, for the N patients. The third descriptor, called *area*, computes the standard deviation of area under the ROC curve for the N patients. Finally, the last descriptor, called *threshold*, assess the variability of the threshold around the closest point to upper left corner for the N patients. To do so, we search for the left and right points to the closest point to upper left corner that are equal to the minimum distance to the upper left corner multiplied by a factor of square root of two. If the normalization strategy is effective, the thresholds corresponding to these two points should not vary significantly.

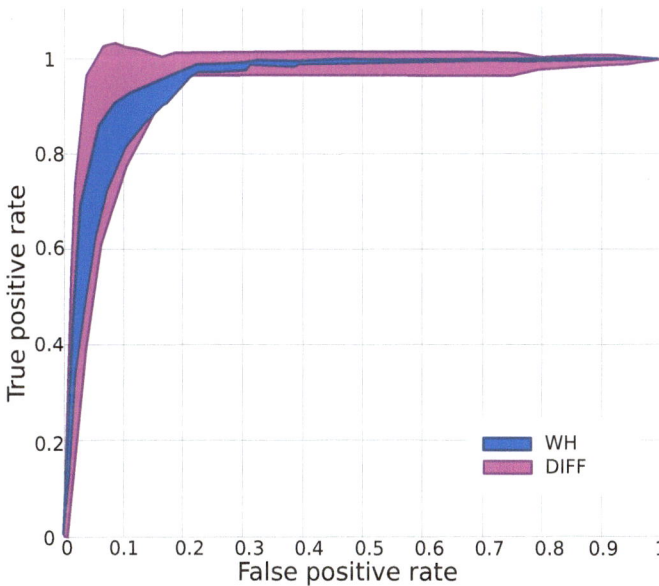

**Fig. (5).** Variability of ROC curves for SS normalization level in DIFF and WM ROI descriptor. Shade areas represent standard deviations along the ROC curves for the 13 human patients.

The smaller these descriptors for the N patients are and the more robust the normalization strategy for the prediction of the final infarct lesion is. Indeed, it means that there is less disparity between patients and so, a common behavior between the patients exists to predict the final lesion infarct after thresholding a specific perfusion parametric map type. Fig. (**5**) shows for illustration a comparison of two normalization strategies for a given perfusion parametric map. The ROC curves for the set of tested patients show a smaller standard deviation for one of the normalization strategies identified as better. A good normalization strategy should give similar results for several descriptors of the ROC curve.

In addition to the test of normalization strategies on real data, we performed the normalization study on simulated perfusion MRI data. The contrast-agent concentration-time images and their ground truth after deconvolution were simulated from a 3D label image – extracted from a real image database – that determines the tissue type of each voxel: white and healthy tissue, gray and healthy tissue, ischemic tissue or background voxels. The contrast-agent concentration associated to each voxel v, Cv(t) (mM), is modelled as the convolution of a global arterial input function, Ca(t) (mM), and of an impulse response function specific to each voxel, fv(t), which corresponds to our ground truth after deconvolution and contains the information on the state of perfusion of clinical interest;

$$ C_v(t) \sim \int_0^t C_a(\tau) f_v(t - \tau) d\tau, $$

where $C_a(t)$ is a gamma function and fv(t) = CBFv for t< MTTv and fv(t) = 0 for t >MTTv, with CBFv the cerebral blood flow and MTTv the mean transit time. The values of CBFv and MTTv are specific to each voxel v and depend on its tissue type. We consider four classes of voxels: white matter, grey matter, lesion and background. Background voxels are simply set to 0 for all time points. The CBFv and MTTv associated to each voxel v is modeled as a random variable that follows a truncated normal distribution specific to the tissue type of the voxel. The mean CBF values were set to 60 mL/100g/min, 25 mL/100g/min and 10 mL/100g/min respectively for the healthy gray, healthy white and ischemic tissues. The mean CBV values were set to 4 mL/100g, 2 mL/100g and 1.5 mL/100g respectively for the healthy gray, healthy white and ischemic tissues. This resulted in mean MTT values of 4.2 s, 5.2 s and 9.4 s respectively for the healthy gray, healthy white and ischemic tissues. Background voxels are simply set to 0 for all time points. A Gaussian noise, meant to model the fluctuations in the MRI acquisition system, is finally added to the images in order to obtain a mean peak signal to noise ratio over the brain voxels of 22.6 dB, typical of the noise level observed in clinical data. The interest of such a simulation approach is that it will be possible to quantify the importance of each source of variability in the normalization strategy.

## RESULTS

The best normalization strategies are highlighted in green while the one giving the worst performances in terms of variability are in red in Table **1**. As visible in Table **1**, all the values are of the same order of magnitude, in the sense of the same decade, for each ROC curve descriptor. There are nonetheless differences and choosing one normalization strategy over another can affect the variability up to a factor of 6 (in TTP map with the *area* ROC descriptor).

Inside this variability, one can identify some invariants. Some ROC descriptors are not sensitive to the ROI of normalization (WH, WM or DIFF) for a specific normalization level such as on the whole volume or reference slice. When comparing the normalization levels (*i.e.* V, SS and RS), the smallest variability of prediction in temporal maps (TTP and MTT) and in maps associated to the blood volume (CBF and CBV) were observed for the normalization level corresponding to slice by slice (SS). This is obtained in Table **1** because multiple ROC descriptors are simultaneously smaller for SS normalization level. An alternative choice of normalization level can lead to an increase of the variability up to a factor of 6 for certain ROC descriptors, as computed in Table **1** by calculating the ratio of the value highlighted in green over the value highlighted in red for each ROC descriptor. The smallest ROC curve variations are observed for the *min* and the *threshold* ROC descriptors. This is a very important result since these descriptors really determine the possibility to use the ROC curve in order to select the best threshold to be applied on perfusion parametric map. It therefore appears that the choice of the normalization is not critically dependent on the type of PWI map to be analyzed. But, choosing one normalization strategy over another can affect the variability. Concerning the ROI of the normalization, here again some interesting results are obtained with smaller variability quasi systematically observed with a normalization taken in the whole hemisphere for all perfusion parametric maps.

We performed similar analysis on the simulated data as given in Table **2**. Interestingly the order of magnitude of the variability descriptors are similar to the one obtained with the experimental data. Also, although the results are not exactly identical, the worst choice of normalization ROI appears to be the DIFF while the optimal normalization strategy in terms of variability appears to be the choice of a slice by slice normalization in the whole hemisphere and this for the two tested perfusion map.

**Table 1. ROC curve descriptors (*min, threshold, area, all ROC*) for each normalization level and ROI for real experimental data from 13 patients. The smallest standard deviation for each PWI map type – highlighted in green – emphasizes the normalization strategy where the smallest inter-individual variability was encountered.**

**TTP**

| ROI | | V | | | | SS | | | | RS | | |
|---|---|---|---|---|---|---|---|---|---|---|---|---|
| | Min | Threshold | Area | All Roc | Min | Threshold | Area | All Roc | Min | Threshold | Area | All Roc |
| WH | 0.07 | 0.17 | 0.02 | 0.05 | 0.06 | 0.15 | 0.02 | 0.05 | 0.07 | 0.17 | 0.02 | 0.05 |
| WM | 0.07 | 0.17 | 0.02 | 0.05 | 0.06 | 0.15 | 0.02 | 0.04 | 0.07 | 0.17 | 0.02 | 0.05 |
| DIFF | 0.07 | 0.17 | 0.02 | 0.05 | 0.07 | 0.16 | 0.03 | 0.06 | 0.07 | 0.17 | 0.07 | 0.05 |

**MTT**

| ROI | | V | | | | SS | | | | RS | | |
|---|---|---|---|---|---|---|---|---|---|---|---|---|
| | Min | Threshold | Area | All Roc | Min | Threshold | Area | All Roc | Min | Threshold | Area | All Roc |
| WH | 0.06 | 0.17 | 0.02 | 0.10 | 0.06 | 0.15 | 0.02 | 0.09 | 0.06 | 0.17 | 0.02 | 0.10 |
| WM | 0.06 | 0.17 | 0.02 | 0.10 | 0.06 | 0.16 | 0.02 | 0.09 | 0.06 | 0.17 | 0.02 | 0.10 |
| DIFF | 0.06 | 0.17 | 0.02 | 0.10 | 0.04 | 0.25 | 0.04 | 0.11 | 0.06 | 0.17 | 0.07 | 0.10 |

**CBF**

| ROI | | V | | | | SS | | | | RS | | |
|---|---|---|---|---|---|---|---|---|---|---|---|---|
| | Min | Threshold | Area | All Roc | Min | Threshold | Area | All Roc | Min | Threshold | Area | All Roc |
| WH | 0.07 | 0.23 | 0.04 | 0.04 | 0.02 | 0.15 | 0.04 | 0.02 | 0.07 | 0.23 | 0.04 | 0.04 |
| WM | 0.07 | 0.23 | 0.04 | 0.04 | 0.07 | 0.16 | 0.04 | 0.03 | 0.07 | 0.23 | 0.04 | 0.04 |
| DIFF | 0.07 | 0.23 | 0.04 | 0.04 | 0.04 | 0.21 | 0.01 | 0.07 | 0.07 | 0.23 | 0.04 | 0.04 |

**CBV**

| ROI | | V | | | | SS | | | | RS | | |
|---|---|---|---|---|---|---|---|---|---|---|---|---|
| | Min | Threshold | Area | All Roc | Min | Threshold | Area | All Roc | Min | Threshold | Area | All Roc |
| WH | 0.07 | 0.23 | 0.04 | 0.04 | 0.02 | 0.15 | 0.04 | 0.02 | 0.07 | 0.23 | 0.04 | 0.04 |
| WM | 0.07 | 0.23 | 0.04 | 0.04 | 0.07 | 0.16 | 0.04 | 0.03 | 0.07 | 0.23 | 0.04 | 0.04 |
| DIFF | 0.07 | 0.23 | 0.04 | 0.04 | 0.04 | 0.21 | 0.01 | 0.07 | 0.07 | 0.23 | 0.04 | 0.04 |

**Table 2. Similar as in Table 1 but with *in-silico* numerical simulations.**

| V | | | | SS (WH) | | | | RS | | | |
|---|---|---|---|---|---|---|---|---|---|---|---|
| Min | Threshold | Area | All Roc | Min | Threshold | Area | All Roc | Min | Threshold | Area | All Roc |
| 0.061 | 0.066 | 0.026 | 0.009 | 0.064 | 0.086 | 0.029 | 0.007 | 0.061 | 0.066 | 0.026 | 0.009 |

| V | | | | SS (WM) | | | | RS | | | |
|---|---|---|---|---|---|---|---|---|---|---|---|
| Min | Threshold | Area | All Roc | Min | Threshold | Area | All Roc | Min | Threshold | Area | All Roc |
| 0.061 | 0.066 | 0.026 | 0.009 | 0.061 | 0.080 | 0.026 | 0.008 | 0.061 | 0.066 | 0.026 | 0.009 |

| V | | | | SS (DIFF) | | | | RS | | | |
|---|---|---|---|---|---|---|---|---|---|---|---|
| Min | Threshold | Area | All Roc | Min | Threshold | Area | All Roc | Min | Threshold | Area | All Roc |
| 0.061 | 0.066 | 0.026 | 0.009 | 0.100 | 0.078 | 0.049 | 0.029 | 0.061 | 0.066 | 0.026 | 0.009 |

CBF

| V | | | | SS (WH) | | | | RS | | | |
|---|---|---|---|---|---|---|---|---|---|---|---|
| Min | Threshold | Area | All Roc | Min | Threshold | Area | All Roc | Min | Threshold | Area | All Roc |
| 0.062 | 0.035 | 0.022 | 0.003 | 0.069 | 0.045 | 0.022 | 0.003 | 0.062 | 0.035 | 0.022 | 0.003 |

| V | | | | SS (WM) | | | | RS | | | |
|---|---|---|---|---|---|---|---|---|---|---|---|
| Min | Threshold | Area | All Roc | Min | Threshold | Area | All Roc | Min | Threshold | Area | All Roc |
| 0.062 | 0.035 | 0.022 | 0.003 | 0.062 | 0.058 | 0.026 | 0.003 | 0.062 | 0.035 | 0.022 | 0.003 |

| V | | | | SS (DIFF) | | | | RS | | | |
|---|---|---|---|---|---|---|---|---|---|---|---|
| Min | Threshold | Area | All Roc | Min | Threshold | Area | All Roc | Min | Threshold | Area | All Roc |
| 0.062 | 0.035 | 0.022 | 0.003 | 0.112 | 0.093 | 0.096 | 0.003 | 0.062 | 0.035 | 0.022 | 0.003 |

CBV

# DISCUSSION AND CONCLUSION

These results quantify the influence of the normalization strategy on quantitative analysis of brain PWI parametric maps. The choice of the normalization method is not too sensitive to the perfusion parametric map to be analyzed. A slice by slice normalization level optimally reduces the variability of the predictive value of the different perfusion maps. Also the normalization with the whole hemisphere on each slice appears as the best strategy concerning the choice of the region of interest. This cohort is rather small. However, interestingly, these experimental results on real data were also found in accordance with the results obtained with numerical simulations of perfusion MRI data. This further confirms the robustness of these findings. The optimality of the slice by slice normalization level could be explained by the fact that this approach enables to compensate for the magnetic field non homogeneity which can cause some grey level shift between each slice. This is particularly interesting in our case since the perfusion data were acquired with rather thick slices. A seemingly surprising result is that the normalization with the contralateral "mirror" volume of the diffusion mask lesion (DIFF) does not end up to be a robust normalization strategy while it could be a priori appearing as the most specifically stroke-based strategy. A possible posteriori interpretation for this may be a consequence of two facts. First, human brains are not purely symmetrical. Second, although in the considered cohort, the lesions are restricted to a single hemisphere of the brain, the patients suffering from stroke do not necessarily have a perfectly healthy contralateral hemisphere. Stroke does not evolve only following a "natural course" linked with inflammation processes but also by taking into account the patient specific state of the brain before stroke. Several biomarkers can be present before acute stroke in the contralateral hemisphere such as microbleeds [21], white matter hyper-intensities [22], lacunar infarct [23], or also cerebral atrophy [24]. These biomarkers may translate into hypo or hyper values perfusion, *i.e.* artefacts if the contralateral is intended to be a healthy reference. Such artefacts could be associated to the increased variability of the predictability when taking the contralateral "mirror" volume of the diffusion mask lesion. A way to minimize the effect of these artefacts, due to the state of the brain before stroke, would be to segment them and to withdraw them from the normalization region of interest. This could be an interesting perspective. However, if the biomarkers correspond to a minor part of the whole hemisphere (as is often the case in practice), another approach consists in normalization with the largest possible part of a given slice, *i.e.* the whole hemisphere. And this whole hemisphere normalization has been found optimal in this study, instead of the contralateral diffusion region which is much smaller.

In this chapter we focused on the question of spatial normalization of perfusion weighted imaging in acute stroke. At another level of perspective, such investigations could be extended in various directions. Perfusion weighted imaging is used to compute hemodynamic maps in the study of other cerebral diseases such as glioma [25 - 29] or multiple sclerosis [30, 31] where the question of normalization has been approached [32, 33] but not yet in informational terms with detection or prediction related to the inter-individual variability as performance measure as proposed here. Hemodynamic maps are also produced with other MRI sequences such as arterial spin labeling [34] and it would here again be interesting to consider the question of the spatial normalization. All these perspectives could be tackled following the general methodology presented in this chapter with DSC PWI imaging applied to acute stroke.

## TAKE HOME MESSAGE

A slice by slice normalization level optimally reduces the variability of the predictive value in perfusion MRI during acute ischemic stroke. The normalization with the whole hemisphere on each slice appears as the best strategy concerning the choice of the region of interest.

## CONFLICT OF INTEREST

The authors confirm that they have no conflict of interest to declare for this publication.

## ACKNOWLEDGEMENTS

This work was supported by the LABEX PRIMES (ANR-11-LABX- 0063) of Université de Lyon, within the program "Investissements d'Avenir" (ANR-1--IDEX-0007) operated by the French National Research Agency (ANR).

## REFERENCES

[1] Østergaard L, Weisskoff RM, Chesler DA, Gyldensted C, Rosen BR. High resolution measurement of cerebral blood flow using intravascular tracer bolus passages. Part I: Mathematical approach and statistical analysis. Magn Reson Med 1996; 36(5): 715-25.
[http://dx.doi.org/10.1002/mrm.1910360510] [PMID: 8916022]

[2] Zaro-Weber O, Moeller-Hartmann W, Heiss WD, Sobesky J. Influence of the arterial input function on absolute and relative perfusion-weighted imaging penumbral flow detection: a validation with $^{15}$O-water positron emission tomography. Stroke 2012; 43(2): 378-85.
[http://dx.doi.org/10.1161/STROKEAHA.111.635458] [PMID: 22135071]

[3] Ibaraki M, Ito H, Shimosegawa E, *et al.* Cerebral vascular mean transit time in healthy humans: a comparative study with PET and dynamic susceptibility contrast-enhanced MRI. J Cereb Blood Flow Metab 2007; 27(2): 404-13.
[http://dx.doi.org/10.1038/sj.jcbfm.9600337] [PMID: 16736045]

[4] Borghammer P, Jonsdottir KY, Cumming P, *et al.* Normalization in PET group comparison studies the importance of a valid reference region. Neuroimage 2008; 40(2): 529-40.
[http://dx.doi.org/10.1016/j.neuroimage.2007.12.057] [PMID: 18258457]

[5] Takasawa M, Jones PS, Guadagno JV, *et al.* How reliable is perfusion MR in acute stroke? Validation and determination of the penumbra threshold against quantitative PET. Stroke 2008; 39(3): 870-7.
[http://dx.doi.org/10.1161/STROKEAHA.107.500090] [PMID: 18258831]

[6] Willats L, Calamante F. The 39 steps: evading error and deciphering the secrets for accurate dynamic susceptibility contrast MRI. NMR Biomed 2013; 26(8): 913-31.
[http://dx.doi.org/10.1002/nbm.2833] [PMID: 22782914]

[7]    Diamant M, Harms MP, Immink RV, Van Lieshout JJ, Van Montfrans GA. Twenty-four-hour non-invasive monitoring of systemic haemodynamics and cerebral blood flow velocity in healthy humans. Acta Physiol Scand 2002; 175(1): 1-9.
[http://dx.doi.org/10.1046/j.1365-201X.2002.00953.x] [PMID: 11982498]

[8]    Helenius J, Perkiö J, Soinne L, *et al.* Cerebral hemodynamics in a healthy population measured by dynamic susceptibility contrast MR imaging. Acta Radiol 2003; 44(5): 538-46.
[http://dx.doi.org/10.1034/j.1600-0455.2003.00104.x] [PMID: 14510762]

[9]    Christensen S, Mouridsen K, Wu O, *et al.* Comparison of 10 perfusion MRI parameters in 97 sub-6-hour stroke patients using voxel-based receiver operating characteristics analysis. Stroke 2009; 40(6): 2055-61.
[http://dx.doi.org/10.1161/STROKEAHA.108.546069] [PMID: 19359626]

[10]   Calamante F. Arterial input function in perfusion MRI: a comprehensive review. Prog Nucl Magn Reson Spectrosc 2013; 74: 1-32.
[http://dx.doi.org/10.1016/j.pnmrs.2013.04.002] [PMID: 24083460]

[11]   Meijs M, Christensen S, Lansberg MG, Albers GW, Calamante F. Analysis of perfusion MRI in stroke: To deconvolve, or not to deconvolve. Magn Reson Med 2016; 76(4): 1282-90.
[PMID: 26519871]

[12]   Frindel C, Robini MC, Rousseau D. A 3-D spatio-temporal deconvolution approach for MR perfusion in the brain. Med Image Anal 2014; 18(1): 144-60.
[http://dx.doi.org/10.1016/j.media.2013.10.004] [PMID: 24184525]

[13]   Singer OC, de Rochemont RduM, Foerch C, *et al.* Relation between relative cerebral blood flow, relative cerebral blood volume, and mean transit time in patients with acute ischemic stroke determined by perfusion-weighted MRI. J Cereb Blood Flow Metab 2003; 23(5): 605-11.
[http://dx.doi.org/10.1097/01.WCB.0000062342.57257.28] [PMID: 12771576]

[14]   Takasawa M, Jones PS, Guadagno JV, *et al.* How reliable is perfusion MR in acute stroke? Validation and determination of the penumbra threshold against quantitative PET. Stroke 2008; 39(3): 870-7.
[http://dx.doi.org/10.1161/STROKEAHA.107.500090] [PMID: 18258831]

[15]   Kosior JC, Smith MR, Kosior RK, Frayne R. Cerebral blood flow estimation *in vivo* using local tissue reference functions. J Magn Reson Imaging 2009; 29(1): 183-8.
[http://dx.doi.org/10.1002/jmri.21605] [PMID: 19097104]

[16]   Arakawa S, Wright PM, Koga M, *et al.* Ischemic thresholds for gray and white matter: a diffusion and perfusion magnetic resonance study. Stroke 2006; 37(5): 1211-6.
[http://dx.doi.org/10.1161/01.STR.0000217258.63925.6b] [PMID: 16574931]

[17]   Sakaie KE, Shin W, Curtin KR, McCarthy RM, Cashen TA, Carroll TJ. Method for improving the accuracy of quantitative cerebral perfusion imaging. J Magn Reson Imaging 2005; 21(5): 512-9.
[http://dx.doi.org/10.1002/jmri.20305] [PMID: 15834910]

[18]   Zopf R, Klose U, Karnath HO. Evaluation of methods for detecting perfusion abnormalities after stroke in dysfunctional brain regions. Brain Struct Funct 2012; 217(2): 667-75.
[http://dx.doi.org/10.1007/s00429-011-0363-4] [PMID: 22124664]

[19]   Karnath HO, Zopf R, Johannsen L, Fruhmann Berger M, Nägele T, Klose U. Normalized perfusion

MRI to identify common areas of dysfunction: patients with basal ganglia neglect. Brain 2005; 128(Pt 10): 2462-9.
[http://dx.doi.org/10.1093/brain/awh629] [PMID: 16150848]

[20]    Calamante F, Connelly A, van Osch MJ. Nonlinear DeltaR*2 effects in perfusion quantification using bolus-tracking MRI. Magn Reson Med 2009; 61(2): 486-92.
[http://dx.doi.org/10.1002/mrm.21839] [PMID: 19161169]

[21]    Greenberg SM, Vernooij MW, Cordonnier C, *et al.* Cerebral microbleeds: a guide to detection and interpretation. Lancet Neurol 2009; 8(2): 165-74.
[http://dx.doi.org/10.1016/S1474-4422(09)70013-4] [PMID: 19161908]

[22]    Prins ND, Scheltens P. White matter hyperintensities, cognitive impairment and dementia: an update. Nat Rev Neurol 2015; 11(3): 157-65.
[http://dx.doi.org/10.1038/nrneurol.2015.10] [PMID: 25686760]

[23]    Koch S, McClendon MS, Bhatia R. Imaging evolution of acute lacunar infarction: leukoaraiosis or lacune? Neurology 2011; 77(11): 1091-5.
[http://dx.doi.org/10.1212/WNL.0b013e31822e1470] [PMID: 21880998]

[24]    Wardlaw JM, Smith EE, Biessels GJ, *et al.* Neuroimaging standards for research into small vessel disease and its contribution to ageing and neurodegeneration. Lancet Neurol 2013; 12(8): 822-38.
[http://dx.doi.org/10.1016/S1474-4422(13)70124-8] [PMID: 23867200]

[25]    Law M, Young R, Babb J, Pollack E, Johnson G. Histogram analysis *versus* region of interest analysis of dynamic susceptibility contrast perfusion MR imaging data in the grading of cerebral gliomas. AJNR Am J Neuroradiol 2007; 28(4): 761-6.
[PMID: 17416835]

[26]    Thomsen H, Steffensen E, Larsson EM. Perfusion MRI (dynamic susceptibility contrast imaging) with different measurement approaches for the evaluation of blood flow and blood volume in human gliomas. Acta Radiol 2012; 53(1): 95-101.
[http://dx.doi.org/10.1258/ar.2011.110242] [PMID: 22114021]

[27]    Bedekar D, Jensen T, Schmainda KM. Standardization of relative cerebral blood volume (rCBV) image maps for ease of both inter- and intrapatient comparisons. Magn Reson Med 2010; 64(3): 907-13.
[http://dx.doi.org/10.1002/mrm.22445] [PMID: 20806381]

[28]    Paulson ES, Schmainda KM. Comparison of dynamic susceptibility-weighted contrast-enhanced MR methods: recommendations for measuring relative cerebral blood volume in brain tumors. Radiology 2008; 249(2): 601-13.
[http://dx.doi.org/10.1148/radiol.2492071659] [PMID: 18780827]

[29]    Jafari-Khouzani K, Emblem KE, Kalpathy-Cramer J, *et al.* Repeatability of cerebral perfusion using dynamic susceptibility contrast MRI in glioblastoma patients. Transl Oncol 2015; 8(3): 137-46.
[http://dx.doi.org/10.1016/j.tranon.2015.03.002] [PMID: 26055170]

[30]    Peruzzo D, Castellaro M, Calabrese M, *et al.* Heterogeneity of cortical lesions in multiple sclerosis: an MRI perfusion study. J Cereb Blood Flow Metab 2013; 33(3): 457-63.
[http://dx.doi.org/10.1038/jcbfm.2012.192] [PMID: 23250108]

[31]   Law M, Saindane AM, Ge Y, *et al.* Microvascular abnormality in relapsing-remitting multiple sclerosis: perfusion MR imaging findings in normal-appearing white matter. Radiology 2004; 231(3): 645-52.
[http://dx.doi.org/10.1148/radiol.2313030996] [PMID: 15163806]

[32]   Ellingson BM, Zaw T, Cloughesy TF, *et al.* Comparison between intensity normalization techniques for dynamic susceptibility contrast (DSC)-MRI estimates of cerebral blood volume (CBV) in human gliomas. J Magn Reson Imaging 2012; 35(6): 1472-7.
[http://dx.doi.org/10.1002/jmri.23600] [PMID: 22281731]

[33]   Prah MA, Stufflebeam SM, Paulson ES, *et al.* Repeatability of standardized and normalized relative CBV in patients with newly diagnosed glioblastoma. AJNR Am J Neuroradiol 2015; 36(9): 1654-61.
[http://dx.doi.org/10.3174/ajnr.A4374] [PMID: 26066626]

[34]   Ferré JC, Bannier E, Raoult H, Mineur G, Carsin-Nicol B, Gauvrit JY. Arterial spin labeling (ASL) perfusion: techniques and clinical use. Diagn Interv Imaging 2013; 94(12): 1211-23.
[http://dx.doi.org/10.1016/j.diii.2013.06.010] [PMID: 23850321]

# Genetic Causes of Ischemic Stroke

Anna Bersano[*] and M. Ranieri

*Cerebrovascular Unit, IRCCS Foundation Neurological Institute "C. Besta", Via Celoria 11, Milan 20133, Italy*

**Abstract:** The pathogenesis of ischemic stroke remains unknown but a better knowledge of its pathogenetic mechanism may help us in identifying more effective therapies to reduce the the disease burden. Family and twin studies support the role of genetic factors in stroke pathophysiology. A number of monogenic conditions presenting with stroke have been described. They account for only a small proportion of strokes, but it is believed they are underestimated and the study of these diseases may provide insight in the pathogenic pathways of stroke, given also the existence of animal models in which examine disease mechanisms. However, in most cases, stroke is believed to be a multifactorial disorder. A number of genetic association studies using the candidate gene approach have failed in demonstrating reliable associations between stroke and genetic variants. Although several molecular variants resulted from GWAS strongly associated with ischemic stroke risk, they account for only a small part of the risk of ischemic stroke. Moreover, the pathogenic significance of many of these genetic variants has yet to be determined by functional studies so that the significance of these findings in clinical practice has been limited. Interestingly, the studies conducted so far demonstrated that the majority of the identified genetic variants found were associated with specific stroke subtypes, supporting the hypothesis that distinct genetic architecture and pathophysiological mechanisms underlie specific stroke subtypes.

## INTRODUCTION

Evidence from epidemiological and twin studies support a genetic predisposition to stroke occurrence and outcome [1 - 4]. Family history data suggest that genetic risk differ by stroke subtype, with greater familial associations for large-artery and

---

[*] **Corresponding author Anna Bersano:** Cerebrovascular Unit; IRCCS Foundation Neurological Institute "C. Besta", Via Celoria 11, Milan, 20133, Italy; Tel: +390223943320; Fax: +390223943581; Email: anna.bersano@istituto-besta.it

**Alberto Radaelli, Giuseppe Mancia, Carlo Ferrarese & Simone Beretta (Eds.)**

small-artery (lacunar) than for cardioembolic stroke [5]. A number of monogenic diseases have been described as responsible for stroke. In some of these strokes may be a part of a systemic disorder and may manifest in late disease phases. However, they are considered rare diseases accounting only for a small percentage of strokes and the genetic contribution to stroke is believed to be polygenic [1, 2]. This case is much more complex since genetic contribution results from the interaction of multiple risk alleles with small effect and genetic factors could act at various levels by predisposing to common risk factors, or, alternatively, by a direct effect on stroke risk occurrence, infarct size and response to ischemic injury [6].

Several methodological difficulties have been highlighted in studies on stroke genetics. The late onset, the difficulty in collecting genealogical trees, the phenotypic heterogeneity, and the presence of confounding risk factors make it difficult to apply linkage-based methods [1, 2].

A number of pathways including hemostatic and inflammatory systems, homocysteine metabolisms, renin-angiotensin-aldosterone system have been explored applying candidate gene approach. Recently, developed advanced high throughput platforms such as genome-wide association studies (GWAS) and Next generation sequencing as well as bioinformatic approaches are considered promising in tools for identification of novel biological mechanisms that underlie the pathogenesis of cerebrovascular diseases. This effort might lead in the future to the development of preventive strategies and individual tailored treatments.

The purpose of this chapter is to provide an update on the most well characterised monogenic disorders associated with stroke and on the most recent advances on genetic variants associated with stroke.

## MONOGENIC STROKE DISORDERS

Despite monogenic diseases are considered rare and believed to account for about 1% to 5% of all strokes, they are probably underestimated. They can be misdiagnosed simply because physicians may not include them in the differential diagnoses or they are difficulty recognised given the pleomorphic phenotypic spectrum in which stroke may be only a part of a systemic disorder [4]. However, although rare, these diseases may have important implication in the comprehension of pathogenic pathways multifactorial stroke [5], given also the existence of animal models in which to examine the disease pathophysiology. Moreover, their identification and diagnosis is an important challenge for clinicians for the implementation of a correct management of these patients, including genetic counseling, preventative and therapeutic measures [5 - 8], since they are usually life-threatening or chronically debilitating diseases. A large number of single-gene disorders is well known as cause of stroke (Table **1**). Interesting progresses have been particularly reported in discovering new heritable entities underlying small vessel diseases.

## Cerebral Autosomal Dominant Arteriopathy with Subcortical Infarcts and Leukoencephalopathy (CADASIL) (OMIM 125310-600276)

Cerebral autosomal dominant arteriopathy with subcortical infarcts and leukoencephalopathy (CADASIL) is an autosomal dominant disease caused by mutations in the NOTCH3 gene on chromosome 19q12 encoding a trans-membrane receptor with an extracellular domain containing 34 epidermal growth factor repeats (EGFRs) with six cysteine residues [9, 10]. Particularly, CADASIL results from mutations, mostly missense although small in-frame deletions or splice-site mutations have also been reported, in exons encoding EGFRs (exons 2-24) altering the number of cysteine and leaving one unpaired. Although a mutation cluster in exons 3 and 4 has been reported, a wider variation in mutational spectrum has been described [11 - 13]. CADASIL is the most common mendelian disorder associated with stroke (estimated prevalence of about 2-4/100000 inhabitants) [14 - 16]. Clinical presentation is essentially characterised by four main clinical features, which are migraine, lacunar strokes, mood disorders and cognitive impairment. Migraine, usually with aura, which has been observed in 20- 40% of patients, is the presenting clinical feature in the 60-75% (onset around the 20s or 30s). The most frequent manifestation are recurrent subcortical ischaemic events (TIA or stroke), which are reported in 60-85% of patients (mean age at onset 46+9.7 years) [17 - 19]. Ischemic strokes are lacunar and occur in most cases in the absence of common cerebrovascular risk factors, although some risk factors such as smoking and high cholesterol level have been recognised to condition an earlier stroke onset [18, 19]. Ischemic events are generally recurrent (from 2 to 5 events) and progressively lead to gait difficulty and pseudobulbar palsy [20, 21]. Cognitive impairment, which involves mostly executive functions and processing speed, occurs early and has been observed in nearly all patients by the age of 50 years [22, 23]. Cognitive decline is commonly progressive leading to dementia and worsens with recurrent stroke. Psychiatric disorders, particularly depression, anxiety and apathy are reported in 20-31% of patients [18, 20, 24, 25]. Other less common clinical manifestations are seizures reported in 5-10% of patients, intracerebral hemorrhages [26, 27], deafness and parkinsonism [22]. Although very rare, spinal cord involvement has been reported in few cases [28, 29]. MRI changes, characterised mostly by leukoencephalopathy and lacunar infarcts, can be detected after the age of 35 years and generally precede the symptoms onset by 10-15 years. The earliest changes are diffuse hyperintense lesions on T2-weighted or FLAIR images affecting the periventricular areas and centrum semiovale leading to confluent leukoaraiosis involving the anterior temporal poles.

Lacunar infarcts, which were observed in 75% of patients aged 30-40 years, increase with age and are located mostly in subcortical white matter, basal ganglia, thalamus, internal capsule and brainstem [30]. However, also cortical microinfarcts have been observed with high resolution MRI [31, 32]. Involvement of the anterior temporal lobe and external capsule is considered highly suggestive of CADASIL [33 - 35]. Other radiological features reported in CADASIL are subcortical microbleeds (CMBs) and cerebral atrophy [36]. Lacunar infarcts and microbleeds have been identified as the most important MRI parameters associated with cognitive dysfunction [37, 38]. Accumulation of granular osmio-philic material (GOM) within the vascular smooth cells of blood vessels is a specific hisotopathological features. GOM deposition occurs in peripheral and CNS arteries, primarily leptomeningeal and small penetrating arteries [39]. Electron microscopy for GOM in skin is considered a diagnostic tool due to the high specificity. However, since the sensitivity of this test is variable [40 - 43], DNA sequencing of exons 2-24 of NOTCH3 remains the gold standard for the diagnosis of CADASIL, having a 100% specificity in detecting a mutation which changes the number of cysteine residues within an EGFR.

**Table 1. Single gene disorders associated with stroke.**

| Monogenic causes of stroke |
|---|
| CADASIL |
| CARASIL |
| Retinal Vasculopathy with Cerebral Leukodystrophy (RVCL) |
| COL4A1 small vessel arteriopathy with haemorrhage |
| Familial hyperlipidaemias |
| Pseudoxanthoma elasticum |
| Neurofibromatosis type I |
| Ehlers-Danlos syndrome type IV |
| Marfan syndrome |
| Fabry disease |
| Homocysteinuria |
| Sickle cell disease |
| Familial cardiomyopathies |
| Familial arrhythmias |
| Hereditary haemorrhagic telangiectasia |
| Mitochondrial disorders (MELAS) |

## Cerebral Autosomal Recessive Arteriopathy with Subcortical Infarcts and Leukoencephalopathy (CARASIL) (OMIM 192315)

Cerebral autosomal recessive arteriopathy with subcortical infarcts and leukoencephalopathy (CARASIL) is an autosomal recessive disorders caused by mutations in HTRA1 gene on chromosome 10q25 [44]. The prevalence of CARASIL is unknown. Approximatively 50 cases have been reported so far mainly in Asian populations [45, 46], with the exception of recent cases of European patients [47, 48]. Head alopecia, which is one of the most frequent and earlier clinical symptoms, has been observed in approximately 90% of patients during adolescence. The second more common manifestation is lacunar stroke mainly in basal ganglia or brainstem with progressive small vessel disease onset from 20 to 44 years (mean 32 years).

Dementia is another common clinical feature developed by age 30- 40 years and is characterised by forgetfulness followed by disorientation in time, calculation deficits, emotional incontinence up to severe memory deficits and abulia [44]. Seizures and psychiatric disorders (personality changes, emotional lability, abulia and phallic syndrome) and attacks of severe back pain with lumbar disc herniation have also been described [49]. Additional manifestations may be pseudobulbar palsy, spondylosis deformans; less commonly ophthalmoplegia, ataxia have been observed. A case of cerebral hemorrhage in advanced disease course [44] has been reported. The disease affects predominantly males (3:1) and the average illness duration is up to 20-30 years, although most of patients became bed ridden within 10 years from onset [49, 50]. T2 weighted cerebral MRI shows by age 20 years diffuse and symmetrical white matter hyperintensities and lacunar infarcts in the basal ganglia and thalamus, which usually precede the symptoms onset [49]. Lesions tent to extend during the disease course into basal ganglia, thalami, brainstem and cerebellum and sometimes involve temporal lobes and external capsule as CADASIL. Histological changes are not disease specific and are characterised by loss of vascular smooth muscle cells and arteriolosclerosis. Differently from CADASIL GOM deposits have not been found.

## Retinal Vasculopathy with Cerebral Leukodystrophy (RVCL) (OMIM 192315)

Retinal vasculopathy with cerebral leukodystrophy (RVCL) is an autosomal dominant disease of the small vessel caused by mutation in the TREX1 gene on chromosome 3p21, that subsumes a number of different entities originally reported as distinct disorders: hereditary endotheliopathy with retinopathy, nephropathy and stroke (HERNS), cerebroretinal vasculopathy (CRV) and hereditary vascular retinopathy (HVR) [51]. The clinical phenotype consists of progressive visual loss in the 4th or 5th decade, due to retinal vasculopathy and microaneurysms. Neurological involvement occurs in the third or fourth decade of life and consists of ischemic stroke/TIA, seizures, migraine, psychiatric disturbances (personality disorders, anxiety, depression) or cognitive impairment leading to death in 5-10 years after the disease onset [52]. In some families a systemic small vessel arteriopathy manifesting with Rayanud's phenomenon, hepatic micronodular cirrhosis, renal failure and osteonecrosis has been described [54]. MRI findings are characterised by multiple subcortical hyperintense lesions on T2-weighted sequences involving the periventricular and deep white matter and corpus callosum but often contrast enhancing pseudotumor lesions surrounded by vasogenic oedema in cerebral and cerebellar deep white matter have been reported [53]. Interestingly, heterozygous TREX1 mutations, sparing the region coding the catalytic function and preserving the exonuclease function, result in RCVL while TREX1 homozygous mutations are associated with a more severe phenotype known as Aicardi- Goutière syndrome (AGS), a rare, familial, early-onset progressive encephalopathy with basal ganglia calcifications and cerebrospinal fluid lymphocytosis.

## Fabry Disease (OMIM #301500)

Fabry disease (FD) [Anderson-Fabry disease, Online Mendelian Inheritance in Man OMIM 301500] is a multisystem X-linked lysosomal storage disorder resulting in lysosomal glycosphingolipid (globotriaosylceramide or Gb3) deposition due to alpha-galactosidase A enzyme (α-Gal A) absence or deficiency, caused by a mutation in the GLA gene [54, 55].

Fabry disease is a rare, although probably underdiagnosed. The reported incidence ranges from 1:40,000 to 1:117,000 worldwide [56]. However, definitive prevalence data are lacking since the available observations are derived from different patient populations (cardiac, renal, or cerebrovascular diseases) Although Gb3 storage begins prenatally, clinical symptoms do not manifest until childhood. Burning pain in the extremities with glove and stock distribution, gastrointestinal disorders and hypohidrosis are the most frequent presenting features.

Usually, renal involvement, ranging from proteinuria to renal failure, cardiac and cerebrovascular disorders, develops after the age of 20 years [57]. The severity of the disease is related to residual α-Gal A enzymatic activity. Even though a clear genotype-phenotype correlation has not been observed, mutations leading to a complete loss of function are more frequently associated with the classical phenotype. The disease primarily occurs among hemizygous males. However, a significant proportion of heterozygous females also may be symptomatic, even if at an older age in comparison to affected males [58, 59]. The presence of symptomatic heterozygous females is not clear. X inactivation mechanism but also the clinical variability due to other genetic or environmental factors have been invoked as possible explanations.

Generally, cerebrovascular complications develop after the 20th with a mean age of onset of 33–46 years in males and 40–52 years in females [60 - 62]. The reported prevalence ranges from 24% to 48% in affected males and from 7% to 32% in affected females [60, 61, 63 - 65]. In 2005 Rolfs *et al.* in a study on 721 patients affected by cryptogenic stroke (aged 18- 55) found mutations in GLA gene in 4.9% of men and in 2.4% of women [66]. GLA mutation was described with a prevalence of about 1% in two other studies investigating the prevalence of FD not only in cryptogenic stroke but in young patients with cerebrovascular disease [67, 68]. This rate increased to 4.6% if ischemic stroke due to small vessel disease (SVD), to 7% in the presence of SVD without associated high blood pressure (BP) and up to 12.5% if a vertebrobasilar stroke coexisted with SVD and normal BP [69]. More recently, SIFAP 1 showed an incidence of definite and probable (at least two biochemical markers including Gb3, lyso-Gb3 o Gb3-24 in the urine) FD of 0.5% and 0.4% respectively in young stroke patients (18-55 yrs) [70]. Ischemic episodes (stroke or TIA), are due to the small and large vessels disease, but also to cardiogenic embolism [62]. The pathophysiology of the cerebral vasculopathy is still poorly understood since cardioembolic pathogenesis probably explains only a small proportion of strokes in FD patients. A more complex mechanism including changes in angiogenesis, endothelial dysfunction and unbalance of blood constituents more likely explains cerebrovascular accidents in these patients [71]. The disease is characterized by a progressive disease course in which cerebrovascular disorders recur and cerebral lesions accumulate gradually.

Another classical clinical manifestation is neuropathic involvement, which can be as high as 80% in FD. Neuropathic involvement in FD may start in childhood may suggest the diagnosis [57, 72, 73]. Patients commonly present a distal length-dependent painful small-fiber sensory neuropathy, characterized by acroparesthesia, burning dysesthesia, sensory loss in hands or feet. Sixty-eighty percent of FD patients refers pain, which may be chronic or episodic (Fabry's crises). Pain may be triggered by stress, physical exercise, fever or temperature variation. Also affected females may present an early-onset neuropathic pain [74].

Multisystemic manifestations include kidney involvement, due to GB3 deposition in the glomerular, mesangial, intersticial cells, which often begins with microalbuminuria and proteinuria in the 2nd and 3rd decade of life. Cardiac symptoms including left ventricular hypertrophy, arrhythmia, valvular abnormalities, conductions disorders, and coronary artery disease are reported in 40-60% of patients [75, 76]. Myocardial fibrosis mostly in posterolateral wall and mild myocardium occurs in later disease course leading to a reduced cardiac function up to congestive heart failure [76]. Other extraneurological frequent manifestations include characteristic small reddish raised skin lesions (angiokeratomas), a corneal opacity that usually does not impair vision and detectable by slit lamp examination (cornea verticillata), which occurs almost in all hemizygous males, and gastrointestinal respiratory and orthopaedic disorders. T2- and FLAIR-weighted images typically show multiple hyperintensities affecting the deep hemispheric white matter and brainstem, which often predate the onset of neurological symptoms and signs [77, 78]. Also hemorrhagic lesions have been reported in FD patients, mostly associated with hypertension [79].

Vessel abnormalities such as tortuosity and abnormal ectasia of large vessels (dolichoectasia) have been also described as additional radiological features. Pulvinar hyperintensities on T1-weighted images, (23% of FD patients) are the only peculiar radiological feature of this disease. The significance of these lesion is still unclear although the hyperdense aspect on cerebral CT support the hypothesis that they may represent calcification and mineralisation induced by increased blood flow in the posterior circulation [80].

## COL4A1/A2 related Arteriopathy (OMIM 605595-120130)

A wide spectrum of conditions with neurological and systemic involvement with infantile or adult onset was attributed to mutations in COL4A1 gene (13q34) encoding for collagen IV, alpha 1 which is an essential component of basal membrane stability. COL4A1 syndrome can manifest in childhood with porencephaly, infantile hemiparesis, cerebral hemorrhage and developmental delay [81]. Recently carriers of COL4A1 mutations have been recognised to present a SVD features with ischemic lacunar infarcts, leukoencephalopathy and brain haemorrhages [82, 83]. Asymptomatic cerebral aneurysms, mostly of the intracranial portion of the internal carotid artery, were observed in 44% of subjects submitted to appropriate investigations, often multiple. Other neurological manifestations include migraine with or without aura, seizures, cognitive impairment, psychiatric disorders, dementia and visual loss due to retinal ischemic changes or haemorrhages and retinal arteriolar tortuosity. Systemic features include nephropathy, Raynaud's syndrome disorders, myopathy with muscle cramps and cardiac disorders [81]. MRI findings include diffuse leukoencephalopathy (63.5%), lacunar infarcts (16.5%), microbleeds (52.8% with GRE sequences), dilated perivascular spaces (19.2%), and deep cerebral haemorrhages. Poroncephalic lesions characterised by fluid filled periventricular cysts may be observed [81].

## Mitochondrial Myopathy, Encephalopathy, Lactic Acidosis and Stroke-Like Episodes (MELAS) (OMIM 540000)

Mitochondrial myopathy, encephalopathy, lactic acidosis and stroke-like episodes (MELAS) syndrome is the most frequent heritable mitochondrial disorder.

In the Caucasian population the estimated prevalence of 3243A>G mutation, accounting for 80% of MELAS cases, ranges from 5 to 236 per 100,000 [84, 85]. The age of onset range usually between 2 and 20 years [85]. Stroke-like episodes (usually characterized by aphasia, cortical blindness, hemianopia, hemiparesis), which are usually transient and not-disabling, are the clinical disease hallmark [85, 86]. Focal and generalized seizures are reported in 85-100% of MELAS patients, often originating from the occipital lobe and during the stroke like episodes. Migraine is another common feature described in 77% of patients and in 15% of cases may be the initial symptom [85]. Additional features include cognitive decline, short stature, hearing loss, psychosis, lactic acidosis, opthalmic disturbance (ophtalmoplegia, pigmentary retinopathy, optic atrophy), short stature, diabetes and myopathy with easy fatigability and exercise intolerance. Cardiac disturbance most likely as cardiomyopathy, conduction defects or chronic heart failure as well as diabetes mellitus and gastrointestinal disturbances are also frequent complications of MELAS syndrome. However, the presentation is variable due at least in part to heteroplasmy phenomenon with different level of mutant and wild type mtDNA in different tissues [87]. Cerebral CT scan revealed aspecific ischemic lesions or bilateral basal ganglia calcifications [88]. Although, there are not neuroradiological specific diagnostic MRI features, the migrating hyperintensities, particularly the T2 and DWI sequences, not strictly related to distinct arterial territories and migrating over time suggest a metabolic disorders. Thalamus may be involved whereas cortical lesions generally spare the deeper white matter, reflecting the high metabolic demand of these regions.

In general, the posterior territories, particularly the temporo-parieto-occipital lobes, are more frequently affected than the anterior regions [89]. MELAS is mostly caused by a point mutation in mitochondrial genome (mtDNA), which is in 80% of cases a mutation (m.3243A>G) of the mitochondrial tRNA Leu (UUR) gene (MTTL1) [85, 90].

Only a minority of subjects with m.3243A>G mutation have clinical symptoms since for the heteroplasmy phenomenon each mitochondrion has many copies of mtDNA but the number of mutated mtDNA is variable. Thus, different amount of abnormal mtDNA characterizes cells and tissues of an individual explaining variable penetrance and clinical expression differences. Another important concept is the threshold effect: a threshold level, variable among individuals and based on the balance of oxygen supply and demand of mutated mtDNA, triggers the expression of disease symptoms. For these peculiar aspects of mitochondrial heritability, the negative genetic test and muscle biopsy do not definitively rule out the diagnosis. Other mtDNA mutations in MTTL1 gene and other transfer RNA genes (MTTF, MTTv, MTTQ), in other complex 1 subunits (MTND1, MTND5 and MTND6) as well as mutations in nuclear genes leading to secondary mtDNA changes (depletions and multiple deletions)have been also described as cause of MELAS [91].

The mutations in MELAS syndrome most lead to a functional impairment of respiratory chain elements and finally to an imbalance between energy requirement and available energy of the cell. Other mechanisms including the abnormal release of reactive oxygen species that are converted in toxic compounds or abnormal calcium levels as well as nitric oxide have been described in the pathogenesis of MELAS. The pathogenesis of stroke-like episodes is still unclear and two possible main mechanisms have been invoked. The mitochondrial cytopathy theory support the idea that leucine transfer RNA mutations decrease protein synthesis and cause oxidative phosphorylation failure, leading to adenosine triphosphate depletion (ATP) and energy failure. Conversely, for the mitochondrial angiopathy theory the cerebral small vessel dysfunction might be due to the accumulation of abnormal mitochondria in the endothelium and smooth muscle. An increased neuronal hyperexcitability, which increases energy demand in a neuronal population with mitochondrial dysfunction has been also proposed as possible alternative pathophysiological mechanism.

A typical pattern of ragged red fibers has been observed on skeletal muscle biopsy, in MELAS patients (80-100% of specimens). Muscle fibers show also positive staining for modified Gomori trichrome but also also cytochrome c oxidase (COX)-negative fibers, succinate dehydrogenase (SDH) hyperreactivity and, at ultrastructural level, abnormally shaped mitochondria with paracristalline inclusions [85].

## Multifactorial Stroke

Most of strokes are believed to be polygenic. In this case the identification of genetic risk is challenging since the genetic basis is probably largely related to multiple genetic variants with small effect sizes but also lifestyle and comorbidities may contribute to the patient phenotype. Historically, polygenic stroke and other complex diseases were explored applying the candidate gene association study approach. In this kind of studies a gene, which is believed to be involved in stroke risk, is identified as a "candidate" and the frequency of genetic variants, usually single nucleotide polymorphisms (SNPs), within that gene is compared between stroke cases and controls. A long list of genes involved in endothelial function and nitric oxide release, the renin–angiotensin– aldosterone system axis, coagulation, haemostasis and inflammation have been investigated in ischaemic stroke. However, the results of most of these studies have been disappointing and the associations were difficultly replicated in independent series [6]. Several issues including the selected genes, the small sample size, the poor characterization of cases and controls have been invoked as possible causes of failure of these studies.

Accordingly, only few genes including methylenetetrahydrofolate reductase (MTHFR), angiotensin-converting enzyme (ACE), factor V Leiden and prothrombin genes were reliably associated with stroke risk by meta-analyses of published data [6, 92, 93]. However, although carefully conducted, also the results of these meta-analyses have to be interpreted with caution given the publication bias of the included studies, which is exacerbated by preferential publication of positive associations. The failure of candidate gene approach induced the development of new hightroughput technologies such as genome-wide association studies (GWAs).

The most important advantage of GWAS approach is that it overcomes the 'a priori' gene selection bias allowing associations between novel chromosomal loci and clinical disorders [94, 95]. Up to date GWAS studies provided the strongest evidence for loci associated with ischemic stroke, in particular for some stroke subtypes. For instance two loci associated with atrial fibrillation have both been observed to be risk factors for cardioembolic stroke. The first is a locus on chromosome 4q25, that is believed to be PITX2, a gene encoding a transcription factor regulated by b-catenin, which is involved in left right asymmetry and differentiation of left atrium. This gene, which was firstly associated with atrial fibrillation [96, 97], was replicated in multiple populations, by several groups belonging to the International Stroke Genetics Consortium (ISGC, www.strokegenetics.com), which found it to be specifically associated with cardioembolic stroke subtype. A second variant in the ZFHX3 gene at 16q22, encoding a zinc-finger protein, has been associated with atrial fibrillation and cardioembolic ischaemic stroke [98]. Lastly, a genetic variant on chromosome 9p21 locus has been associated with myocardial infarction and coronary artery disease (CAD). This variant was also found by a meta-analysis to be associated with large artery stroke independently from any other vascular risk factor including CAD [99]. This region of chromosome 9 includes the cyclin-dependent kinase inhibitor CDK2MA and CDK2MB genes and a non-coding RNA also known as ANRIL, whose function is unclear.

## Stroke Subtypes Associations

Few novel associations have been also observed in ischemic stroke by GWAS. A

GWA study on 1112 Japanese ischaemic stroke patients found an association between a SNP in a PRKCH, a gene encoding for serin-Theonine kinase, which regulates cell differentiation, proliferation and apoptosis, and small-vessel disease stroke [100]. This variant was replicated in two independent Japanese and Chinese populations and also in patients with MRI detected, predominantly lacunar, silent brain infarctions [101, 102]. A molecular variant at chromosome 6p21.1 was found in large-artery atherosclerotic stroke. Another study found a specific association between a variant in the MMP12 gene, which encodes for the matrix metalloproteinase 12, a macrophage metalloelastase, and large-artery atherosclerotic stroke [103].

Recently, a GWAS conducted by the Wellcome Trust Case Control Consortium 2 (WTCCC2) in about 3500 ischaemic stroke cases from four European centres found a new variant associated with large-vessel stroke at chromosome 7p21 (OR1.42) [104]. This result was replicated in further 6000 patients from Europe, US and Australia and in following studies [105 - 107]. The found variant, which was also found in a meta-analysis (METASTROKE), is located in a highly conserved, and probably, functional area, within the introns rather than the coding regions [105].

## Limits of GWAS and Next Generation Studies

Although the GWAS is a comprehensive and unbiased approach, and the results of some still ongoing studies are awaited, this study design is discussed for several reasons. These include 1) the potentially high rates of false-positive results due to multiple testing, 2) the need for large sample sizes that sometimes lack well phenotyping 3) the lack of information of the functions of most found genes, and 4) the difficult detection of rare and structural variants.

The incomplete DNA covering and the high cost of GWAs promoted the development of other advanced technologies such as Next generation sequencing (NGS). It is a highly parallel DNA sequencing technology that can produce many hundreds of thousands or millions of short reads that can be obtained in a short time and at relatively low cost. This technique, which was initially applied in resequencing target sequence identified by GWAS, may include both complete genome (whole genome sequencing-WGS) or coding sequences (whole exome sequencing-WES) and suboxone panels of specific genes [108, 109]. Since NGS presents some advantages in term of cost and time of examination, it is becoming an important research but also diagnostic tool, mostly for the diagnosis of rare inherited disorders and monogenic diseases [110].

## CONCLUSION

Although the identification of the genetic factors contributing to interindividual differences in stroke could lead to new evaluation, treatment and prevention approaches, genetic investigation of stroke is still in its infancy. The diagnosis of monogenic disorders, despite rare, is important for patients and their family for the implementation of careful preventative measures and the possibility of prenatal testing. Furthermore, the improvement of the knowledge in these diseases and the availability of experimental models, contribute to our understanding of pathogenic mechanism of sporadic stroke. However most of stroke have probably a complex genetic aetiology, based on multiple small gene effects. In these cases, the influence of several other genetic factors probably underlying the common risk factors such as hypertension and diabetes has to be considered. To date, despite the development of powerful advanced molecular and analytical tools, only a few molecular variants, detected by candidate gene approach were found in association with stroke risk and have been significantly replicated in independent series. Also the findings from of GWAS, although in some cases strongly associated with stroke, explain only a small proportion of strokes. Moreover, the pathogenic significance of many of the genetic variants associated with ischaemic stroke is yet to be determined as the clinical impact of these results is still limited. Functional studies are needed to assess the pathogenic significance of these variants and to identify possible therapeutic targets. Interestingly, most of the identified associations are specific for stroke subtypes, highlighting the importance of the collection of well phenotyped patients and supporting the development of treatment approaches that take into account the different pathophysiologies of the stroke subtypes. Lastly, findings from novel techniques such as the Next generation sequencing will integrate with GWAS results by identifying rare genetic varients missed by GWAS.

## TAKE HOME MESSAGE

Ischemic stroke is a multi-factorial disease with a complex genetic background. Rare causes of monogenic stroke may help identifying common genetic mechanisms which may also apply in specific stroke subtypes within the general stroke population.

## CONFLICT OF INTEREST

The authors confirm that they have no conflict of interest to declare for this publication.

## ACKNOWLEDGEMENTS

Declared none.

## REFERENCES

[1]     Hassan A, Markus HS. Genetics and ischaemic stroke. Brain 2000; 123: 1784-812.
        [http://dx.doi.org/10.1093/brain/123.9.1784]

[2]     Rubattu S, Giliberti R, Volpe M. Etiology and pathophysiology of stroke as a complex trait. Am J Hypertens 2000; 13: 1139-48.
        [http://dx.doi.org/10.1016/S0895-7061(00)01249-8]

[3]     Jerrard-Dunne P, Cloud G, Hassan A, Markus HS. Evaluating the genetic component of ischemic stroke subtypes: a family history study. Stroke 2003; 34: 1364-9.
        [http://dx.doi.org/10.1161/01.STR.0000069723.17984.FD]

[4]     Meschia JF, Worrall BB, Rich SS. Genetic susceptibility to ischemic stroke. Nat Rev Neurol 2011; 7: 369-78.
        [http://dx.doi.org/10.1038/nrneurol.2011.80]

[5]     Markus HS. Stroke genetics. Hum Mol Genet 2011; 20(R2): R124-31.
        [http://dx.doi.org/10.1093/hmg/ddr345]

[6]     Bersano A, Ballabio E, Bresolin N, Candelise L. Genetic polymorphisms for the study of multifactorial stroke. Hum Mutat 2008; 29(6): 776-95.
        [http://dx.doi.org/10.1002/humu.20666]

[7]     Ballabio E, Bersano A, Bresolin N, Candelise L. Monogenic vessel diseases related to ischemic stroke: a clinical approach. J Cereb Blood Flow Metab 2007; 27: 1649-62.
        [http://dx.doi.org/10.1038/sj.jcbfm.9600520]

[8]     Bersano A, Baron P, Lanfranconi S, *et al.* Lombardia GENS: a collaborative registry for monogenic diseases associated with stroke. Funct Neurol 2012; 27(2): 107-17.

[9]     Joutel A, Corpechot C, Ducros A, *et al.* Notch3 mutations in CADASIL, a hereditary adult-onset

condition causing stroke and dementia. Nature 1996; 383(6602): 707-10.
[http://dx.doi.org/10.1038/383707a0]

[10]    Joutel A, Corpechot C, Ducros A, *et al.* Notch3 mutations in cerebral autosomal dominant arteriopathy with subcortical infarcts and leukoencephalopathy (CADASIL), a mendelian condition causing stroke and vascular dementia. Ann N Y Acad Sci 1997; 826: 213-7. [Review].
[http://dx.doi.org/10.1111/j.1749-6632.1997.tb48472.x]

[11]    Dotti MT, Federico A, Mazzei R, *et al.* The spectrum of Notch3 mutations in 28 Italian CADASIL families. J Neurol Neurosurg Psychiatry 2005; 76: 736-8.
[http://dx.doi.org/10.1136/jnnp.2004.048207]

[12]    Cappelli A, Ragno M, Cacchiò G, Scarcella M, Staffolani P, Pianese L. High recurrence of the R1006C NOTCH3 mutation in central Italian patients with cerebral autosomal dominant arteriopathy with subcortical infarcts and leukoencephalopathy (CADASIL). Neurosci Lett 2009; 462: 176-8.
[http://dx.doi.org/10.1016/j.neulet.2009.06.087]

[13]    Bianchi S, Rufa A, Ragno M, *et al.* High frequency of exon 10 mutations in the NOTCH3 gene in Italian CADASIL families: phenotypic peculiarities. J Neurol 2010; 257: 1039-42.
[http://dx.doi.org/10.1007/s00415-010-5481-z]

[14]    Razvi SS, Davidson R, Bone I, Muir KW. The prevalence of cerebral autosomal dominant arteriopathy with subcortical infarcts and leucoencephalopathy (CADASIL) in the west of Scotland. J Neurol Neurosurg Psychiatry 2005; 76: 739-41.
[http://dx.doi.org/10.1136/jnnp.2004.051847]

[15]    Kalimo H, Ruchoux MM, Viitanen M, Kalaria RN. CADASIL: a common form of hereditary arteriopathy causing brain infarcts and dementia. Brain Pathol 2002; 12: 371-84.
[http://dx.doi.org/10.1111/j.1750-3639.2002.tb00451.x]

[16]    Narayan SK, Gorman G, Kalaria RN, Ford GA, Chinnery PF. The minimum prevalence of CADASIL in northeast England. Neurology 2012; 78: 1025-7.
[http://dx.doi.org/10.1212/WNL.0b013e31824d586c]

[17]    Bousser M, Tournier-Lasserve E. Cerebral autosomal dominant arteriopathy with subcortical infarcts and leukoencephalopathy: from stroke to vessel wall physiology. J Neurol Neurosurg Psychiatry 2001; 70: 285-7S.
[http://dx.doi.org/10.1136/jnnp.70.3.285]

[18]    Singhal S, Bevan S, Barrick T, Rich P, Markus HS. The influence of genetic and cardiovascular risk factors on the CADASIL phenotype. Brain 2004; 127: 2031-8.
[http://dx.doi.org/10.1093/brain/awh223]

[19]    Adib-Samii P, Brice G, Martin RJ, Markus HS. Clinical spectrum of CADASIL and the effect of cardiovascular risk factors on phenotype: study in 200 consecutively recruited individuals. Stroke 2010; 41: 630-4.
[http://dx.doi.org/10.1161/STROKEAHA.109.568402]

[20]    Dichgans M, Mayer M, Uttner I, *et al.* The phenotypic spectrum of CADASIL: clinical findings in 102 cases. Ann Neurol 1998; 44: 731-9.
[http://dx.doi.org/10.1002/ana.410440506]

[21]   Opherk C, Peters N, Herzog J, Luedtke R, Dichgans M. Long-term prognosis and causes of death in CADASIL: a retrospective study in 411 patients. Brain 2004; 127: 2533-9.
[http://dx.doi.org/10.1093/brain/awh282]

[22]   Chabriat H, Joutel A, Dichgans M, Tournier-Lasserve E, Bousser MG. Cadasil. Lancet Neurol 2009; 8: 643-53.
[http://dx.doi.org/10.1016/S1474-4422(09)70127-9]

[23]   Dichgans M. Cognition in CADASIL. Stroke 2009; 40: S45-7.
[http://dx.doi.org/10.1161/STROKEAHA.108.534412]

[24]   Chabriat H, Vahedi K, Iba-Zizen MT, *et al.* Clinical spectrum of CADASIL: a study of 7 families. Cerebral autosomal dominant arteriopathy with subcortical infarcts and leukoencephalopathy. Lancet 1995; 346: 934-9.
[http://dx.doi.org/10.1016/S0140-6736(95)91557-5]

[25]   Razvi SS, Davidson R, Bone I, Muir KW. The prevalence of cerebral autosomal dominant arteriopathy with subcortical infarcts and leucoencephalopathy (CADASIL) in the west of Scotland. J Neurol Neurosurg Psychiatry 2005; 76: 739-41.
[http://dx.doi.org/10.1136/jnnp.2004.051847]

[26]   Choi JC, Kang SY, Kang JH, Park JK. Intracerebral hemorrhages in CADASIL. Neurology 2006; 67: 2042-4.
[http://dx.doi.org/10.1212/01.wnl.0000246601.70918.06]

[27]   Lee YC, Liu CS, Chang MH, *et al.* Population-specific spectrum of NOTCH3 mutations, MRI features and founder effect of CADASIL in Chinese. J Neurol 2009; 256: 249-55.
[http://dx.doi.org/10.1007/s00415-009-0091-3]

[28]   Hinze S, Goonasekera M, Nannucci S, *et al.* Longitudinally extensive spinal cord infarction in CADASIL. Pract Neurol 2015; 15(1): 60-2.
[http://dx.doi.org/10.1136/practneurol-2014-000870]

[29]   Bentley P, Wang T, Malik O, *et al.* CADASIL with cord involvement associated with a novel and atypical NOTCH3 mutation. J Neurol Neurosurg Psychiatry 2011; 82(8): 855-60.
[http://dx.doi.org/10.1136/jnnp.2010.223297]

[30]   Choi JC. Cerebral autosomal dominant arteriopathy with subcortical infarcts and leukoencephalopathy: a genetic cause of cerebral small vessel disease. J Clin Neurol 2010; 6: 1-9.
[http://dx.doi.org/10.3988/jcn.2010.6.1.1]

[31]   Jouvent E, Poupon C, Gray F, *et al.* Intracortical infarcts in small vessel disease: a combined 7-T postmortem MRI and neuropathological case study in cerebral autosomal-dominant arteriopathy with subcortical infarcts and leukoencephalopathy. Stroke 2011; 42: e27-30.
[http://dx.doi.org/10.1161/STROKEAHA.110.594218]

[32]   Benjamin P, Viessmann O, MacKinnon AD, Jezzard P, Markus HS. 7 Tesla MRI in cerebral small vessel disease. Int J Stroke 2015; 10(5): 659-64.
[http://dx.doi.org/10.1111/ijs.12490]

[33]   Pantoni L, Pescini F, Nannucci S, *et al.* Comparison of clinical, familial, and MRI features of CADASIL and NOTCH3-negative patients. Neurology 2010; 74: 57-63.

[http://dx.doi.org/10.1212/WNL.0b013e3181c7da7c]

[34]   Jacqmin M, Hervé D, Viswanathan A, *et al.* Confluent thalamic hyperintensities in CADASIL. Cerebrovasc Dis 2010; 30: 308-13.
[http://dx.doi.org/10.1159/000319607]

[35]   Singhal S, Rich P, Markus HS. The spatial distribution of MR imaging abnormalities in cerebral autosomal dominant arteriopathy with subcortical infarcts and leukoencephalopathy and their relationship to age and clinical features. AJNR Am J Neuroradiol 2005; 26(10): 2481-7.

[36]   Peters N, Holtmannspötter M, Opherk C, *et al.* Brain volume changes in CADASIL: a serial MRI study in pure subcortical ischemic vascular disease. Neurology 2006; 66: 1517-22.
[http://dx.doi.org/10.1212/01.wnl.0000216271.96364.50]

[37]   Liem MK, van der Grond J, Haan J, *et al.* Lacunar infarcts are the main correlate with cognitive dysfunction in CADASIL. Stroke 2007; 38: 923-8.
[http://dx.doi.org/10.1161/01.STR.0000257968.24015.bf]

[38]   Liem MK, Lesnik Oberstein SA, Haan J, *et al.* MRI correlates of cognitive decline in CADASIL: a 7-year follow-up study. Neurology 2009; 72: 143-8.
[http://dx.doi.org/10.1212/01.wnl.0000339038.65508.96]

[39]   Morroni M, Marzioni D, Ragno M, *et al.* Role of electron microscopy in the diagnosis of cadasil syndrome: a study of 32 patients. PLoS One 2013; 8(6): e65482.
[http://dx.doi.org/10.1371/journal.pone.0065482]

[40]   Markus HS, Martin RJ, Simpson MA, *et al.* Diagnostic strategies in CADASIL. Neurology 2002; 59: 1134-8.
[http://dx.doi.org/10.1212/WNL.59.8.1134]

[41]   Ruchoux MM, Chabriat H, Bousser MG, Baudrimont M, Tournier-Lasserve E. Presence of ultrastructural arterial lesions in muscle and skin vessels of patients with CADASIL. Stroke 1994; 25: 2291-2.
[http://dx.doi.org/10.1161/01.STR.25.11.2291]

[42]   Tikka S, Mykkänen K, Ruchoux MM, *et al.* Congruence between NOTCH3 mutations and GOM in 131 CADASIL patients. Brain 2009; 132: 933-9.
[http://dx.doi.org/10.1093/brain/awn364]

[43]   Lesnik Oberstein SA, van Duinen SG, van den Boom R, *et al.* Evaluation of diagnostic NOTCH3 immunostaining in CADASIL. J Cereb Blood Flow Metab 2003; 23: 599-604.

[44]   Fukutake T. Cerebral autosomal recessive arteriopathy with subcortical infarcts and leukoencephalopathy (CARASIL): from discovery to gene identification. J Stroke Cerebrovasc Dis 2011; 20: 85-93.
[http://dx.doi.org/10.1016/j.jstrokecerebrovasdis.2010.11.008]

[45]   Zheng DM, Xu FF, Gao Y, Zhang H, Han SC, Bi GR. A Chinese pedigree of cerebral autosomal recessive arteriopathy with subcortical infarcts and leukoencephalopathy (CARASIL): clinical and radiological features. J Clin Neurosci 2009; 16: 847-9.
[http://dx.doi.org/10.1016/j.jocn.2008.08.031]

[46]   Yanagawa S, Ito N, Arima K, Ikeda S. Cerebral autosomal recessive arteriopathy with subcortical

infarcts and leukoencephalopathy. Neurology 2002; 58: 817-20.
[http://dx.doi.org/10.1212/WNL.58.5.817]

[47] Mendioroz M, Fernández-Cadenas I, Del Río-Espinola A, *et al.* A missense HTRA1 mutation expands CARASIL syndrome to the Caucasian population Neurolog 2010; 75: 2033-5.

[48] Menezes Cordeiro I, Nzwalo H, Sá F, *et al.* Shifting the CARASIL paradigm: report of a non-Asian family and literature review. Stroke 2015; 46(4): 1110-2.
[http://dx.doi.org/10.1161/STROKEAHA.114.006735]

[49] Fukutake T, Hirayama K. Familial young-adult-onset arteriosclerotic leukoencephalopathy with alopecia and lumbago without arterial hypertension. Eur Neurol 1995; 35: 69-79.
[http://dx.doi.org/10.1159/000117096]

[50] Hara K, Shiga A, Fukutake T, *et al.* Association of HTRA1 mutations and familial ischemic cerebral small-vessel disease. N Engl J Med 2009; 360: 1729-39.
[http://dx.doi.org/10.1056/NEJMoa0801560]

[51] Richards A, van den Maagdenberg AM, Jen JC, *et al.* C-terminal truncations in human 3'-5' DNA exonuclease TREX1 cause autosomal dominant retinal vasculopathy with cerebral leukodystrophy. Nat Genet 2007; 39: 1068-70.
[http://dx.doi.org/10.1038/ng2082]

[52] Ophoff RA, DeYoung J, Service SK, *et al.* Hereditary vascular retinopathy cerebroretinal vasculopathy and hereditary endotheliopathy with retinopathy nephropathy and stroke map to a single locus on chromosome 3p211-p213. Am J Hum Genet 2001; 69: 447-53.
[http://dx.doi.org/10.1086/321975]

[53] DiFrancesco JC, Novara F, Zuffardi O, *et al.* TREX1 C-terminal frameshift mutations in the systemic variant of retinal vasculopathy with cerebral leukodystrophy. Neurol Sci 2015; 36(2): 323-30.
[http://dx.doi.org/10.1007/s10072-014-1944-9]

[54] Pastores GM, Lien YH. Biochemical and molecular genetic basis of Fabry disease. J Am Soc Nephrol 2002; 13: S130-3.

[55] Schäfer E, Baron K, Widmer U, Deegan P, Neumann HP, Sunder-Plassmann G, *et al.* Thirty-four novel mutations of the GLA gene in 121 patients with Fabry disease. Hum Mutat 2005; 25: 412.
[http://dx.doi.org/10.1002/humu.9327]

[56] Hoffmann B, Mayatepek E. Fabry disease-often seen, rarely diagnosed. Dtsch Arztebl Int 2009; 106: 440-7.

[57] Bersano A, Lanfranconi S, Valcarenghi C, Bresolin N, Micieli G, Baron P. Neurological features of Fabry disease: clinical, pathophysiological aspects and therapy. Acta Neurol Scand 2012; 126(2): 77-97.
[http://dx.doi.org/10.1111/j.1600-0404.2012.01661.x]

[58] Macdermot KD, Holmes A, Miners AH. Anderson- Fabry disease: clinical manifestations and impact of disease in a cohort of 60 obligate carrier females. J Med Genet 2001; 38: 769-71.
[http://dx.doi.org/10.1136/jmg.38.11.769]

[59] Wendrich K, Whybra C, Ries M, Gal A, Beck M. Neurological manifestation of Fabry disease in females. Contrib Nephrol 2001; 136: 241-4.

[http://dx.doi.org/10.1159/000060195]

[60]    Mitsias P, Levine SR. Cerebrovascular complications of Fabry disease. Ann Neurol 1996; 40: 8-17.
        [http://dx.doi.org/10.1002/ana.410400105]

[61]    Vedder AC, Linthorst GE, Van Breemen MJ, *et al.* The DutchFabry cohort: diversity of clinical
        manifestations and Gb3 levels. J Inherit Metab Dis 2007; 30: 68-78.
        [http://dx.doi.org/10.1007/s10545-006-0484-8]

[62]    Kolodny EH, Pastores GM. Anderson–Fabry disease: extrarenal, neurologic manifestations. J Am Soc
        Nephrol 2002; 13: S3-S150.

[63]    Sims K, Politei J, Banikazemi M, Stroke LE. in Fabry disease frequently occurs before diagnosis and
        in the absence of other clinical events: natural history data from the Fabry Registry. Stroke 2009; 40:
        788-94.
        [http://dx.doi.org/10.1161/STROKEAHA.108.526293]

[64]    Grewal RP. Stroke in Fabry disease. J Neurol 1994; 241: 153-6.
        [http://dx.doi.org/10.1007/BF00868342]

[65]    Mehta A, Ginsberg L, Investigators FO. Natural history of the cerebrovascular complications of Fabry
        disease. Acta Paediatr 2005; 94: 24-7.
        [http://dx.doi.org/10.1080/08035320510028076]

[66]    Rolfs A, Böttcher T, Zschiesche M, *et al.* Prevalence of Fabry disease in patients with cryptogenic
        stroke: a prospective study. Lancet 2005; 366(9499): 1794-6.
        [http://dx.doi.org/10.1016/S0140-6736(05)67635-0]

[67]    Brouns R, Sheorajpanday R, Braxel E, *et al.* Middelheim Fabry Study (MiFaS): a retrospective
        Belgian study on the prevalence of Fabry disease in young patients with cryptogenic stroke. Clin
        Neurol Neurosurg 2007; 109(6): 479-84.
        [http://dx.doi.org/10.1016/j.clineuro.2007.03.008]

[68]    Baptista MV, Ferreira S, Pinho-E-Melo T, *et al.* PORTuguese Young STROKE Investigators.
        Mutations of the GLA gene in young patients with stroke: the PORTYSTROKE study-screening
        genetic conditions in Portuguese young stroke patients. Stroke 2010; 41(3): 431-6.
        [http://dx.doi.org/10.1161/STROKEAHA.109.570499]

[69]    Brouns R, Thijs V, Eyskens F, *et al.* BeFaS Investigators. Belgian Fabry study: prevalence of Fabry
        disease in a cohort of 1000 young patients with cerebrovascular disease. Stroke 2010; 41(5): 863-8.
        [http://dx.doi.org/10.1161/STROKEAHA.110.579409]

[70]    Rolfs A, Fazekas F, Grittner U, *et al.* Stroke in Young Fabry Patients (sifap) Investigators. Acute
        cerebrovascular disease in the young: the Stroke in Young Fabry Patients study. Stroke 2013; 44(2):
        340-9.
        [http://dx.doi.org/10.1161/STROKEAHA.112.663708]

[71]    Testai FD, Gorelick PB. Inherited metabolic disorders and stroke part 1: Fabry disease and
        mitochondrial myopathy, encephalopathy, lactic acidosis, and stroke like episodes. Arch Neurol 2010;
        67: 19-24.
        [http://dx.doi.org/10.1001/archneurol.2009.309]

[72]    Valeriani M, Mariotti P, Le Pera D, *et al.* Functional assessment of A delta and C fibers in patients

with Fabry's disease. Muscle Nerve 2004; 30: 708-13.
[http://dx.doi.org/10.1002/mus.20174]

[73]   Kocen RS, Thomas PK. Peripheral nerve involvement in Fabry's disease. Arch Neurol 1970; 22(1):
81-8.
[http://dx.doi.org/10.1001/archneur.1970.00480190085014]

[74]   Whybra C, Wendrich K, Ries M, Gal A, Beck M. Clinical manifestation in female Fabry disease
patients. Contrib Nephrol 2001; 136: 245-50.
[http://dx.doi.org/10.1159/000060196]

[75]   Linhart A, Lubanda JC, Palecek T, *et al.* Cardiac manifestations in Fabry disease. J Inherit Metab Dis
2001; 24 (Suppl. 2): 75-83.
[http://dx.doi.org/10.1023/A:1012428009627]

[76]   Schiffmann R, Warnock DG, Banikazemi M, *et al.* Fabry disease: progression of nephropathy, and
prevalence of cardiac and cerebrovascular events before enzyme replacement therapy. Nephrol Dial
Transplant 2009; 24(7): 2102-11.
[http://dx.doi.org/10.1093/ndt/gfp031]

[77]   Fellgiebel A. Mu¨ ller MJ, Ginsberg L. CNS manifestations of Fabry disease. Lancet Neurol 2005; 5:
791-5.
[http://dx.doi.org/10.1016/S1474-4422(06)70548-8]

[78]   Jardim L, Vedolin L, Schwartz IV, *et al.* CNS involvement in Fabry disease: clinical and imaging
studies before and after 12 months of enzyme replacement therapy. J Inherit Metab Dis 2004; 27: 229-
40.
[http://dx.doi.org/10.1023/B:BOLI.0000028794.04349.91]

[79]   Nakamura K, Sekijima Y, Nakamura K, *et al.* Cerebral hemorrhage in Fabry's disease. J Hum Genet
2010; 55(4): 259-61.
[http://dx.doi.org/10.1038/jhg.2010.18]

[80]   Moore DF, Ye F, Schiffmann R, Butman JA. Increased signal intensity in the pulvinar on T1-
weighted images: a pathognomonic MR imaging sign of Fabry disease. AJNR Am J Neuroradiol 2003;
24: 1096-101.

[81]   Lanfranconi S, Markus HS. COL4A1 mutations as a monogenic cause of cerebral small vessel disease:
a systematic review. Stroke 2010; 41(8): e513-8.
[http://dx.doi.org/10.1161/STROKEAHA.110.581918]

[82]   Gould DB, Phalan FC, van Mil SE, *et al.* Role of COL4A1 in small-vessel disease and hemorrhagic
stroke. N Engl J Med 2006; 354(14): 1489-96.
[http://dx.doi.org/10.1056/NEJMoa053727]

[83]   van der Knaap MS, Smit LM, Barkhof F, *et al.* Neonatal porencephaly and adult stroke related to
mutations in collagen IV A1. Ann Neurol 2006; 59(3): 504-11.
[http://dx.doi.org/10.1002/ana.20715]

[84]   Manwaring N, Jones MM, Wang JJ, *et al.* Population prevalence of the MELAS A3243G mutation.
Mitochondrion 2007; 7: 230-3.
[http://dx.doi.org/10.1016/j.mito.2006.12.004]

[85]    Pavlakis SG, Phillips PC, DiMauro S, De Vivo DC, Rowland LP. Mitochondrial myopathy, encephalopathy, lactic acidosis and stroke-like episodes: a distinctive clinical syndrome. Ann Neurol 1984; 16: 481-8.
[http://dx.doi.org/10.1002/ana.410160409]

[86]    Iizuka T, Sakai F. Pathogenesis of stroke-like episodes in MELAS: analysis of neurovascular cellular mechanisms. Curr Neurovasc Res 2005; 2: 29-45.
[http://dx.doi.org/10.2174/1567202052773544]

[87]    Sproule DM, Kaufmann P. Mitochondrial myopathy, encephalopathy, lactic acidosis and stroke-like episodes: basic concepts,clinical phenotype, and therapeutic management of MELAS syndrome. Ann N Y Acad Sci 2008; 1142: 133-58.
[http://dx.doi.org/10.1196/annals.1444.011]

[88]    Ito H, Mori K, Kagami S. Neuroimaging of stroke-like episodes in MELAS. Brain Dev 2011; 33: 283-8.
[http://dx.doi.org/10.1016/j.braindev.2010.06.010]

[89]    Yoneda M, Maeda M, Kimura H, Fujii A, Katayama K, Kuriyama M. Vasogenic edema on MELAS: a serial study with diffusion-weighted MR imaging. Neurology 1999; 53: 2182-4.
[http://dx.doi.org/10.1212/WNL.53.9.2182]

[90]    Sato W, Hayasaka K, Komatsu K, *et al.* Genetic analysis of three pedigrees of mitochondrial myopathy, encephalopathy, lactic acidosis, and strokelike episodes (MELAS). Am J Hum Genet 1992; 50: 655-7.

[91]    Kirby DM, McFarland R, Ohtake A, *et al.* Mutations of the mitochondrial ND1 gene as a cause of MELAS. J Med Genet 2004; 41: 784-9.
[http://dx.doi.org/10.1136/jmg.2004.020537]

[92]    Casas JP, Hingorani AD, Bautista LE, Sharma P. Meta-analysis of genetic studies in ischemic stroke: thirty-two genes involving approximately 18,000 cases and 58,000 controls. Arch Neurol 2004; 61: 1652-61.
[http://dx.doi.org/10.1001/archneur.61.11.1652]

[93]    Ariyaratnam R, Casas JP, Whittaker J, Smeeth L, Hingorani AD, Sharma P. Genetics of ischaemic stroke among persons of non- European descent: a meta-analysis of eight genes involving approximately 32,500 individuals. PLoS Med 2007; 4: e131.
[http://dx.doi.org/10.1371/journal.pmed.0040131]

[94]    Markus HS. Wellcome Trust Genome-Wide Association Study of Ischemic Stroke. Stroke 2013; 44: S20-2.
[http://dx.doi.org/10.1161/STROKEAHA.112.680652]

[95]    Bevan S, Markus HS. Genetics of common polygenic ischaemic stroke: Current understanding and future challenges, Stroke Res. Treat 2011; 2011: 179061.

[96]    Gudbjartsson DF, Arnar DO, Helgadottir A, *et al.* Variants conferring risk of atrial fibrillation on chromosome 4q25. Nature 2007; 448: 353-7.
[http://dx.doi.org/10.1038/nature06007]

[97]    Gretarsdottir S, Thorleifsson G, Manolescu A, *et al.* Risk variants for atrial fibrillation on chromosome

4q25 associate with ischemic stroke. Ann Neurol 2008; 64: 402-9.
[http://dx.doi.org/10.1002/ana.21480]

[98] Gudbjartsson DF, Holm H, Gretarsdottir S, *et al.* A sequence variant inZFHX3on 16q22 associates with atrial fibrillation and ischemic stroke. Nat Genet 2009; 41: 876-8.
[http://dx.doi.org/10.1038/ng.417]

[99] Gudbjartsson DF, Holm H, Gretarsdottir S, *et al.* A sequence variant in ZFHX3 on 16q22 associates with atrial fibrillation and ischemic stroke. Nat Genet 2009; 41: 876-8.
[http://dx.doi.org/10.1038/ng.417]

[100] Gschwendtner A, Bevan S, Cole JW, *et al.* Sequence variants on chromosome 9p21.3 confer risk for atherosclerotic stroke. Ann Neurol 2009; 65: 531-9.
[http://dx.doi.org/10.1002/ana.21590]

[101] Kubo M, Hata J, Ninomiya T, *et al.* A nonsynonymous SNP in PRKCH (protein kinase C eta) increases the risk of cerebral infarction. Nat Genet 2007; 39(2): 212-7.
[http://dx.doi.org/10.1038/ng1945]

[102] Serizawa M, Nabika T, Ochiai Y, *et al.* Association between PRKCH gene polymorphisms and subcortical silent brain infarction. Atherosclerosis 2008; 199(2): 340-5.
[http://dx.doi.org/10.1016/j.atherosclerosis.2007.11.009]

[103] Wu L, Shen Y, Liu X, *et al.* The 1425G/A SNP in PRKCH is associated with ischemic stroke and cerebral hemorrhage in a Chinese population. Stroke 2009; 40(9): 2973-6.
[http://dx.doi.org/10.1161/STROKEAHA.109.551747]

[104] Traylor M, Mäkelä KM, Kilarski LL, *et al.* A novel MMP12 locus is associated with large artery atherosclerotic stroke using a genome-wide age-at-onset informed approach. PLoS Genet 2014; 10(7): e1004469.
[http://dx.doi.org/10.1371/journal.pgen.1004469]

[105] Bellenguez C, Bevan S, Gschwendtner A, *et al.* International Stroke Genetics Consortium (ISGC), Wellcome Trust Case Control Consortium 2 (WTCCC2). Genome-wide association study identifies a variant in HDAC9 associated with large vessel ischemic stroke. Nat Genet 2012; 44(3): 328-33.

[106] Traylor M, Farrall M, Holliday Elizabeth G, *et al.* Genetic risk factors for ischaemic stroke and its subtypes (the METASTROKE collaboration): a meta-analysis of genome-wide association studies. Lancet Neurol 2012; 11(11): 951-62.
[http://dx.doi.org/10.1016/S1474-4422(12)70234-X]

[107] Han Y, Sun W, Wang L, *et al.* HDAC9 gene is associated with stroke risk in a Chinese population. Exp Biol Med (Maywood) 2013; 238(7): 842-7.
[http://dx.doi.org/10.1177/1535370213494650]

[108] Ng SB, Buckingham KJ, Lee C, *et al.* Exome sequencing identifies the cause of a mendelian disorder. Nat Genet 2010; 42: 30-5.
[http://dx.doi.org/10.1038/ng.499]

[109] Boycott KM, Vanstone MR, Bulman DE, MacKenzie AE. Rare-disease genetics in the era of next-generation sequencing: discovery to translation. Nat Rev Genet 2013; 14: 681-91.
[http://dx.doi.org/10.1038/nrg3555]

[110]  Tan RY, Markus HS. Monogenic causes of stroke: now and the future. J Neurol 2015; 262(12): 2601-16.
[http://dx.doi.org/10.1007/s00415-015-7794-4]

# CHAPTER 9

# Diagnostic Challenges: Cryptogenic Ischemic Stroke

**Antonio Vincenti**[*]

*Electrophysiology Unit, Multimedica IRCCS Sesto San Giovanni, Milan, Italy*

**Abstract:** Cryptogenic ischemic stroke defines the situation where the cause of the thromboembolic event is not evident. Atrial fibrillation (AF) is a possible cause of cryptogenic stroke, even if asymptomatic. AF is the most common arrhythmia, and its incidence increases with age. AF is associated with an increased risk of ischemic stroke and systemic embolism, independent of the type of AF and also of the symptoms caused by the arrhythmia. The thromboembolic risk is associated to some clinical variables like age, hypertension, heart failure, diabetes, previous stroke, vascular diseases and gender. The mechanism of thrombosis in AF is complex, and comprises blood stasis in the left atrial appendage, but also atrial and endothelial damage, alteration of the extracellular matrix, and activation of humoral factors with prothrombotic significance.

AF is often asymptomatic or "silent", as demonstrated in many clinical situations. Silent AF may be a frequent cause of otherwise unexplained stroke. The association between stroke and silent AF was demonstrated in many trials, especially in patients with an implanted device, like pacemakers, implantable cardiac defibrillators (ICD) and cardiac resynchronisation therapy (CRT) devices, where a reliable report of the arrhythmia is available. The best system to discover if a patient with cryptogenic stroke has AF is the continuous monitoring with an implantable loop recorder. However, the temporal relationship between AF and stroke is not often evident, so that the decision to prevent thromboembolisms in patients with silent AF should be based on the evaluation of risk with the appropriate score index. In the secondary prevention of stroke and transient ischemic attack (TIA), however, anticoagulation is generally indicated if a silent AF is demonstrated.

[*] **Corresponding author Antonio Vincenti:** Electrophysiology Unit, Multimedica IRCCS Sesto San Giovanni, Milan, Italy; Tel: +39 330237357; Email: antvince@tin.it

Alberto Radaelli, Giuseppe Mancia, Carlo Ferrarese & Simone Beretta (Eds.)

**Keywords:** Atrial fibrillation, Cryptogenic stroke, Implantable defibrillators, Implantable loop recorder, Left atrial appendage, Pacemaker, Silent atrial fibrillation, Thromboembolic risk score, Thromboembolism.

Cryptogenic ischemic stroke (CIS) is defined as the situation where, after the examinations of the acute phase, including an electrocardiogram (EKG), a transthoracic and transesophageal echocardiogram, a 24 hour EKG monitoring, or a telemetric EKG recording, and after assessing the regular neurologic and neurovascular exams, the origin of the ischemic event is not evident.

Epidemiological studies document that between 50 and 60% of strokes are due to cardiovascular documented problems; among them about 15% are due to documented atrial fibrillation, but in about 25-40% of ischemic strokes, no etiologic factor is evident [1 - 5]. A portion of these cerebral ischemic episodes is often attributed to subclinic or silent atrial fibrillation (AF) as the etiologic cause, that is one or more arrhythmic episodes elapsed without symptoms before the index episode [6].

## ATRIAL FIBRILLATION: PREVALENCE AND THROMBOEMBOLIC RISK

Atrial fibrillation is the most common sustained arrhythmia, with a prevalence of between 1 and 2% in the general population, increasing with age, reaching and exceeding 8% in subjects over 80 years of age. AF is associated, as an independent factor, to an increased risk of stroke. Stroke risk is about 5-fold in AF patients compared with controls [7].

The cause of ischemic strokes is AF in about 15-17% of all cases. It is relevant to point out that AF related strokes show a higher mortality and higher disability level than non AF related strokes [8].

It is well known that AF can be classified as *paroxysmal* (when spontaneously ceases, usually within 48 hours from onset, and anyway within 7 days), *persistent* (when it lasts more than 7 days, or can be interrupted with drugs or electrical cardioversion) and *long lasting persistent* or *permanent* (when it lasts a long period and/or is considered not possible to be further interrupted). In spite of what is often considered, the thromboembolic risk does not depend on the type of AF, and, with some limitation that will be discussed later on, neither on the duration of episodes of paroxysmal AF [9, 10].

Conversely, the thromboembolic risk depends on a series of clinical variables, used to construct specific scores to evaluate the risk: the first score was the "$CHADS_2$" [11] (Fig. **1**), which considers congestive heart failure, hypertension, age, diabetes and previous stroke or TIA, the last scoring two points; more recently the "$CHA_2DS_2VASc$" score [12] (Fig. **2**), where age > 74, with double score, the vascular peripheral or coronary disease, and female sex were added (female gender is considered only for more advanced age). As shown in Fig. (**2**), the $CHA_2DS_2VASc$ score is capable to stratify the risk even for the lowest levels, and in particular to identify, for subjects with score 0, a group of patients with a very low risk, similar to patients without AF.

| Stroke Risk Factor | Score |
|---|:---:|
| **C**ongestive Heart Failure | 1 |
| **H**ypertension | 1 |
| **A**ge (> 75 years) | 1 |
| **D**iabetes | 1 |
| Prior **S**troke / TIA | 2 |
| *Max Score* | 6 |

Fig. (**1**). $CHADS_2$ score for calculation of thromboembolic risk in non-valvular atrial fibrillation.

## MECHANISM OF THROMBOSIS AND THROMBO-EMBOLI IN NON-VALVULAR ATRIAL FIBRILLATION

Non-valvular atrial fibrillation (NVAF) is defined as AF in the absence of significant mitral valve disease (stenosis) and mechanical prosthetic valves. The definition is not negligible, inasmuch as the mechanism of atrial thrombosis may be partly different in these situations comparing to NVAF.

| CHA$_2$DS$_2$-VASc criteria | Score | CHA$_2$DS$_2$-VASc total score | Rate of stroke/other TE (%/year) (95% CI)* | |
|---|---|---|---|---|
| **C**ongestive heart failure/ left ventricular dysfunction | 1 | 0 | 0 | (0–0) |
| **H**ypertension | 1 | 1 | 0.6 | (0.0–3.4) |
| **A**ge ≥75 yrs | 2 | 2 | 1.6 | (0.3–4.7) |
| **D**iabetes mellitus | 1 | 3 | 3.9 | (1.7–7.6) |
| **S**troke/transient ischaemic attack/TE | 2 | 4 | 1.9 | (0.5–4.9) |
| | | 5 | 3.2 | (0.7–9.0) |
| **V**ascular disease (prior myocardial infarction, peripheral artery disease or aortic plaque) | 1 | 6 | 3.6 | (0.4–12.3) |
| | | 7 | 8.0 | (1.0–26.0) |
| **A**ge 65–74 yrs | 1 | 8 | 11.1 | (0.3–48.3) |
| **S**ex **c**ategory (i.e. female gender) | 1 | 9 | 100 | (2.5–100) |

**Fig. (2).** CHA$_2$DS$_2$VASc score for calculation of thromboembolic risk in non-valvular atrial fibrillation. Rate of stroke and other thromboembolic events according to the score.

The mechanism of thrombosis in NVAF is somewhat complex: it is true that modifications in the blood flow in the atria in AF play a relevant role, this is applied in particular for inflow and outflow from the left atrial appendage. However, other mechanisms are also involved, such as modifications in the endothelial wall of the atrium, and changes in plasmatic factors involved in the coagulation cascade [13].

The left atrial appendage (LAA) is an accessory chamber of the atrium, whose function is not yet clearly explained; one of the possible functions could be the involvement in neuroendocrine homeostasis. Its shape and dimension vary greatly, and the shape partly determines the formation of thrombi internally, in association with the presence of pectinate muscles that may render its internal surface particularly rough [14, 15].

During sinus rhythm, the atrial-auricular flow is quadriphasic, which is observable when evaluated with transesophageal echocardiogram (TEE), but this kind of flow is lost during AF episodes.

With TEE, the presence of spontaneous echo-contrast, also called "smoke" is often evident; this can be considered a pre-thrombotic situation. This phenomenon is ascribed to the interaction between erythrocytes and fibrinogen that in turn depends on the relative concentration in the blood of the two components. It is highly favored by flow reduction, and it is observable even in sinus rhythm, particularly for a variable period after cardioversion.

In addition to flow modifications, even structural alterations of the atrial wall, particularly at the level of the endocardium in the LAA, may participate in the development of thrombosis. Endocardial damage, with micro-interruptions of the endocardium, and platelet aggregation have been described with electron microscopy, but also with conventional microscopy; and again myocitic hypertrophy and necrosis, and mononuclear cells infiltrates may be evident [16, 17].

Moreover, alterations in the extracellular matrix may be involved in the process, as documented by the increased presence of various metalloproteinases in the bloodstream, their inhibitors and their grown factors: all these factors are involved in the turnover of the collagen matrix. These factors have a discrete relevance in the structural and electrical remodeling of the atrium with AF, and they may also play a role in the coagulation process.

Moreover a lot of data are available, that underline the activation of many humoral factors with prethrombotic significance, generally related to fibrin turnover [13]. In fact, in AF patients high levels of fragments of prothrombin 1 and 2, and of thrombin-prothrombin complexes are found.

The presence and the level of a quite simple prothrombotic index like D-dimer of fibrin was shown to be associated with auricular thrombosis, and its absence has been proposed as an indicator of the absence of thrombosis. An increased D-dimer level is particularly found in AF associated strokes [18].

In the field of biohumoral activation, an increased activity of von Willebrand factor, the activation of fibrinolysis, and platelet activation were described, again leading to the prothrombotic. Many elements may lead to biohumoral modifications in the prothrombotic direction: which include the activation of inflammation factors, of growth factors, the reduction of nitric oxide turnover, and the activation of the renin-angiotensin system.

Actually the combination of factors related to blood flow, of factors related to endothelial lesions and of prothrombotic elements of the blood, fully satisfies the theory of the Virchow Triad, and makes atrial fibrillation a situation of real predisposition to thrombosis [19].

As a confirmation of these statements, it has been shown that the incidence of AF related ischemic stroke is reduced by 60-70% with the use of antithrombotic agents, in particular to warfarin and to the new direct thrombin or Xa-factor inhibitors [20, 21].

## CRYPTOGENIC STROKE AND ATRIAL FIBRILLATION

Actually from 25 to 40% of the ischemic strokes have no explanation [1 - 5]: patent AF is one of the known etiologic causes, both when it is present at the moment of the index event, and when it is reported as anamnestic episode. The patent AF is associated with about 15% of ischemic strokes.

Atrial fibrillation is usually symptomatic, determining palpitations, dyspnoea, fatigue, angina, dizziness and syncope. The presence of symptoms can be classified. In the guidelines of the European Society of Cardiology [22], the classification of symptoms of AF was introduced, expressed in EHRA classes: class I is referred to as the absolute absence of symptoms, while class IV corresponds to the presence of disabling symptoms, such as normal daily activities that need to be interrupted.

Not rarely AF can be asymptomatic or "silent". Although it may happen with high heart rate, it is exactly the heart rate that primarily determinate the degree of perceived symptoms, as is demonstrated by the evidence that many AF episodes may be perceived or not by the same subject, depending on mean heart rate.

The portion of patients with asymptomatic AF is variable according to the clinical context and to the method used to detect it. According to the EURObservational Research Programme - AF (EORP-AF) - Pilot General Registry [23], almost 40% of AF patients visited in the cardiology ambulatory were completely asymptomatic, and another 30% were only slightly symptomatic. In patients who underwent transcatheter ablation like pulmonary vein isolation, the percentage of symptomatic AF recurrences ranged from 0 to 31%, and this variability depends, as in general, on the method used to detect the presence of the arrhythmia, being the highest when it is possible to use continuous monitoring systems, like implantable loop recorders [24, 25].

Even in the case of execution of an EKG for various reasons, it is possible to find silent AF, as an occasional finding, in 16-25% of cases [26]. The treatment with anti-arrhythmic drugs used for rhythm control is often associated with symptom suppression, but quite often this does not correspond to the abolition of the arrhythmia, that may recur without symptoms [27, 28].

However, the real determination of the frequency of silent AF may be obtained only when a prolonged and continuous monitoring system is available. This is the case of subjects with implantable devices (like pacemakers, implantable cardiac defibrillators [ICD] and/or resynchronization devices, and implantable loop recorders). In these situations, from 51 to 74% of the patients show supraventricular tachyarrhythmia, whose recognition is made easier (for most pacemakers and ICDs) by the presence of an atrial lead, making it easy to record the rapid atrial AF potentials [29, 30].

We have pathophysiological assumptions to speculate that AF, even if silent, is the cause of thromboembolism. Actually, all the mechanisms leading to thrombosis are active, even if AF is not sensed. Moreover, from the theoretic point of view, if the arrhythmia is not felt — and this depends essentially on the heart rate and cardiac function — the intervention to interrupt it and the anticoagulation could be delayed, favoring the thrombus formation in this way.

In summary, one of the explanations of cryptogenic stroke is silent atrial fibrillation.

Many studies point out that silent AF is present in cryptogenic strokes with a frequency ranging from 5 and 20% of cases. It is obvious that the chance of discovering silent AF in these patients may not depend only on the EKG recorded at the hospitalization for the index stroke: many experiences indicate that a long lasting monitoring period is needed to obtain an acceptable sensibility in detecting silent AF. In a recent meta-analysis [31], it was confirmed that the chance of detecting silent AF in patients with cryptogenic stroke essentially depends on monitoring duration. The analysis included 31 different studies, 3 of which were randomized, that fulfilled the inclusion criteria of the meta-analysis. The overall proportion of newly detected AF was 7.4%, but it was 5.1% for short monitoring periods (< 3 days) and 15% for monitoring periods longer than 7 days. Prolonging the monitoring period from 24 hours to 30 days and 180 days, the AF was detected in 4.2%, 15.3% and 29.2% of cases, respectively.

According to these evidences, both the guidelines on atrial fibrillation [22] and those on the secondary prevention of stroke and TIA [32] suggest a monitoring period of 30 days or more, for a reliable chance of detecting silent AF.

In patients with cryptogenic stroke, the best performance in terms of detecting silent AF is given by implantable loop recorders (ILR), capable of giving a precise idea of the AF burden, by monitoring EKG up to 36 months. These devices are generally equipped with a software able to recognize AF on the basis of the great variability of the RR interval; even if there is a great amount of false positive readings in this kind of analysis, and an accurate validation of episodes is requested, the false positive readings are absolutely rare. In the prospective randomized Crystal AF study [33], AF was detected in 8.9%, 12.4% and 30% of patients with cryptogenic stroke after 6, 12 and 36 months of monitoring with ILR, respectively. In patients randomized to standard monitoring, AF was detected during the same time periods in 1.4%, 2% and 3% of cases.

A shorter period of monitoring with an event-triggered external recorder was used in the EMBRACE study [34], where an episode of AF ≥ 30" within 90 days was detected in 16.1% of patients in the event recorder group *vs* 2.5% of the control arms.

The rationale is to effectively treat all patients with cryptogenetic stroke or TIA with anticoagulants agents, when the silent AF is documented.

This rationale is not fully unquestionable, first of all for the great heterogeneity of the studies on the incidence of silent AF in cryptogenic stroke, even if the general tendency toward a greater incidence of the arrhythmia with a prolonged monitoring period is maintained.

A second source of uncertainty is the question of what is the shortest duration of an AF episode that can be considered significant as a possible cause of ischemic strokes.

In spite of these doubts, it is ascertained that silent AF is a common finding in patients with cryptogenic stroke (up to 30% of cases if a prolonged monitoring system is used). However, the clinical and prognostic impact of silent AF is yet completely clarified.

Scientific literature provides us only data related to patients with implanted devices, like pacemakers, defibrillators and cardiac resynchronization therapy (CRT) devices; these are the best instruments to give reliable data on the presence of a silent arrhythmia. Obviously these subjects represent only a portion of patients at risk of stroke; however, in these patients, silent AF is associated to an increased risk of thromboembolic events with a hazard ratio ranging from 2.2 to 9.4 [35]. An asymptomatic AF could be associated even to an increased mortality [36]. According to the above mentioned EURObservational Research Programme - AF (EORP-AF) Pilot General Registry [23], the mortality is even doubled when silent AF is present, compared to symptomatic arrhythmia.

Regarding the minimum duration of an arrhythmic episode determining an increased risk, this depends on the definition of "arrhythmic event" given in each individual study considered.

In the Ancillary MOST (Mode Selection Trial), an increased risk was determined with episodes longer than 5' [29]. In the ASSERT study [37], the risk was increased in the presence of arrhythmic episodes longer than 6' (we are dealing with a quite low level of risk, *i.e.*, 1.69% per year in patients with AF episodes *vs* 0.69% per year in those non presenting arrhythmic episodes).

And again, in the index episodes, the expression of an increased risk was longer than 1 hour in the SOS-AF Project (Stroke prevention Strategies Based on Information From Implanted Device) [38], longer than 3.8 hours in the Home Monitor CRT trial [39], longer than 5.5 hours in the TRENDS trial [40], up to the longest duration of 24 hours in the "Registro Italiano di AT500" [30].

From these data it is evident that, if it is definite that the presence of AF episodes is associated with an increased risk of thromboembolic events, the critical duration of the episodes in order to establish a real risk is still debatable.

The issue has been better clarified by the work of Botto and coworkers [41], where the authors, again by analyzing the data stored in the implanted devices, identified patients with AF episodes longer than 5', and those with episodes longer than 24 hours. At the same time patients were stratified according to the CHADS$_2$ score: patients with a higher score presented a high risk of thromboembolic events (5%) even without AF episodes. On the contrary patients with a CHADS$_2$ score 0 presented a low risk (0, 8%), even with episodes longer than 24 hours.

In other words, it seems that there is not a critical duration of the episodes determining an increased risk, but it is advisable to consider these data — when available — together with the general risk of thromboembolic events (Fig. **3**).

# Risk of thromboembolic events

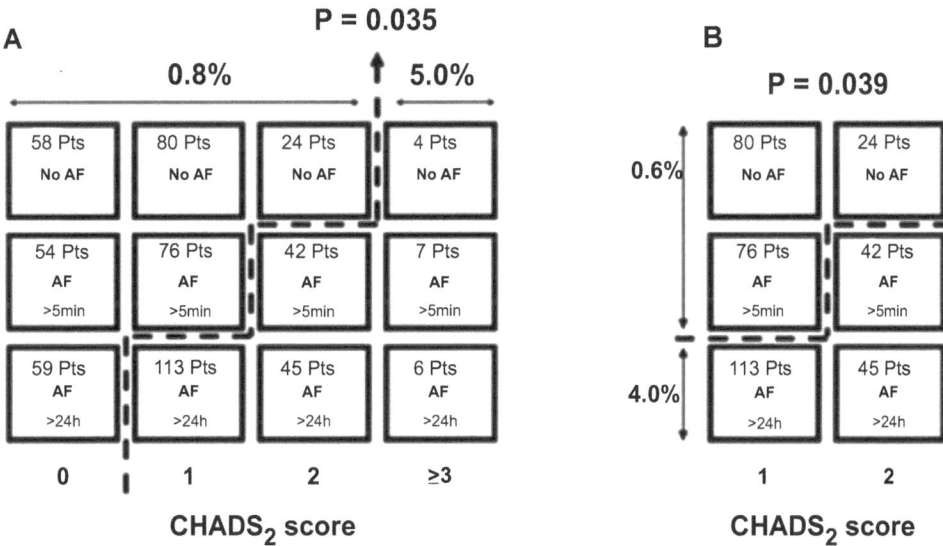

**Fig. (3).** from Botto GL *et al.* [41]. Combining the data on atrial fibrillation (AF), AF duration and CHADS2 score enabled the whole population to be separated (dashed line) in two groups with different risks of thromboembolic events.

Moreover, in view of these data, one issue remains unresolved: it is not clear if silent arrhythmia is the direct cause of thromboembolism, or only a marker of its increased risk. Many studies at this regard analyzed the time relationship between the arrhythmia onset and the thromboembolic event. In the ASSERT study [42], among 51 patients with an implanted device, who had a stroke or a thromboembolic event, 26 (51%) showed episodes of asymptomatic AF, but only 18 of them (35%) just before the event, and only 4 (8%) in the 30 days before the event.

In the TRENDS study [43] 40 patients with an implanted device had a stroke or systemic thromboembolism: only 50% of them showed AF or a trial tachyarrhythmias before the event, but 9 of them had no episode in the 30 days before the stroke. Therefore, in summary, 73% of patients with thromboembolic events did not show any arrhythmic episodes in the 30 days before the index event.

In the IMPACT study [44], among 69 patients with an implanted device and thromboembolic events, only 20 (29%) showed tachyarrhythmic episodes 1-489 days before the event, while in the remaining 71% of patients no AF episode preceding the clinical event was found.

Although the association between supra-ventricular tachyarrhythmias and thromboembolic events is quite evident, the relation of cause and effect is not completely proved.

In addition to these considerations, in the IMPACT study [44], in which patients with implanted devices showing tachyarrhythmias were randomized to receive anticoagulant agents (mainly anti vitamin K agents) only when AF was detected, or in the traditional way; it was necessary to interrupt the study after 2 years of follow-up, because it was impossible to demonstrate any outcome differences between patients taking anticoagulants "on demand" or in the regular way (total number of events, major haemorrhagic events, thromboembolic events).

These data, even if partial, make the basic assumption of an absolute indication to anticoagulation in subjects with silent AF and a high risk of thromboembolic events debatable. It is likely that further large, prospective and randomized studies are needed to fully clarify the problem. Moreover, one has to keep in mind that all the reported data only concern patients with implanted devices, and they represent a selected population.

For patients with silent AF and previous thromboembolic events, it is useful to remember that the mechanisms leading to stroke may be multiple. In some cases the blood stasis provoked in the atrium by AF may play a determinant role, but in other cases the structural atrial and endothelial modifications, caused by previous and repeated AF episodes, may be important. Finally, in some cases the stroke mechanism may not be related to AF at all.

In many cases, the presence of AF episodes may simply be a marker of an increased risk of thromboembolic recurrence, and it may interact with other factors, like hypertension, diabetes, heart failure and other vascular diseases. The level of risk is then determined by score systems such as the $CHA_2DS_2$-VASc, which includes all these elements.

While the indication to anticoagulant therapy is still debatable in patients with silent AF, as concluded trials demonstrating its advantage are lacking, in the presence of cryptogenetic stroke or TIA that *"per se"* implies a score of 2 points in the $CHA_2DS_2$-VASc system, the indication to anticoagulant therapy being reasonably determined, according to the common opinion and to the current guidelines [22, 32].

## CONCLUSION

Atrial fibrillation, even if asymptomatic, is a frequent cause of ischemic stroke. The time relationship between the arrhythmia and the neurologic event is often lacking, so that atrial fibrillation is more easily considered a marker of thromboembolic risk rather than a direct cause of the ischemic stroke.

Therefore, unless there are absolute contraindications, treatment with anticoagulant drugs is indicated in secondary prevention of ischemic stroke, when atrial fibrillation is demonstrated.

Long duration EKG monitoring is recommended to examine the presence of silent atrial fibrillation episodes, if these are not evident at the basal EKG or in anamnestic reports.

## TAKE HOME MESSAGE

Atrial fibrillation, even if asymptomatic, is a frequent cause of ischemic stroke. Long duration EKG monitoring is recommended to examine the presence of silent atrial fibrillation episodes. Unless there are absolute contraindications, treatment with anticoagulant drugs is indicated in secondary prevention of ischemic stroke, when atrial fibrillation is demonstrated.

## CONFLICT OF INTEREST

The author confirms that the author has no conflict of interest to declare for this publication.

## ACKNOWLEDGEMENTS

Declared none.

## REFERENCES

[1]   Wolf PA, Dawber TR, Thomas HE Jr, Kannel WB. Epidemiologic assessment of chronic atrial fibrillation and risk of stroke: the Framingham study. Neurology 1978; 28(10): 973-7.
[http://dx.doi.org/10.1212/WNL.28.10.973] [PMID: 570666]

[2]   Tayal AH, Tian M, Kelly KM, *et al.* Atrial fibrillation detected by mobile cardiac outpatient telemetry in cryptogenic TIA or stroke. Neurology 2008; 71(21): 1696-701.
[http://dx.doi.org/10.1212/01.wnl.0000325059.86313.31] [PMID: 18815386]

[3]   Jabaudon D, Sztajzel J, Sievert K, Landis T, Sztajzel R. Usefulness of ambulatory 7-day ECG monitoring for the detection of atrial fibrillation and flutter after acute stroke and transient ischemic attack. Stroke 2004; 35(7): 1647-51.
[http://dx.doi.org/10.1161/01.STR.0000131269.69502.d9] [PMID: 15155965]

[4]   Ionita CC, Xavier AR, Kirmani JF, Dash S, Divani AA, Qureshi AI. What proportion of stroke is not explained by classic risk factors? Prev Cardiol 2005; 8(1): 41-6.
[http://dx.doi.org/10.1111/j.1520-037X.2005.3143.x] [PMID: 15722693]

[5]   Sacco RL, Ellenberg JH, Mohr JP, *et al.* Infarcts of undetermined cause: the NINCDS Stroke Data Bank. Ann Neurol 1989; 25(4): 382-90.
[http://dx.doi.org/10.1002/ana.410250410] [PMID: 2712533]

[6]   Liao J, Khalid Z, Scallan C, Morillo C, ODonnell M. Noninvasive cardiac monitoring for detecting paroxysmal atrial fibrillation or flutter after acute ischemic stroke: a systematic review. Stroke 2007;

38(11): 2935-40.
[http://dx.doi.org/10.1161/STROKEAHA.106.478685] [PMID: 17901394]

[7]     Wolf PA, Abbott RD, Kannel WB. Atrial fibrillation as an independent risk factor for stroke: the Framingham Study. Stroke 1991; 22(8): 983-8.
[http://dx.doi.org/10.1161/01.STR.22.8.983] [PMID: 1866765]

[8]     Lamassa M, Di Carlo A, Pracucci G, *et al.* Characteristics, outcome, and care of stroke associated with atrial fibrillation in Europe: data from a multicenter multinational hospital-based registry (The European Community Stroke Project). Stroke 2001; 32(2): 392-8.
[http://dx.doi.org/10.1161/01.STR.32.2.392] [PMID: 11157172]

[9]     Hart RG, Pearce LA, Rothbart RM, McAnulty JH, Asinger RW, Halperin JL. Stroke with intermittent atrial fibrillation: incidence and predictors during aspirin therapy. J Am Coll Cardiol 2000; 35(1): 183-7.
[http://dx.doi.org/10.1016/S0735-1097(99)00489-1] [PMID: 10636278]

[10]    Hohnloser SH, Pajitnev D, Pogue J, *et al.* Incidence of stroke in paroxysmal *versus* sustained atrial fibrillation in patients taking oral anticoagulation or combined antiplatelet therapy: an ACTIVE W Substudy. J Am Coll Cardiol 2007; 50(22): 2156-61.
[http://dx.doi.org/10.1016/j.jacc.2007.07.076] [PMID: 18036454]

[11]    Gage BF, Waterman AD, Shannon W, Boechler M, Rich MW, Radford MJ. Validation of clinical classification schemes for predicting stroke: results from the National Registry of Atrial Fibrillation. JAMA 2001; 285(22): 2864-70.
[http://dx.doi.org/10.1001/jama.285.22.2864] [PMID: 11401607]

[12]    Lip GY, Nieuwlaat R, Pisters R, Lane DA, Crijns HJ. Refining clinical risk stratification for predicting stroke and thromboembolism in atrial fibrillation using a novel risk factor-based approach: the euro heart survey on atrial fibrillation. Chest 2010; 137(2): 263-72.
[http://dx.doi.org/10.1378/chest.09-1584] [PMID: 19762550]

[13]    Watson T, Shantsila E, Lip GY. Mechanisms of thrombogenesis in atrial fibrillation: Virchows triad revisited. Lancet 2009; 373(9658): 155-66.
[http://dx.doi.org/10.1016/S0140-6736(09)60040-4] [PMID: 19135613]

[14]    Blackshear JL, Odell JA. Appendage obliteration to reduce stroke in cardiac surgical patients with atrial fibrillation. Ann Thorac Surg 1996; 61(2): 755-9.
[http://dx.doi.org/10.1016/0003-4975(95)00887-X] [PMID: 8572814]

[15]    Pollick C, Taylor D. Assessment of left atrial appendage function by transesophageal echocardiography. Implications for the development of thrombus. Circulation 1991; 84(1): 223-31.
[http://dx.doi.org/10.1161/01.CIR.84.1.223] [PMID: 2060098]

[16]    Boldt A, Wetzel U, Lauschke J, *et al.* Fibrosis in left atrial tissue of patients with atrial fibrillation with and without underlying mitral valve disease. Heart 2004; 90(4): 400-5.
[http://dx.doi.org/10.1136/hrt.2003.015347] [PMID: 15020515]

[17]    Frustaci A, Chimenti C, Bellocci F, Morgante E, Russo MA, Maseri A. Histological substrate of atrial biopsies in patients with lone atrial fibrillation. Circulation 1997; 96(4): 1180-4.
[http://dx.doi.org/10.1161/01.CIR.96.4.1180] [PMID: 9286947]

[18]   Turgut N, Akdemir O, Turgut B, *et al.* Hypercoagulopathy in stroke patients with nonvalvular atrial fibrillation: hematologic and cardiology investigations. Clin Appl Thromb Hemost 2006; 12(1): 15-20.
[http://dx.doi.org/10.1177/107602960601200104] [PMID: 16444430]

[19]   Brotman DJ, Deitcher SR, Lip GY, Matzdorff AC. Virchows triad revisited. South Med J 2004; 97(2): 213-4.
[http://dx.doi.org/10.1097/01.SMJ.0000105663.01648.25] [PMID: 14982286]

[20]   Hart RG, Pearce LA, Aguilar MI. Meta-analysis: antithrombotic therapy to prevent stroke in patients who have nonvalvular atrial fibrillation. Ann Intern Med 2007; 146(12): 857-67.
[http://dx.doi.org/10.7326/0003-4819-146-12-200706190-00007] [PMID: 17577005]

[21]   Ruff CT, Giugliano RP, Braunwald E, *et al.* Comparison of the efficacy and safety of new oral anticoagulants with warfarin in patients with atrial fibrillation: a meta-analysis of randomised trials. Lancet 2014; 383(9921): 955-62.
[http://dx.doi.org/10.1016/S0140-6736(13)62343-0] [PMID: 24315724]

[22]   Camm AJ, Lip GY, De Caterina R, *et al.* 2012 focused update of the ESC Guidelines for the management of atrial fibrillation: an update of the 2010 ESC Guidelines for the management of atrial fibrillation. Developed with the special contribution of the European Heart Rhythm Association. Eur Heart J 2012; 33(21): 2719-47.
[http://dx.doi.org/10.1093/eurheartj/ehs253] [PMID: 22922413]

[23]   Boriani G, Laroche C, Diemberger I, *et al.* Asymptomatic atrial fibrillation: clinical correlates, management and outcome in the EURObservational Research Program - AF (EORP-AF) - Pilot General Registry. Am J Med 2014 Dec 19; pii: S0002-9343(14)01207-.
[http://dx.doi.org/10.1016/j.amjmed.2014.11.026]

[24]   Steven D, Rostock T, Lutomsky B, *et al.* What is the real atrial fibrillation burden after catheter ablation of atrial fibrillation? A prospective rhythm analysis in pacemaker patients with continuous atrial monitoring. Eur Heart J 2008; 29(8): 1037-42.
[http://dx.doi.org/10.1093/eurheartj/ehn024] [PMID: 18263865]

[25]   Manganiello S, Anselmino M, Amellone C, *et al.* Symptomatic and asymptomatic long-term recurrences following transcatheter atrial fibrillation ablation. Pacing Clin Electrophysiol 2014; 37(6): 697-702.
[http://dx.doi.org/10.1111/pace.12387] [PMID: 24665920]

[26]   Nieuwlaat R, Capucci A, Camm AJ, *et al.* Atrial fibrillation management: a prospective survey in ESC member countries: the Euro Heart Survey on Atrial Fibrillation. Eur Heart J 2005; 26(22): 2422-34.
[http://dx.doi.org/10.1093/eurheartj/ehi505] [PMID: 16204266]

[27]   Patten M, Maas R, Bauer P, *et al.* Suppression of paroxysmal atrial tachyarrhythmiasresults of the SOPAT trial. Eur Heart J 2004; 25(16): 1395-404.
[http://dx.doi.org/10.1016/j.ehj.2004.06.014] [PMID: 15321697]

[28]   Fetsch T, Bauer P, Engberding R, *et al.* Prevention of atrial fibrillation after cardioversion: results of the PAFAC trial. Eur Heart J 2004; 25(16): 1385-94.
[http://dx.doi.org/10.1016/j.ehj.2004.04.015] [PMID: 15302102]

[29]  Glotzer TV, Hellkampt AS, Zimmerman J, *et al.* MOST Investigators. Atrial high rate episodes detected by pacemaker diagnostics predict death and stroke: report of the Atrial Diagnostic Ancillary Study of the Mode Selection Trial (MOST). Circulation 2003; 107: 1614-9.
[http://dx.doi.org/10.1161/01.CIR.0000057981.70380.45] [PMID: 12668495]

[30]  Capucci A, Santini M, Padeletti L, *et al.* Monitored atrial fibrillation duration predicts arterial embolic events in patients suffering from bradycardia and atrial fibrillation implanted with antitachycardia pacemakers. J Am Coll Cardiol 2005; 46(10): 1913-20.
[http://dx.doi.org/10.1016/j.jacc.2005.07.044] [PMID: 16286180]

[31]  Dussault C, Toeg H, Nathan M, Wang ZJ, Roux JF, Secemsky E. Electrocardiographic monitoring for detecting atrial fibrillation after ischemic stroke or transient ischemic attack: systematic review and meta-analysis. Circ Arrhythm Electrophysiol 2015; 8(2): 263-9.
[http://dx.doi.org/10.1161/CIRCEP.114.002521] [PMID: 25639643]

[32]  Kernan WN, Ovbiagele B, Black HR, *et al.* Guidelines for the prevention of stroke in patients with stroke and transient ischemic attack: a guideline for healthcare professionals from the American Heart Association/American Stroke Association. Stroke 2014; 45(7): 2160-236.
[http://dx.doi.org/10.1161/STR.0000000000000024] [PMID: 24788967]

[33]  Choe WC, Passman RS, Brachmann J, *et al.* CRYSTAL AF Investigators. A comparison of atrial fibrillation monitoring strategies after Cryptogenic stroke (from the Cryptogenic stroke and underlying AF trial). Am J Cardiol 2015; 116(6): 889-93.
[http://dx.doi.org/10.1016/j.amjcard.2015.06.012] [PMID: 26183793]

[34]  Gladstone DJ, Spring M, Dorian P, *et al.* Atrial fibrillation in patients with cryptogenic stroke. N Engl J Med 2014; 370(26): 2467-77.
[http://dx.doi.org/10.1056/NEJMoa1311376] [PMID: 24963566]

[35]  Glotzer TV, Ziegler PD. Cryptogenic stroke: Is silent atrial fibrillation the culprit? Heart Rhythm 2015; 12(1): 234-41.
[http://dx.doi.org/10.1016/j.hrthm.2014.09.058] [PMID: 25285649]

[36]  Martinez C, Katholing A, Freedman SB. Adverse prognosis of incidentally detected ambulatory atrial fibrillation. A cohort study. Thromb Haemost 2014; 112: 276-86.
[http://dx.doi.org/10.1160/TH4-04-0383] [PMID: 24953051]

[37]  Healey JS, Connolly SJ, Gold MR, *et al.* Subclinical atrial fibrillation and the risk of stroke. N Engl J Med 2012; 366(2): 120-9.
[http://dx.doi.org/10.1056/NEJMoa1105575] [PMID: 22236222]

[38]  Boriani G, Glotzer TV, Santini M, *et al.* Device-detected atrial fibrillation and risk for stroke: an analysis of >10,000 patients from the SOS AF project (Stroke preventiOn Strategies based on Atrial Fibrillation information from implanted devices). Eur Heart J 2014; 35(8): 508-16.
[http://dx.doi.org/10.1093/eurheartj/eht491] [PMID: 24334432]

[39]  Shanmugam N, Boerdlein A, Proff J, *et al.* Detection of atrial high-rate events by continuous home monitoring: clinical significance in the heart failure-cardiac resynchronization therapy population. Europace 2012; 14(2): 230-7.
[http://dx.doi.org/10.1093/europace/eur293] [PMID: 21933802]

[40]   Glotzer TV, Daoud EG, Wyse DG, *et al.* The relationship between daily atrial tachyarrhythmia burden from implantable device diagnostics and stroke risk: the TRENDS study. Circ Arrhythm Electrophysiol 2009; 2(5): 474-80.
[http://dx.doi.org/10.1161/CIRCEP.109.849638] [PMID: 19843914]

[41]   Botto GL, Padeletti L, Santini M, *et al.* Presence and duration of atrial fibrillation detected by continuous monitoring: crucial implication for the risk of thromboembolic events. J Cardiovasc Electrophysiol 2009; 20: 241-8.

[42]   Brambatti M, Connolly SJ, Gold MR, *et al.* Temporal relationship between subclinical atrial fibrillation and embolic events. Circulation 2014; 129(21): 2094-9.
[http://dx.doi.org/10.1161/CIRCULATIONAHA.113.007825] [PMID: 24633881]

[43]   Daoud EG, Glotzer TV, Wyse DG, *et al.* Temporal relationship of atrial tachyarrhythmias, cerebrovascular events, and systemic emboli based on stored device data: a subgroup analysis of TRENDS. Heart Rhythm 2011; 8(9): 1416-23.
[http://dx.doi.org/10.1016/j.hrthm.2011.04.022] [PMID: 21699833]

[44]   Martin DT, Bersohn MM, Waldo AL, *et al.* Randomized trial of atrial arrhythmia monitoring to guide anticoagulation in patients with implanted defibrillator and cardiac resynchronization devices. Eur Heart J 2015; 36(26): 1660-8.
[http://dx.doi.org/10.1093/eurheartj/ehv115] [PMID: 25908774]

# CHAPTER 10

# Emerging Concepts for Neuroprotection

**Barbara Casolla, Serena Candela, Giuliano Sette** and **Francesco Orzi**[*]

*NESMOS (Neuroscience Mental Health and Sensory Organs) Department, School of Medicine and Psychology, Sapienza University, Rome, Italy*

**Abstract:** Following an ischemic insult, the early damage associated with the energy defect gives rise to molecular events, which may occur even during reperfusion to sustain a progression of the damage in the ensuing hours or days. *Neuroprotection* refers to interventions that are supposed to beneficially interfere with the maturation of the ischemic damage. The post-ischemic molecular events embrace a huge variety of mechanisms. Each mechanism is entangled with others, to configure a pathogenic process that has the characteristics of a near-chaotic phenomenon. To add to the complexity, the ischemic process includes both mechanisms that fuel the pathogenic process promoting cell death, and mechanisms reflecting the effort of the organism to oppose the process.

Interventions aimed to oppose the maturation process activate brain repair and epigenetic mechanisms to promote survival pathways. Examples of potential neuroprotective approaches are: pre- and post-conditioning, hypothermia, and a number of drugs. All the treatments, however, that were proven to be effective in animal models, failed in clinical trials. No unique explanation accounts for the gap between laboratory animal and clinical studies.

**Keywords:** Acute ischemic stroke, Clinical trials, Experimental stroke models, Ischemic cascade, Ischemic conditioning, Mynocycline, Neuroprotection, Therapeutic hypothermia.

[*] **Corresponding author Francesco Orzi:** NESMOS (Neuroscience Mental Health and Sensory Organs) Department, School of Medicine and Psychology, Sapienza University, Rome, Italy; Tel: 06 3377 5829; Fax: 06 3377 5902; Email: francesco.orzi@uniroma1.it

Alberto Radaelli, Giuseppe Mancia, Carlo Ferrarese & Simone Beretta (Eds.)

.

# INTRODUTION

In a classical experimental set up, 5 minutes of bilateral occlusion of the carotid arteries in the gerbil causes no apparent, immediate brain tissue damage. The animal survives the transient loss of blood flow to the entire brain without evident behavioral abnormality or structural tissue damage. Parts of the brain, however, eventually dye hours or days following the ischemic insult. Typically, following the 5-minute occlusion the animals develop a focal lesion in the CA1 section of the hippocampus. The lesion becomes structurally evident 3 or 4 days post ischemia. Remarkably, the pathogenic process that eventually leads to cell death occurs under conditions of normal cerebral blood flow (CBF), as the perfusion returns back to normal in a few minutes after the release of the occlusion. Two phenomena, therefore, characterize the 2-vessel 5-minute occlusion in the gerbil: 1) an interval of time during which there is no structural change before the damage eventually becomes apparent, 2-4 days following recirculation (*maturation phenomenon*); 2) a focal distribution of the damage in spite of the whole brain ischemia (*selective vulnerability*).

If the vessel occlusion lasts just 2-minutes, the animal survives to the insult without any apparent lesion to be observed in the ensuing days. The non-lethal 2-minutes occlusion, however, makes the animal tolerant to the 5-minute insult. Thus, performing a 2-minute vessel occlusion in the gerbil 2 days before a subsequent 5-minute occlusion makes the typically lethal insult ineffective. This is to say that a subliminal, or non-lethal, insult acts as a *preconditioning* stimulus, which makes the animal tolerant to ischemia (*ischemic tolerance*).

The findings (*maturation phenomenon*, and *preconditioning*) indicate that the ischemic insult triggers a number of changes, which have a progress over time. The changes seem to include mechanisms that promote the ischemic damage and, at the same time, mechanisms that counteract the insult. In addition, the *selective vulnerability* phenomenon clearly suggests that intrinsic tissue factors contribute heavily to the damage, as the same blood flow reduction (in terms of intensity and duration) causes tissue damage in certain areas of the brain and not in others. Severe hypoxia or hypoglycemia as well may produce brain injuries limited to specific brain areas, consistently with the notion that variables other than blood flow, both local and systemic, are relevant in determining the vulnerability to the energy deprivation.

The report of the maturation phenomenon has boosted research in the field, as it became evident that ischemic damage is not just a sudden event causing necrosis. It can be a process triggered, but not sustained, by the initial ischemic insult. In the last three decades a huge amount of data and high number of reports have characterized the mechanisms associated with the ischemic insult. The findings all together depict a complex picture in which several variables interact in a conflicting mode. It is worth stressing that deleterious mechanisms may coexist with protective mechanisms. As a whole the post-ischemic event configures a sort of chaotic system, which is affected by both local and systemic variables. Dissecting the different components is an impossible task. We might grossly consider two conceptual frameworks to describe the ischemic pathogenic process, as suggested by experimental observations [1].

One aspect refers to the hemodynamic abnormalities, which cause a defect in supply of energy substrates to the brain. Following an ischemic insult, the mismatch between energy demand and supply from blood circulation is the main mechanism involved in causing an early damage and in triggering the maturation process. The initial mismatch is obviously related to the low residual blood flow. In absence of energy deposits, the brain tissue uniquely relies on continuous supply of oxygen and nutrients. Within minutes after ischemia loss of ATP results in decreased function of the ion pumps and consequent break-down of the ion gradient, which is the basic mechanism for the electrochemical force that drives the neuronal signaling. Under physiological conditions, a partial decrease of the electrochemical energy is restored by a transient increase of the local blood flow (*functional hyperemia*). During ischemia, the lack of fuel causes a sustained failure of the sodium pumps and sustained depolarization. Such a depolarization is characterized by near-complete break-down of the ion gradient across the membrane, loss of electrical activity and neuronal swelling (*cytotoxic edema*). The depolarization may spread to the surrounding naive tissue (*spreading depolarization*). Neuronal depolarization causes glutamate release. Both NMDA and AMPA/kainate receptors contribute to the excitotoxic neuronal response, which amplifies the initial energy mismatch. All these phenomena occur in the early post-ischemia phase. The initial energy/supply mismatch may be as deep as to cause an irreversible process, which brings the tissue to death in a few minutes. Such a short interval occurs for instance in conditions in which the residual blood flow is lower that 20-30% of normal. The interval may be longer and the tissue may die in 1-2 hours if the entity of the residual blood is not as low. This condition is best modeled in animals with permanent vessel occlusion.

A second framework conceptualizes the biochemical changes that occur under restored blood flow. In cases in which the ischemia is followed by efficient reperfusion the mismatch subdues to events that are not directly related to the energy defect. Indeed the events may require energy or protein synthesis. Thus, these events are triggered, but not sustained, by the initial energy defect. They consist in a cascade process, which eventually brings the cells to death, in spite of the recovered blood flow. In these cases cells may die hours or days following the insult. Other cells may instead lose their function to recover in a late stage. This is a phase that might be defined *molecular* more than *haemodynamic*, in order to stress the relevance of biochemical processes that occur under conditions of restored blood flow. This phase operationally defines the time during which neuroprotective interventions potentially unwind the molecular cascade of event that drive the cells to dysfunction or death. Such a phase is modeled in animals submitted to temporary vessel occlusion, followed by reperfusion. In models of focal ischemia such molecular events are peripheral with respect to the ischemic core and characterize the dynamic features of the so-called *penumbra*. Intuitively, different ischemic conditions distribute along a continuum at the extremes of which is the complete-permanent ischemia that causes cell death in a few minute, and the incomplete-temporary occlusion that may end up in delayed recovery.

## Neuroprotection

Interventions aimed to oppose the energy mismatch are essentially addressed to reduce the energy demand or improve the blood flow. These interventions are conceptually effective only if carried out in the early phase of the ischemia. How early it is mostly determined by the entity of the residual blood flow and duration of the ischemia and by a number of variables, which include age, diabetes, hypertension, local or systemic inflammations, and body temperature. In conditions of near-zero blood flow without reperfusion the "therapeutic window" might be as short as few minutes, as previously mentioned. Theoretically, the interventions aimed to oppose the pathogenic mechanisms associated with no-reflow include administration of drugs to suppress the spreading depolarization, or hypothermia in order to reduce the metabolic demand of the ischemic tissue. Considerable interest has been recently devoted to the improvement of collateral blood supply in order to elude the vessel obstruction causing the ischemia [2]. Experimental techniques that supposedly increase blood flow mediated by collaterals include volume expansion, partial aortic occlusion or external pressure cuffs and, stimulation of the sphenopalatine ganglion [3]. As part of the parasympathetic cerebrovascular innervation the sphenopalatine ganglion receives preganglionic neurons from the superior salivatory nucleus. Postganglionic neurons provide nitroxidergic innervation to the cerebral vasculature. Innervation of the carotid and intracerebral arteries is extensive, and several neurotransmitters (such as acetylcholine, vasoactive intestinal polypeptide, and nitrous oxide) are involved in vasodilation. Stimulation of the sphenopalatine ganglion (in rats, cats, or humans) results in ipsilateral vasodilatory response, consisting in a sensible (up to 40%) increase in blood flow.

The term *neuroprotection* best addresses the effects of interventions that are supposed to beneficially interfere with the "metabolic" processes. These are the mechanisms that (in our schematic, simplified approach) follow the initial mismatch phase and occur during reperfusion and are triggered but not sustained by the energy defect. Thus, objective of neuroprotection is to contrast the pathogenic molecular events that determine the maturation of the ischemic damage. Obviously the dichotomy between energy defect and "molecular" events refers to a hyper-simplified scheme. The two mechanisms may coexist. Still they might represent different distribution in space and time. For instance, if the reperfusion is present but it is partial (in extent or late in time) the energy defect and molecular phases partially overlap. Areas of early damage or necrosis, mainly located in the central ischemic core, may coexist with areas of dysfunctional brain, which may evolve in late cell death or tissue damage, or recovery [1].

Molecular events that follow the ischemic insult embrace a huge variety of mechanisms. Each mechanism is entangled with others, so to configure a pathogenic process that has the characteristics of a near-chaotic phenomenon. To add to the complexity, the ischemic process includes mechanisms that seem to fuel the pathogenic process and promote the cell deaths and, at the same time, mechanisms reflecting the effort of the organism to oppose the process. The different mechanisms are reviewed elsewhere [4, 5].

The "molecular" phase is better described in terms of interactions among blood cells, endothelial cells, immune cells, neurons, glia and other components of the neurovascular unit. The endothelium releases factors that can influence the proliferation and differentiation of adjacent cells. Adhesion molecules (such as P-selectin) are translocated to the surface membrane of platelets and endothelial cells, and pro-inflammatory signals are rapidly generated. Activated platelets release cytokines (IL-1a). Neutrophils, macrophages, mast cells and lymphocytes can enter the brain, mainly as a result of disruption of the BBB. The surface receptors on neutrophils and macrophages activate cell signaling that enhances inflammatory processes. Dendritic cells (DCs), macrophages and microglia behave as antigen-presenting cells (APCs). These cells transport the antigen to the regional lymph nodes and present it to lymphocytes. Pathogen recognition is accomplished by a series of surface receptors, which respond to two major classes of molecules: pathogen-associated patterns (PAMPs) and damage-associated patterns (DAMPs). DAMPs include molecules released by damaged neurons. DAMPs, as well PAMPs, bind to cell receptors called pattern recognition receptors (PRRs). PRRs include the toll-like receptors (TLRs) and the nucleotide-binding domain leucine-rich repeat–containing receptors (NLRs). DAMPs mainly activate TLRs, which reside on the plasma membrane or in endosomal compartments. The engagement of TLRs activates NF-κB, resulting in increased transcription of over 150 genes, mainly encoding IL-1 family cytokines. ATP and UTP activate NLRs, whose function is dependent on the assembly of large (~700-kDa) complexes termed "inflammasomes". TLRs and NLRs are therefore highly effective at sensing and responding to non-infectious sterile tissue injury, as observed in stroke or trauma.

**Double Sword Process**

Superimposed to mechanism that drive cells and tissue to necrosis or delayed death are a number of processes directed at preserving the tissue or promoting repair [6]. Examples of intracellular mechanisms include protein synthesis inhibition [7], activation of anti-apoptotic pathways, release of neurotransmitters that oppose the glutamate-driven excitotoxicity, increased expression of growth factors (such as VEGF, EPO) and of antioxidant response, upregulation of chaperon proteins and production of anti-inflammatory and neuroprotective cytokines such as interleukin-10 and transforming growth factor-$\beta$.

The very same mechanisms or pathways, however that contribute to cell survival or tissue repair may also promote cellular death, depending on a number of local or systemic variables. For instance, over-activation of NMDA receptors induces acute excitotoxicity [8], but without NMDA signaling, chronic neuronal remodeling cannot take place [9]. NMDA receptor location and subunit composition differentially regulate neuronal survival or death. Selective enhancement of synaptic receptors (in which NR2A peptide subunits predominate over NR2B) promotes neuronal survival [10]. The finding clearly indicates the risk of a therapeutic approach based on indiscriminate pharmacological manipulation of the NMDA function, one that doesn't take into account the pro-survival in addition to the excitotoxic role of these receptors. Matrix metalloproteinases degrade and damage neurovascular substrates in the acute phase [11], but the same proteases may promote the recovery phase [12]. The intracellular mediator HMGB1 promotes necrosis [13] but released from reactive astrocytes it may promote angiogenesis and synaptic plasticity in the recovery phase [14].

A large body of data has grown in the last decade to demonstrate that inflammation is a central component in the pathophysiology of cerebral ischemia. Neuroprotective strategies aimed to manipulate different aspects of the inflammation have, however, given contradictory results, in experimental animal models [15]. Where the immune response (especially the early, innate one) contributes to the post-ischemic injury, the same response may enhance tissue repair and function recovery. Trying to determine whether inflammation is good or bad for stroke reflects a naive question. Inflammation embraces a number of different mechanisms within a complex scenario, where deleterious events are counteracted by protective mechanisms, in a very reciprocally connected way.

## Systemic Variables

The entire scenario represent a complex system, influenced by a large number of variables, which seem to exceed the boundaries of just a central nervous system event [16, 17]. Recent findings have contributed to appreciate the relevance of systemic variables in determining the outcome of an ischemic insult.

The association between stroke and antecedent inflammatory states, or between stroke and chronic inflammatory diseases, has been known for long time. The clinical observations are consistent with recent experimental data suggesting that systemic inflammation may have a role in causing stroke, or in modifying the tissue response to the ischemic injury. For instance, microglia represent a key element of the inflammatory response to ischemia. Microglia are not uniform in their activity. Under pathological conditions microglia can proliferate and migrate. Activated microglia can assume a primarily cytotoxic phenotype called M1, or an anti-inflammatory, protective phenotype called M2. Likely, during the evolving ischemic process, microglia activation fluctuates along a continuum, which represents at the extremes the M1 and M2 phenotypes. Such a fluctuation follows the influence of a number of local mechanisms. Systemic variables are also involved. Microglia can in fact be primed to preferentially assume one phenotype with respect to the other. Comorbidities, such as hyperlipidemia, may prime peripheral monocytes/macrophages to mediate a proinflammatory response to stroke and thus to enhance the post-ischemic maturation process [18]. There is growing evidence that an underlying inflammatory status, or possibly other systemic conditions, drive the postischemic immune response towards a detrimental effect [19]. It is, therefore, a substantial hypothesis that different systemic variables may affect the susceptibility of the brain tissue to ischemic damage and the property of the tissue to respond to the insult. The issue has considerable consequences on prevention, therapy and rehabilitation of stroke. Table 1 shows examples of therapeutic approaches.

Clinical trials, aimed to modify the immune response after stroke [20, 21], have been ineffective. The failure probably reflects the complexity, redundancy or double-edge sword effect of post-stroke inflammation. In addition, the stroke-immune response relationship is bidirectional. Stroke is consistently associated with post-stroke immune-depression, represented by lymphopenia, up-regulation of anti-inflammatory cytokines, and splenic atrophy [22]. The immune-depression seems to be mediated by catecholamines and steroids released by sympathetic activation after stroke. One may wonder whether the immune-depression represents one of the mechanisms selected during evolution to reduce the immuno-mediated damage associated with the ischemic insult.

**Table 1. Examples of therapeutic approaches.**

| Treatments | Target |
|---|---|
| **Experimental Approaches** | |
| Preconditioning | Improvement of energy metabolism; activation of epigenetic mechanisms; inflammation |
| Hematopoietic growth factors (EPO; G-CSF; GM-CSF) | Both central and peripheral protective mechanisms; brain repair mechanisms |
| Administration of NADPH | Antioxidant systems; ATP production |
| **Clinical Approaches** | |
| Hypothermia | Reduction of the energy demand; promotion of survival mechanisms |
| Minocycline | Early inflammatory signal |
| Sex hormones | anti-apoptotic, anti-inflammatory and anti-oxidant properties |

## Examples of Potential Neuroprotective Approaches

### *Preconditioning and Ischemic Tolerance*

Preconditioning (PC) is an alternative pathway to provide neuroprotection from cerebral ischemia. The list of PC stimuli resulting in ischemic tolerance includes hypoxia, cortical spreading depression, administration of inflammatory mediators, and of course short episodes of transient focal or global cerebral ischemia. The preconditioning stimulus thus activates different pathways to increase the resistance to ischemia. The so-called "early" tolerance develops within few minutes from the preconditioning stimulus. It is a protein synthesis independent mechanism and it leads to the activation of mediators that act directly on effectors to improve energy metabolism. The "delayed" tolerance occurs 12-72 hours following the subliminal insult. It requires the synthesis of transcription factors and activation of epigenetic mechanisms, which reprogram gene expression. Preconditioning may also modulate the post-ischemic immune response [23] and the proinflammatory gene expression [24, 25].

The protective effect of preconditioning, despite its proven potency in several experimental models, has not reached widespread clinical application because of the difficulties in applying the stimulus to the brain. Considerable interest has been devoted to the remote preconditioning. It was originally showed that preconditioning of one coronary territory induces protection from ischemia in other parts of the heart. Subsequently, in animal models, preconditioning of one organ was observed to induce protection in other organs. Furthermore, there are preclinical data confirming that mild ischemia of skeletal limb muscles protects the heart and lungs against ischemia-reperfusion injury [26]. Obviously, applying a stimulus before ischemia has no clinical practicability. There are data, however, showing that the protective effect of the sub-liminal, remote stimulus may remain even if the stimulus is applied just after the lethal ischemia. Thus remote postconditioning may enhance the neuroprotective mechanisms associated with the ischemic insult. Inflating a standard blood pressure cuff applied to a limb may represent a suitable means for inducing remote ischemic conditioning. This is a simple, inexpensive approach. And it is safe enough to be carried out even if the diagnosis of ischemic stroke is uncertain, for instance during ambulance transportation. The effectiveness of the procedure needs to be proved [27].

## *Hypothermia*

Hypothermia is probably the most effective neuroprotective treatment in animal models. Originally the rationale for use of hypothermia was based on the observation that lowering body temperature reduces the energy demand. A number of recent data suggests that cooling interferes with most of the pathogenic mechanisms that cause ischemic damage [28]. An issue is whether hypothermia interferes also with the neuroprotective mechanisms. A number of reports have dealt with such an issue, and although results are not always consistent [29, 30], cooling seems to promote survival mechanisms, by increasing expression of the brain-derived neurotrophic factor (BDNF) [31], glial-derived neurotrophic factor (GDNF) [32], and neurotrophins [33], in animal models of ischemia. The balance seems, therefore, in favor of the neuroprotection. In any case, lowering the body (brain) temperature is likely to extend the therapeutic window. Hypothermia it is the only neuroprotective approved therapy to improve neurological outcome for hypoxic brain injury after cardiac arrest [34] and it has been introduced in the clinical practice as a therapeutic opportunity in infant born at (or near) term with moderate to severe hypoxic-ischemic encephalopathy [35]. Most of the supportive data on the therapeutic hypothermia were obtained in animal models of ischemia [14]. By means of different mechanisms, hypothermia reduces brain energy metabolism, by about 5%/°C (Steen *et al.*, 1983), decreasing the metabolic needs and slowing depletion of ATP (Yenari 2008). In addition, lowering temperature influences the progression of the tissue damage by reducing some key players of the neuroinflammatory response such as MM-P2, MMP-9, NF-κB, interleukin-1β, tumor necrosis factor-α, and interlukin-6. In addition hypothermia reduces free radical formation and excitotoxic neurotransmitter release [36 - 38]. By interfering with both the intrinsic and extrinsic pathway, cooling can also delay apoptotic processes, including the mitochondrial regulatory pathways [35]. Hypothermia can also modify the expression of the BCL2 family members [39] and the activity of pro-death signaling substances such as p53 and NAD depletion [40].

Thus, a large body of experimental data indicates that hypothermia affects both early and late phases of the ischemic damage maturation, providing theoretical background for applying cooling even several hours after the ischemic insult.

The potent neuroprotective effects of hypothermia give new insight into the field of the combination therapies. According to the proven efficacy of fibrinolysis, a question was to determine whether cooling could be mostly effective if combined with recanalization and reperfusion. A reason for concern is that thrombolysis involves temperature-dependent enzymes, and the hypothermia may lessen the efficacy of the tPA. Furthermore, hypothermia is associated with hematologic abnormalities (coagulopathy, platelet dysfunction) and a question is whether the association with thrombolytic drugs is safe. Experimental data are limited. A number of reports and small trials support the feasibility and safety of the association between thrombolysis and hypothermia.

Thus mild hypothermia (34-35 °C), carried out in the early (typically within 6 hours) post stroke phase, is feasible and safe. It may require treatments to minimize discomfort and shivering especially if the hypothermia is induced and maintained by surface cooling by means of cold blankets. Endovascular cooling is better tolerated than surface cooling and it is more effective in cooling the brain. However endovascular cooling is invasive as it requires insertion of a flexible cooling catheter into the inferior vena cava. Shivering is probably the main disadvantage of mild hypothermia, both because of the discomfort and of the vasoconstriction, which slows down the time to reach target temperature. Other potential complications include diuresis and consequent hypovolemia, vasoconstriction, infections (especially pneumonia) [41], coagulopathy or cardiac arrhythmia. Rapid rewarming (faster than 0.5°C/h) should be avoided to preserve the intracranial pressure.

**Table 2. Principal Clinical Trials for Therapeutic Hypothermia.**

| Study name | N | °C | S | E | Adverse events | Results |
|---|---|---|---|---|---|---|
| Copenhagen Stroke Study 2000 | 17+56 | 35.5 | + | | infections (18%), mortality 6 months (12%) | "no poor outcome" (SSS) |
| COOL-AID 2001 | 10+9 | 32 | + | | sinus bradycardia, 3 deaths, not due to the treatment | "feasible and safe" (mRS at 90 days) |
| COOL-AID II 2004 | 18+22 | 33 | | + | 5 deaths, 2 symptomatic hemorrhagic transformation, 2 cardiac events, 5 pulmonary events | "feasible and safe" (mRS at 30 days) |
| ICTuS 2005 | 18+0 | 33 | | + | 4 DVT, 3 bradycardia, 3 nausea/vomiting due to meperidine, 3 hemorrhagic transformations | "feasible" |
| Martin-Shild 2009 | 20+0 | 33-34.5 | + | + | Pneumonia, 1 reduced respiratory drive, 3 deaths (not due to the treatment) | 70% of patients improved of 4 points or more (NIHSS) |
| ICTuS-L 2010 | 28+30 | 33 | | + | pneumonia (50%), intracerebral hemorrhage (28.5%), | no difference in outcome or mortality (NIHSS 90 days) |
| N= number of subjects + control; °C = target temperature; S = Surface Cooling; E = Endovascular Cooling; SSS = Scandinavian Stroke Scale score; mRS = modified Rankin Scale; DVT = Deep Venous Thrombosis; NIHSS = National Institutes of Health Stroke Scale | | | | | | |

Table **2** shows early clinical trial assessing the safety of hypothermia during acute ischemic stroke. Two randomized controlled trial are still ongoing, ICTuS ⅔ and Euro-HYP1.

## Minocycline

Minocycline is a semisynthetic tetracycline, which has been clinically used as an antibiotic and anti-inflammatory drug. Accumulating experimental evidence has demonstrated that minocycline is neuroprotective in multiple neurological disorders, including ischemic and hemorrhagic stroke. Clinical trials suggest (but do not prove) that minocycline may be safe and potentially beneficial in humans [42]. Although its underlying molecular mechanisms remain to be fully defined, minocycline possesses a wide array of anti-inflammatory, antiapoptotic, antioxidative, and vascular protective properties, which might account for the apparent neuroprotective effect.

## CONCLUSION

Comprehensive treatment for acute ischaemic stroke should include both recanalization therapies and neuroprotective therapies, initiated as early as possible. Many neuroprotective drugs have failed to show benefit in the treatment of acute ischaemic stroke, despite apparent success in preclinical stroke models. Increased quality of preclinical testing and appropriate selection of study participants in clinical trials might overcome the barriers to progress in stroke research and allow to discover robustly effective neuroprotective therapies in the near future. Relevant areas of interest for neuroprotection in acute ischemic stroke include therapeutic hypothermia, minocycline and ischemic conditioning.

## TAKE HOME MESSAGE

The term *Neuroprotection* refers to interventions that are supposed to beneficially interfere with the complexity of the post ischemic molecular events. The effectiveness of a number of potential neuroprotective procedures still needs to be proved in clinical studies.

## CONFLICT OF INTEREST

The authors confirm that they have no conflict of interest to declare for this publication.

## ACKNOWLEDGEMENTS

Declared none.

## REFERENCES

[1]    Hossmann KA. The two pathophysiologies of focal brain ischemia: implications for translational stroke research. J Cereb Blood Flow Metab 2012; 32(7): 1310-6.
[http://dx.doi.org/10.1038/jcbfm.2011.186] [PMID: 22234335]

[2]    Sheth SA, Sanossian N, Hao Q, *et al.* Collateral flow as causative of good outcomes in endovascular stroke therapy. J Neurointerv Surg 2016; 8(1): 2-7.
[http://dx.doi.org/10.1136/neurintsurg-2014-011438] [PMID: 25378639]

[3]    Shuaib A, Butcher K, Mohammad AA, Saqqur M, Liebeskind DS. Collateral blood vessels in acute ischaemic stroke: a potential therapeutic target. Lancet Neurol 2011; 10(10): 909-21.
[http://dx.doi.org/10.1016/S1474-4422(11)70195-8] [PMID: 21939900]

[4]    Iadecola C, Anrather J. Stroke research at a crossroad: asking the brain for directions. Nat Neurosci 2011; 14(11): 1363-8.
[http://dx.doi.org/10.1038/nn.2953] [PMID: 22030546]

[5]    Moskowitz MA, Lo EH, Iadecola C. The science of stroke: mechanisms in search of treatments. Neuron 2010; 67(2): 181-98.
[http://dx.doi.org/10.1016/j.neuron.2010.07.002] [PMID: 20670828]

[6]    Iadecola C, Anrather J. The immunology of stroke: from mechanisms to translation. Nat Med 2011; 17(7): 796-808.
[http://dx.doi.org/10.1038/nm.2399] [PMID: 21738161]

[7]    Paschen W. Shutdown of translation: lethal or protective? Unfolded protein response *versus* apoptosis. J Cereb Blood Flow Metab 2003; 23(7): 773-9.
[http://dx.doi.org/10.1097/01.WCB.0000075009.47474.F9] [PMID: 12843781]

[8]    Besancon E, Guo S, Lok J, Tymianski M, Lo EH. Beyond NMDA and AMPA glutamate receptors: emerging mechanisms for ionic imbalance and cell death in stroke. Trends Pharmacol Sci 2008; 29(5): 268-75.
[http://dx.doi.org/10.1016/j.tips.2008.02.003] [PMID: 18384889]

[9]    Young MM, Smith ME, Coote JH. Effect of sympathectomy on the expression of NMDA receptors in the spinal cord. J Neurol Sci 1999; 169(1-2): 156-60.
[http://dx.doi.org/10.1016/S0022-510X(99)00239-7] [PMID: 10540025]

[10]   Chen Q, He S, Hu XL, *et al.* Differential roles of NR2A- and NR2B-containing NMDA receptors in activity-dependent brain-derived neurotrophic factor gene regulation and limbic epileptogenesis. J

Neurosci 2007; 27(3): 542-52.
[http://dx.doi.org/10.1523/JNEUROSCI.3607-06.2007] [PMID: 17234586]

[11]    Yang Y, Candelario-Jalil E, Thompson JF, *et al.* Increased intranuclear matrix metalloproteinase activity in neurons interferes with oxidative DNA repair in focal cerebral ischemia. J Neurochem 2010; 112(1): 134-49.
[http://dx.doi.org/10.1111/j.1471-4159.2009.06433.x] [PMID: 19840223]

[12]    Zhao H, Sapolsky RM, Steinberg GK. Phosphoinositide-3-kinase/akt survival signal pathways are implicated in neuronal survival after stroke. Mol Neurobiol 2006; 34(3): 249-70.
[http://dx.doi.org/10.1385/MN:34:3:249] [PMID: 17308356]

[13]    Qiu J, Nishimura M, Wang Y, *et al.* Early release of HMGB-1 from neurons after the onset of brain ischemia. J Cereb Blood Flow Metab 2008; 28(5): 927-38.
[http://dx.doi.org/10.1038/sj.jcbfm.9600582] [PMID: 18000511]

[14]    Hayakawa K, Nakano T, Irie K, *et al.* Inhibition of reactive astrocytes with fluorocitrate retards neurovascular remodeling and recovery after focal cerebral ischemia in mice. J Cereb Blood Flow Metab 2010; 30(4): 871-82.
[http://dx.doi.org/10.1038/jcbfm.2009.257] [PMID: 19997116]

[15]    Stocchetti N, Taccone FS, Citerio G, *et al.* Neuroprotection in acute brain injury: an up-to-date review. Crit Care 2015; 19: 186.
[http://dx.doi.org/10.1186/s13054-015-0887-8] [PMID: 25896893]

[16]    Dénes A, Humphreys N, Lane TE, Grencis R, Rothwell N. Chronic systemic infection exacerbates ischemic brain damage *via* a CCL5 (regulated on activation, normal T-cell expressed and secreted)-mediated proinflammatory response in mice. J Neurosci 2010; 30(30): 10086-95.
[http://dx.doi.org/10.1523/JNEUROSCI.1227-10.2010] [PMID: 20668193]

[17]    Langdon KD, Maclellan CL, Corbett D. Prolonged, 24-h delayed peripheral inflammation increases short- and long-term functional impairment and histopathological damage after focal ischemia in the rat. J Cereb Blood Flow Metab 2010; 30(8): 1450-9.
[http://dx.doi.org/10.1038/jcbfm.2010.23] [PMID: 20332799]

[18]    Kim E, Febbraio M, Bao Y, Tolhurst AT, Epstein JM, Cho S. CD36 in the periphery and brain synergizes in stroke injury in hyperlipidemia. Ann Neurol 2012; 71(6): 753-64.
[http://dx.doi.org/10.1002/ana.23569] [PMID: 22718544]

[19]    Vogelgesang A, May VE, Grunwald U, *et al.* Functional status of peripheral blood T-cells in ischemic stroke patients. PLoS One 2010; 5(1): e8718.
[http://dx.doi.org/10.1371/journal.pone.0008718] [PMID: 20090932]

[20]    del Zoppo GJ. Acute anti-inflammatory approaches to ischemic stroke. Ann N Y Acad Sci 2010; 1207: 143-8.
[http://dx.doi.org/10.1111/j.1749-6632.2010.05761.x] [PMID: 20955437]

[21]    Use of anti-ICAM-1 therapy in ischemic stroke: results of the Enlimomab Acute Stroke Trial. Neurology 2001; 57(8): 1428-34.
[http://dx.doi.org/10.1212/WNL.57.8.1428] [PMID: 11673584]

[22]    Offner H, Vandenbark AA, Hurn PD. Effect of experimental stroke on peripheral immunity: CNS

ischemia induces profound immunosuppression. Neuroscience 2009; 158(3): 1098-111.
[http://dx.doi.org/10.1016/j.neuroscience.2008.05.033] [PMID: 18597949]

[23]   Gesuete R, Stevens SL, Stenzel-Poore MP. Role of circulating immune cells in stroke and preconditioning-induced protection. Acta Neurochir Suppl (Wien) 2016; 121: 39-44.
[PMID: 26463920]

[24]   Garcia-Bonilla L, Benakis C, Moore J, Iadecola C, Anrather J. Immune mechanisms in cerebral ischemic tolerance. Front Neurosci 2014; 8: 44.
[http://dx.doi.org/10.3389/fnins.2014.00044] [PMID: 24624056]

[25]   Gesuete R, Christensen SN, Bahjat FR, *et al.* Cytosolic receptor melanoma differentiation-associated protein 5 mediates preconditioning-induced neuroprotection against cerebral Ischemic injury. Stroke 2016; 47(1): 262-6.
[http://dx.doi.org/10.1161/STROKEAHA.115.010329] [PMID: 26564103]

[26]   Kilian JG, Nakhla S, Griffith K, Harmer J, Skilton M, Celermajer DS. Reperfusion injury in the human forearm is mild and not attenuated by short-term ischaemic preconditioning. Clin Exp Pharmacol Physiol 2005; 32(1-2): 86-90.
[http://dx.doi.org/10.1111/j.1440-1681.2005.04163.x] [PMID: 15730440]

[27]   Hess DC, Hoda MN, Bhatia K. Remote limb perconditioning [corrected] and postconditioning: will it translate into a promising treatment for acute stroke? Stroke 2013; 44(4): 1191-7.
[http://dx.doi.org/10.1161/STROKEAHA.112.678482] [PMID: 23339961]

[28]   Yenari MA, Han HS. Neuroprotective mechanisms of hypothermia in brain ischaemia. Nat Rev Neurosci 2012; 13(4): 267-78.
[PMID: 22353781]

[29]   Kanagawa T, Fukuda H, Tsubouchi H, *et al.* A decrease of cell proliferation by hypothermia in the hippocampus of the neonatal rat. Brain Res 2006; 1111(1): 36-40.
[http://dx.doi.org/10.1016/j.brainres.2006.06.112] [PMID: 16904084]

[30]   Bennet L, Roelfsema V, George S, Dean JM, Emerald BS, Gunn AJ. The effect of cerebral hypothermia on white and grey matter injury induced by severe hypoxia in preterm fetal sheep. J Physiol 2007; 578(Pt 2): 491-506.
[http://dx.doi.org/10.1113/jphysiol.2006.119602] [PMID: 17095565]

[31]   DCruz BJ, Fertig KC, Filiano AJ, Hicks SD, DeFranco DB, Callaway CW. Hypothermic reperfusion after cardiac arrest augments brain-derived neurotrophic factor activation. J Cereb Blood Flow Metab 2002; 22(7): 843-51.
[http://dx.doi.org/10.1097/00004647-200207000-00009] [PMID: 12142569]

[32]   Schmidt KM, Repine MJ, Hicks SD, DeFranco DB, Callaway CW. Regional changes in glial cell line-derived neurotrophic factor after cardiac arrest and hypothermia in rats. Neurosci Lett 2004; 368(2): 135-9.
[http://dx.doi.org/10.1016/j.neulet.2004.06.071] [PMID: 15351435]

[33]   Boris-Möller F, Kamme F, Wieloch T. The effect of hypothermia on the expression of neurotrophin mRNA in the hippocampus following transient cerebral ischemia in the rat. Brain Res Mol Brain Res 1998; 63(1): 163-73.
[http://dx.doi.org/10.1016/S0169-328X(98)00286-1] [PMID: 9838092]

[34]    Bernard SA, Gray TW, Buist MD, *et al.* Treatment of comatose survivors of out-of-hospital cardiac arrest with induced hypothermia. N Engl J Med 2002; 346(8): 557-63.
[http://dx.doi.org/10.1056/NEJMoa003289] [PMID: 11856794]

[35]    Wu TC, Grotta JC. Hypothermia for acute ischaemic stroke. Lancet Neurol 2013; 12(3): 275-84.
[http://dx.doi.org/10.1016/S1474-4422(13)70013-9] [PMID: 23415567]

[36]    Busto R, Globus MY, Dietrich WD, Martinez E, Valdés I, Ginsberg MD. Effect of mild hypothermia on ischemia-induced release of neurotransmitters and free fatty acids in rat brain. Stroke 1989; 20(7): 904-10.
[http://dx.doi.org/10.1161/01.STR.20.7.904] [PMID: 2568705]

[37]    Kil HY, Zhang J, Piantadosi CA. Brain temperature alters hydroxyl radical production during cerebral ischemia/reperfusion in rats. J Cereb Blood Flow Metab 1996; 16(1): 100-6.
[http://dx.doi.org/10.1097/00004647-199601000-00012] [PMID: 8530542]

[38]    Yenari MA, Han HS. Influence of therapeutic hypothermia on regeneration after cerebral ischemia. Front Neurol Neurosci 2013; 32: 122-8.
[http://dx.doi.org/10.1159/000346428] [PMID: 23859971]

[39]    Liu L, Yenari MA. Therapeutic hypothermia: neuroprotective mechanisms. Front Biosci 2007; 12: 816-25.
[http://dx.doi.org/10.2741/2104] [PMID: 17127332]

[40]    Ji X, Luo Y, Ling F, *et al.* Mild hypothermia diminishes oxidative DNA damage and pro-death signaling events after cerebral ischemia: a mechanism for neuroprotection. Front Biosci 2007; 12: 1737-47.
[http://dx.doi.org/10.2741/2185] [PMID: 17127418]

[41]    Gupta R, Jovin TG, Krieger DW. Therapeutic hypothermia for stroke: do new outfits change an old friend? Expert Rev Neurother 2005; 5(2): 235-46.
[http://dx.doi.org/10.1586/14737175.5.2.235] [PMID: 15853493]

[42]    Fagan SC, Waller JL, Nichols FT, *et al.* Minocycline to improve neurologic outcome in stroke (MINOS): a dose-finding study. Stroke 2010; 41(10): 2283-7.
[http://dx.doi.org/10.1161/STROKEAHA.110.582601] [PMID: 20705929]

# CHAPTER 11

# Pharmacological and Endovascular Recanalization Therapy

**E.C. Agostoni**[*] and **M. Longoni**

*Department of Neuroscience, Neurology and Stroke Unit of the ASST: "Grande Ospedale Metropolitano Niguarda", Milan, Italy*

**Abstract:** The major aim of acute stroke treatment is to save the hypoperfused cerebral parenchyma in order to minimize residual disability. Early recanalization of occluded arteries with thrombolytic therapy is the most efficient procedure for protecting the brain parenchyma which is not yet infarcted.

Intravenous administration of Alteplase (recombinant tissue-type plasminogen activator – rtPA) has proven to be effective in reducing disability at 90 and 180 days after stroke in patients treated within 4.5 hours from symptoms onset.

Recently, striking results have been provided by the endovascular treatment, unless in a selected population. The use of the stent-retrievers or direct thrombus aspiration is now a good option for acute stroke treatment giving the opportunity of an effective multimodal therapeutic approach.

**Keywords:** Actilyse, Acute therapy, Alteplase, Endovascular, Pharmacological, Recanalization, Stent retrievers, Stroke, Thrombectomy, Thrombolysis.

## INTRODUCTION

The major aim of acute stroke treatment is to save the hypoperfused cerebral parenchyma in order to minimize residual disability in the medium and long term after the acute event. Therefore, the main goals of treatment in the acute phase of

[*] **Corresponding author E.C. Agostoni:** Department of Neuroscience, Neurology and Stroke Unit of the ASST: "Grande Ospedale Metropolitano Niguarda", Milan, Italy; Tel: +39 02-64442348; Fax: + 39 02-64442189; Emails: marco.longoni@ospedaleniguarda.it, elioclemente.agostoni@ospedaleniguarda.it

Alberto Radaelli, Giuseppe Mancia, Carlo Ferrarese & Simone Beretta (Eds.)

ischemic stroke concern two main aspects: 1. The attempt to bring the situation of arterial occlusion back to its previous condition of vessel patency, improving the supply of oxygen and glucose correlated to artery reperfusion; 2. To block dysmetabolic processes which, in an anaerobic environment, contribute to the increase in volume of the infarction of brain parenchyma. In the acute phase of stroke, vascular reperfusion and neuroprotection treatments should be practiced respecting the concept of maximum urgency of intervention. The scenario of the therapy offered also includes more invasive procedures requiring surgery. Very briefly, these interventions (*e.g.*: carotid thromboendarterectomy) are aimed at reducing the risk of early recurrence of stroke and preventing deterioration of the anatomical and clinical situation. Another range of surgical procedures (decompressive hemicraniectomy, placement of external ventricular deviation) aim at preventing clinical deterioration in the presence of intracranial hypertension due to the "mass" effect of the lesion

Early recanalization of occluded arteries with thrombolytic therapy is the most efficient procedure for protecting the brain parenchyma which is not yet infarcted. While lysis of the thrombus occluding the vessel is the immediate result that is pursued through this procedure, improvement in terms of clinical outcome is the final objective of such treatment. An earlier meta-analysis published in 2002, which analyzed the data of 2006 patients, confirmed the positive predictive role of recanalization in achieving a positive outcome after 3 months (OR: 4.43; 95% CI: 3.32 – 5.91), as well as in reducing death (OR: 0.24; 95% CI: 0.16 – 0.35) [1]. In the same meta-analysis, 24.1% of the patients showed spontaneous recanalization. However, the highest percentages of reperfusion were observed in the group of patients treated with mechanical thrombectomy (83.6%), followed by a combination of systemic and loco regional therapies (67.5%) and the intra-arterial procedure (63.2%). Several factors are associated with favourable recanalization. First of all, size and location of the thrombus: higher volumes of thrombus, or thrombosis of the large vessels of previous atherosclerotic stenosis, seem to be factors for resistance to thrombolysis, as well as involvement of the extra-cranial internal carotid, occlusions in the carotid artery or the T basilar artery [2, 3]. The status of pial collateral circulation is also a factor that affects the success of reperfusion of the artery [4]. Thrombolytic treatment can be delivered in a well-defined time window, beyond which its effectiveness is significantly reduced at the expenses of safety [5]. Patient management in the hyper acute phase of stroke must provide a quick pathway leading to prompt treatment. In addition to drug therapy, recent findings have meant that therapeutic potentials can be increased by giving a positive presentation of using different devices to offer mechanical recanalization techniques to selected patients [6].

## Systemic Thrombolysis

Intravenous administration of Alteplase (recombinant tissue-type plasminogen activator – rtPA) has proven effective in reducing disability at 90 and 180 days after stroke [5, 7]. However, the benefit of the drug tends to decrease significantly as time goes by, and the time window currently applied is 4.5 hours [8]. At first, Alteplase was administered within three hours from onset of symptoms because of evidence in previous studies such as NINDS, in which 38% of the treated patients reached a favourable outcome compared to 21% of the placebo group, with no significant increase in the risk of mortality [9]. ECASS III assessed the efficacy of the treatment by extending the time window to 4.5 hours. The main result of the study was the effectiveness of Alteplase compared to placebo (OR: 1.34; 95% CI: 1.02 – 1.76; number needed to treat [NNT]: 14), with no significant difference between the two groups regarding mortality and symptomatic haemorrhages [10]. Further evidence emerged from the SITS-ISTR observational study that confirmed data already presented in a previous randomized trial [11]. To date no evidence has emerged from literature concerning the efficacy and safety of rtPA between 4.5 and 6 hours. IST-3 is the most important trial that has taken this therapeutic window into consideration and has enrolled more than 3,000 patients [12]. In particular, the sub analysis of 1,007 patients treated within 4.5 and 6 hours has shown a significant difference between the groups of treated and untreated patients (47% *versus* 43%; OR: 1.31; but with a confidential interval across the line of 1 (95% CI: 0.89 – 1.93). A previous meta-analysis published in 2012 involved over 7,000 patients treated within 6 hours [7]. Globally, the results showed that thrombolytic treatment was superior to placebo (OR: 1.17; 95% CI: 1.06 – 1.29), with a net benefit for those who were treated within 3 hours. In fact, the patients treated between 3 and 6 hours did not benefit significantly from the treatment (OR: 1.07; 95% CI: 0.96 – 1.20). In conclusion, a recent meta-analysis has taken into consideration the trials previously published and has analyzed the outcomes of almost 7,000 patients [13]. The main observations emerging from this analysis concern the clear benefit of receiving thrombolytic therapy within 3 hours (OR: 1.75; 95% CI: 1.35 – 2.27). The benefit is maintained between 3 and 4.5 hours (OR: 1.26; 95% CI: 1.05 – 1.51), whereas it decreases between 4.5 and 6 hours (OR: 1.15; 95% CI: 0.95 – 1.40). An important finding shows that the observed benefit does not depend on the patient's age or clinical severity.

To date other thrombolytic drugs were used in the past with controversial results, among them tenecteplase seems to provide a favourable benefit to risk profile [14]. Moreover a recent data from ENCHANTED trial has shown the rt-PA at a reduced dosage of 0.6mg pro kg seems to be safer in terms of risk of bleeding, while the efficacy is lower [15]. However in a subgroup analysis of patients taking antiplatelets before the ischemic event (data not published) the reduced rt-PA regimen is not inferior in terms of efficacy and significantly safer. Thus can probably lead to a "tailored" strategy of rt-PA administration for the next future.

Finally the combined use of ultrasound together with actilyse, that has previously shown to be more effective than rt-PA alone in terms of rates of recanalization [16, 17] has been recently tested in a randomized control trial that was prematurely terminated for futility [18].

Taking into consideration the data mentioned above, the most relevant message for a clinician can be summarized in one general concept: early intervention in the therapeutic window is the determining factor for the effectiveness of systemic thrombolytic treatment.

**Indications for Intravenous Reperfusion Therapy**

Intravenous reperfusion treatment with Alteplase is indicated for acute ischemic stroke (dosage 0.9 mg/kg - maximum 90 mg, of which 10% administered initially as a bolus. and the remaining quantity over a period of 60 minutes) within 4.5 hours from symptoms onset.

However the FDA (Food and Drug Administration), in contrast to EMA (European Medicines Agency) and AIFA (Agenzia Italiana del Farmaco), has not accepted the extension of the therapeutic window to 4.5 hours derived from the ECASS III trial [10]. Thus the American heart association/American stroke association (AHA/ASA) guidelines [19], unlike the European stroke organization (ESO) [20] and the Italian stroke organization (ISO) guidelines [21], assign an indication of Level B and not of Level A to the administration of Alteplase for treatment of acute stroke within 4.5 hours, with the recommendation that a more restrictive approach be adopted regarding the other criteria if the thrombolytic is administered between 3 and 4.5 hours.

All the guidelines agree on recommending administration of the drug as early as possible, given the inverse linear relation existing between the efficacy of reperfusion therapy and the time the therapy is administered [13]. The AHA/ASA guidelines indicate a precise timing: the therapy should be delivered within 60 minutes of the patient's arrival at the Emergency Department.

According to AHA/ASA, the absolute exclusion criteria for intravenous thrombolytic therapy are as follows:

- **Age below 18 years.**
- **Recent severe trauma or stroke in the last 3 months.** According to the most recent updating of Italian guidelines by the ISO, dated March 2015, stroke in the previous 3 months actually represents a relative contraindication, to be assessed according to times, extension of the previous stroke, age of the patient (the older the patient, the higher the risk of bleeding and the shorter the life expectancy) and potential severity of the ongoing event.
- **Puncture of a non-compressible blood vessel** (<7 days).
- **History of intracranial haemorrhage.**
- **Neoplasms, aneurysm or intracranial arteriovenous malformation.**
- **Recent major intracranial or spinal neurosurgery.**
- **Blood pressure >185/110 mmHg.** In the ISO recommendations dated March 2015, it is stated that the therapy is in any case indicated once the therapeutic target has been achieved. No limitations are mentioned regarding the therapy needed in order to reach the therapeutic target.
- **Severe active or recent bleeding** (last 3 months).
- **Haemorrhagic diathesis,** along with (but not only) platelet count inferior to

$100,000/mm^3$; intravenous administration of heparin in the last 48 hours and aPTT values exceeding the upper limit. Administration of Warfarin with INR >1.7 or PT >15 sec. Use of direct thrombin inhibitor drugs or of Xa factor with significant increase in laboratory test values (aPTT, INR, platelet count, Ecarin time, thrombin time (TT) or other specific tests of Xa factor activity).

Intravenous thrombolysis is indicated if the patient has not been on anticoagulant therapy with direct thrombin inhibitors or Xa factor for at least two days and renal function is not altered.

In patients with PT INR is ≤1.7 American and Italian guidelines are favourable with the use of rt-PA while EMA recommendations contraindicate it. It has been demonstrated that patients on oral anticoagulant therapy (OAT) with sub-therapeutic INR who receive intravenous thrombolysis are more likely to suffer a symptomatic haemorrhagic transformation of the ischaemic lesion, but there is no evidence of worse outcome or increased mortality when compared to patients who are not treated with Warfarin [22]. However, with patients on anticoagulants and who have INR ≤1.7, AHA/ASA guidelines restrict the indication of therapy to administration within 3 hours from onset of symptoms. With patients on anticoagulant therapy, thrombolytic therapy is always contraindicated between 3 and 4.5 hours. This restriction is not mentioned in the Italian guidelines.

Patients who do not use oral anticoagulants or heparin, and who are not known for haemorrhagic diathesis, can start receiving thrombolytic treatment before blood test results are available. Such treatment will be interrupted if PT becomes longer or a thrombocytopenia value of below $100,000/mm^3$ emerges.

- **Glycaemia below 50 mg/dl:** ISO recommendations mention the possibility of treating patients whose focal neurological deficit does not change after correcting glycaemia (Evidence Level GPP (Good Practice Point)). Hyperglycemia is not specifically mentioned as a contraindication to the treatment. According to the latest update of ISO guidelines, when glycaemia is >400 mg/dl thrombolytic treatment is recommended if glycaemia decreases to <200 mg/dl within 4.5 hours from onset of symptoms (Evidence Level GPP).
- **Hypodensity on CT brain scan extending to >1/3 of MCA territory.**

According to EMA and AIFA recommendations, there are further contraindications to intravenous administration of thrombolytic drug which are not directly connected to its use in treating ischemic acute stroke, but to its general use:

- **Strong suspicion of a subarachnoid haemorrhage even when bleeding does not appear on the CT scan** (*i.e.* in presence of strong headache and rigor).
- **Haemorrhagic retinopathy caused by diabetes.**
- **Recent (less than 10 days) external traumatic cardiac massage or delivery.**
- **Bacterial endocarditis, pericarditis.**
- **Acute pancreatitis.**
- **Ulcerous disease of the gastrointestinal tract in the last 3 months, oesophageal varices, arterial aneurysm, arterial or venous malformations.**
- **Neoplasms with increased risk of haemorrhage.**
- **Severe hepatopathy, including hepatic insufficiency, cirrhosis, portal hypertension, and active hepatitis (oesophageal varices).**
- **Recent major surgery or recent severe trauma (<3 months for EMA, <14 days for AHA/ASA).**

AHA/ASA guidelines include some "relative" contraindications, which were originally absolute and have subsequently been revised on the basis of data derived from clinical experience and trials carried out after NINDS

- Mild impairment or rapidly improving impairment: This contraindication was revised with reference to the fact that in an aphasic, hemianopsia patient with strength impairment, a low NIHSS score can also be particularly disabling and with reference to some other studies that have shown how some patients with mild impairment at onset of symptoms and who were therefore not treated with thrombolytic therapy, often had a negative outcome [23 - 25]. The recently updated ISO guidelines confirm recommendation for thrombolytic treatment in patients with mild impairment or rapid improvement, provided that it is still detectable when treatment is started (recommendation B).
- Pregnancy: Alteplase does not pass through the placenta because of its molecular size, it therefore has no teratogenic effects; the most serious risk is placenta abrupto and most of the cases reported in literature had a positive

outcome [26]. Therefore, the administration of Alteplase in pregnancy remains an off-label option to be assessed case by case on the basis of the risk-benefit ratio.

- Seizures at onset of symptoms: In this case treatment is indicated when there is clinical evidence that seizure is a consequence of focal deficit and is not a post-critical status. According to new ISO recommendations it is possible to use neuroimaging and CT angiogram alongside clinical criteria to highlight occlusion of an intracranial vessel; MRI with DWI sequences to highlight an acute ischemic lesion (GPP recommendations).
- Recent bleeding in the gastrointestinal or urinary tract (in the previous 21 days).
- Recent acute myocardial infarct (AMI) (in the last 3 months): In this case the indication is justified by the potential risk of intra-cardiac bleeding, but depending on assessment of the risk/benefit ratio, it is however possible to deliver therapy.

The upper age limit of 80 years is no longer mentioned in AHA/ASA and ISO recommendations. In fact, the patients in this age group still benefit significantly from intravenous thrombolytic therapy [7, 12, 13]. For the same reason, according to the results of IST-3 which were confirmed in the meta-analysis of patients' individual data deriving from randomized studies [13], the upper severity limit of the contraindication has been eliminated (NIHSS >25), because it has been proved that these patients benefit in any case from reperfusion therapy [7].

ISO guidelines explicitly states that recommendation for administering intravenous reperfusion therapy with Alteplase within 4.5 hours from onset of symptoms does not have any age or upper severity limits (recommendation Level A).

Both in the ISO and AHA/ASA guidelines, the contraindication for patients with previous stroke and diabetes has been removed.

Age and upper severity limits, stroke and diabetes mellitus as well as oral anticoagulant therapy are still valid contraindications in AHA/ASA guidelines for patients treated between 3 and 4.5 hours - independently of INR values. This is because, when faced with the risk/benefit ratio, it was considered adequate to select patients with better profiles in terms of other factors which are predictive of the treatment results. However, this restriction is not mentioned in the ESO and ISO guidelines.

## Endovascular Treatment of Stroke (Thrombolysis, Thrombectomy, Thrombus Aspiration)

Although intra-arterial rtPA treatment has always shown promising potential benefits in terms of clinical outcome, its effectiveness remains unproven. The positive aspects of this procedure include the possibility of administering a lower dose of drug than with systemic thrombolysis, direct visualization of vessel recanalization and above all the possibility for the patient to be treated where there are contraindications to intravenous administration of thrombolytic drugs [27]. PROACT II was the first study carried out on a large patient population to give positive results [28]. In 2010, a meta-analysis [29] that assessed trials comparing intra-arterial thrombolysis with other treatments (including endovenous heparin) on a total of 395 patients, showed a clear benefit to clinical outcomes (OR: 2.1), even in the presence of an increase in symptomatic brain haemorrhages (OR: 2.9). More recent studies, such as the Italian randomized study 'SYNTHESIS Expansion' that compared endovenous rtPA and intra-arterial rtPA, have shown that pharmacological endovascular treatment is no more effective than endovenous treatment (OR: 0.71; 95% CI: 0.44 – 1.14) [30]. The combined thrombolytic treatment (endovenous and intra-arterial), known also as bridging therapy, is based on two positive factors which are valid for both treatments: on the one hand, speedy administration of endovenous therapy is widely available; on the other hand intra-arterial treatment is highly effective in obtaining vessel recanalization and, consequently, a better clinical outcome. Although the theory involves the potential added value of intra-arterial therapy, the IMS III study [31] did not find this combined approach beneficial if compared to intravenous treatment. A drastic change in the treatment of acute stroke has occurred recently, with intravascular use of mechanical devices producing a marked improvement in the patients' clinical outcome. In fact, in early 2015, the results of a series of trials which have some common characteristics were published: 1. The combined approach, endovascular and systemic; 2. The use of mechanical thrombectomy (also referred to as *stentrievers*) [32]; 3. Careful and rigorous selection of the patients based on the integration of radiological investigations aimed at identifying the site of the occlusion; 4. A well-defined time limit (which varies in the different trials) within which it is possible to administer endovenous rtPA and perform the endovascular procedure of mechanical thrombectomy. These trials resulted in the updated indications and recommendations [33] for treating acute ischemic stroke: for patients with ischemic stroke in the territory of the anterior circulation and documented occlusion of a major vessel, intra-arterial mechanical thrombectomy is recommended by means of a stentriever device [34]. This treatment can be preceded or not by a standard treatment with intravenous rtPA. In particular, the following criteria seem to be of critical importance for this procedure: 1. Basic neuroimaging must exclude bleeding and must identify at most a small ischemic lesion; 2. Radiological examinations with contrast medium must demonstrate the proximal occlusion of a major vessel of anterior circulation; 3. The therapeutic procedure must be carried out in centres with proven experience [35], above all in using stentriever devices; 4. Mechanical thrombectomy must be performed as early as possible and potentially within 6 hours from onset of symptoms. Below is the description of the most important trials that evaluated the efficacy of additional treatment with mechanical thrombectomy by means of stentriever. The MR CLEAN study [36] included 500 patients with evidence of an arterial proximal occlusion of the anterior circulation, which were chosen at random for mechanical thrombectomy within 6 hours from the onset of symptoms, *versus* standard treatment. Approximately 90% of the patients included in the study had previously received intravenous thrombolytic therapy. The final results have demonstrated the superiority of mechanical thrombectomy compared to standard treatment, when the clinical outcome is assessed 3 months after the event (OR: 1.67; 95% CI: 1.21 – 2.30), with a NNT 7.4. There were no significant increases in mortality rates or in symptomatic haemorrhages in the group of patients submitted to mechanical thrombectomy when compared with standard care. The ESCAPE study [37] enrolled 316 patients with occlusion of a major artery of the anterior circulation and possibility of execution of mechanical thrombectomy up to 12 hours from onset of symptoms. This trial also recognized the same randomization of arms. However, the patients with a big ischemic core on their CT Scan and those with ineffective collateral circulation were excluded. The follow-up results after 3 months showed the superiority of mechanical thrombectomy (OR: 2.6; 95% CI: 1.7 – 3.8) with NNT of 4.2. The SWIFT PRIME study [38] enrolled 196 patients aged between 18 and 80 years with ischemic stroke caused by the occlusion of a large vessel of anterior circulation, established through radiological examination. All patients were treated with endovenous rtPA within 4.5 hours from onset of symptoms. Randomization provided possible mechanical thrombectomy through the Solitaire FR device. After 3 months, thrombectomy achieved a positive outcome in 60% of the patients, *versus* 35% in the control group, with NNT of 4. The EXTEND-IA trial [39] included 70 patients. Excluded from randomization were patients with an ischemic core of over 70 ml or with no brain parenchyma which could potentially be saved. Two groups were created for randomization: one with standard treatment only and the other one with mechanic thrombectomy by means of Solitaire FR. Also in this case, 3 months after the event the patients treated with mechanical thrombectomy benefitted from a more favourable outcome (71% v 40%) with NNT of 3.2, with no significant difference in mortality or symptomatic brain haemorrhages. The REVASCAT [40] study randomized 206 ischemic stroke patients to mechanical thrombectomy within 8 hours *versus* medical treatment only. Endovascular procedure significantly reduced the rate of disability after 3 months from the event, with an improvement of the clinical outcome (44% *versus* 28% with NNT: 6.3), without significantly increasing the risk of mortality or symptomatic brain haemorrhages. On the whole, previous studies provide evidence that an early mechanical thrombectomy procedure with stentriever devices, in addition to intravenous thrombolytic treatment, is effective in reducing disability in patients with stroke caused by large arterial vessel occlusion in anterior circulation. The value of NNT needed to obtain functional independence thus varies between 3 and 7.5. Unlike previous experiences and trials, careful selection of the patients to be treated with mechanical thrombectomy, in addition to systemic thrombolysis, is a key factor in achieving maximum benefit with minimum risk. In particular, a basal CT scan showing evidence of occlusion of intracranial main artery (distal carotid artery, sections M1/M2 MCA or sections A1/A2 of anterior cerebral artery) and the absence of large ischemic infarctions, are two key factors in selecting patients for mechanical thrombectomy. Even in the absence of any validation indicated by the results of randomized trials and only in the light of several clinical series, another kind of arterial recanalization procedure - direct thrombus aspiration [41] - is rapidly spreading to many centres. This therapeutic procedure consists in intracranial navigation with special intracranial catheters, which are soft but wide-lumen (newly marketed), which are brought close to the thrombus. The thrombus, is then sucked manually (by creating a negative pressure in the lumen) or *via* external mechanical aspiration pumps connected to the catheter. According to some authors, this therapeutic procedure allows a high rate of recanalization with extreme rapidity of execution.

A recent meta-analysis on thrombectomy trials has provided interesting data demonstrating the absence of difference in terms of clinical outcome between patients treated or not with rt-PA before the endovascular procedure. This weak evidence is now under investigation with a new RCT (SWIFT PRIME II).

Another interesting issue still debate is the kind of anaesthesia during the procedure. A recent trial (SIESTA) has shown that general anaesthesia instead of conscious sedation are equally efficient (data under publication).

**Indications for Endovascular Therapy**

In June 2015 an update of the 2013 AHA/ASA guidelines was published, regarding endovascular treatment in the acute phase of stroke [33]. The update included the results of 8 trials on endovascular therapy in the acute stroke phase, the results of which were published between 2013 and 2015: SYNTHESIS, IMS III, MR RESCUE, MR CLEAN, ESCAPE, SWIFT PRIME, EXTEND IA, REVASCAT [30, 31, 36 - 40, 42].

Level 'A' indication for endovascular therapy was given to patients over 18 years of age, starting from a good neurological status (mRS pre-event 0 or 1), with occlusion of the internal carotid artery or of the proximal segment (M1) of the middle cerebral artery MCA, with an NIHSS score of ≥6 and an ASPECTS score [43] of ≥6. These restrictions are due to the fact that most of the trials were carried out on randomly selected patients who had these characteristics, thus data is not sufficient to determine whether clinical benefit is preserved also in patients with a more serious clinical status or for patients with early ischemic signs which are more extensive.

Puncture of the arterial vessel can be performed up to 6 hours from onset of symptoms. This time limit is linked to the fact that the thrombectomy procedure could be started within 6 hours for most of the patients involved in these trials, and that data regarding patients treated within 8 and 12 hours, which was collected in REVASCAT and ESCAPE [37, 40], was insufficient to determine the effectiveness of this time window. Furthermore, sub-analysis of MR CLEAN results showed that when therapy was started later than 6 hours from onset of symptoms, patients did not significantly benefit from the treatment [44].

All patients who are eligible must first be treated with endovenous thrombolysis. Contrary to what was stated in the 2013 guidelines, indication for endovascular therapy is not limited to patients who are unresponsive to endovenous therapy: in fact, it is explicitly stated that it is not necessary to observe the patients and candidate them for endovascular treatment only if they do not improve with intravenous treatment [33]. If the patient has criteria which make them eligible for endovascular therapy, they must be treated as soon as possible. In fact, as regards intravenous treatment, the best results are obtained by treating patients as early as possible [44, 45]. Similarly, it is not necessary to repeat CT angiography to confirm arterial occlusion before starting endovascular treatment. In fact this strategy was used in REVASCAT and there was no evidence of better clinical results [40]. The indication for endovascular therapy is Level C in patients with occlusion of: most of the distal segment of the MCA (M2 or M3), anterior cerebral arteries (ACA), posterior cerebral arteries (PCA) and vertebral or basilar arteries. The same level (C) is also assigned to endovascular therapy for patients aged <18 years and for patients who cannot be treated with endovenous thrombolysis because of specific contraindications.

Finally, a Level C recommendation is assigned to angioplasty and/or stenting treatments in acute stenosis of the internal neck carotid artery when thrombectomy is performed.

The ISO recommendations [21] highlights that endovenous thrombolytic treatment if indicated has no alternative treatment. Evidence Level B is assigned to endovascular treatment of stroke with internal carotid occlusion, MCA in segments M1 and M2 and ACA in the proximal segment that do not respond to, or do not have any indications for, intravenous thrombolysis and do not have any indications about possible improvements after endovenous thrombolysis.

Where there is an occlusion of major vessels of the posterior circulation (vertebral, basilar, cerebral arteries in the proximal segment) a GPP indication level is assigned to endovascular treatment on patients who do not respond to or do not have any indications for endovenous thombolytic treatment [46]. New ESO guidelines (under publication) assign a Level A recommendation to endovascular treatment of MCA occlusion within 6 hours from onset of symptoms, and a grade B of basilar artery beyond 3 hours, without time limits.

**Post Treatment Phase**

Patients receiving systemic rt-PA and/or endovascular thrombectomy according to the AHA/ASA guideline indications need to be [33]:

- Admitted to stroke unit for monitoring of vital parameters.
- Assessed for blood pressure and neurological status every 15 minutes during intravenous thrombolysis and in the two hours following it, then every 30 minutes for 6 hours, and then every 60 minutes for 24 hours. If blood pressure exceeds 180/105 mmHg in the 24 hours following thrombolysis, blood pressure must be measured more frequently and the patient must be treated with intravenous agents to keep blood pressure under the values mentioned above.
- Free of antiplatelets and anticoagulants for at least 24 hours if treated with rt-PA
- Well looked for the risk of the development of orolingual angioedema that can cause obstruction of the airways. It is generally a transient and mild reaction, reported in approximately 5% of the patients treated, and its risk increases with the use of ACE inhibitors [47].

If possible, defer insertion of urinary catheter, nasogastric tube or intra-arterial catheter to monitor blood pressure.

**CONCLUSION**

Early recanalization of occluded arteries with thrombolytic therapy is the most efficient procedure for protecting the brain parenchyma which is not yet infarcted. While lysis of the thrombus occluding the vessel is the immediate result that is pursued through this procedure, improvement in terms of clinical outcome is the final objective of such treatment. Intravenous reperfusion treatment with Alteplase is indicated for acute ischemic stroke (dosage 0.9 mg/kg - maximum 90 mg, of which 10% administered initially as a bolus. and the remaining quantity over a period of 60 minutes) within 4.5 hours from symptoms onset and still remain the best medical treatment for stroke patients. Considering the striking results of the recently published endovascular trials, with use of mechanical devices, the combined approach for patients with ischemic stroke in the territory of the anterior circulation and documented occlusion of a major vessel is now the best therapeutic strategy.

Future questions to be answer are:

1. What is the best clinical and neuroradiological modality to select eligible patients?
2. which is the best pathway ("mothership" *versus* "drip and ship" model) for acute stroke patients?
3. Which is the best endovascular approach (stentrievers *versus* direct aspiration)?

Randomized controlled trials addressing these issues are needed.

## TAKE HOME MESSAGE

The main objective of acute stroke treatment is the early recanalization of the occluded artery. Whether intravenous administration of Alteplase has proven to be effective in reducing disability at 90 and 180 days after stroke, new endovascular devices for mechanical clot retrieval have recently shown better results in terms of recanalization rates and outcome in selected patients thus leading to a multimodal therapeutic approach.

## CONFLICT OF INTEREST

The authors confirm that they have no conflict of interest to declare for this publication.

# ACKNOWLEDGEMENTS

Declared none.

# REFERENCES

[1]   Rha JH, Saver JL. The impact of recanalization on ischemic stroke outcome: a meta-analysis. Stroke 2007; 38(3): 967-73.
[http://dx.doi.org/10.1161/01.STR.0000258112.14918.24] [PMID: 17272772]

[2]   Alejandro M. Hounsfield unit value and clot length in the acutely occluded vessel and time required to achieve thrombectomy, complications and outcome J NeuroIntervent Surg 2014; 6: 423-7.

[3]   Zangerle A, Kiechl S, Spiegel M, *et al.* Recanalization after thrombolysis in stroke patients: predictors and prognostic implications. Neurology 2007; 68(1): 39-44.
[http://dx.doi.org/10.1212/01.wnl.0000250341.38014.d2] [PMID: 17200490]

[4]   Ribo M, Flores A, Rubiera M, *et al.* Extending the time window for endovascular procedures according to collateral pial circulation. Stroke 2011; 42(12): 3465-9.
[http://dx.doi.org/10.1161/STROKEAHA.111.623827] [PMID: 21960574]

[5]   Lees KR, Bluhmki E, von Kummer R, *et al.* ECASS, ATLANTIS, NINDS and EPITHET rt-PA Study Group. Time to treatment with intravenous alteplase and outcome in stroke: an updated pooled analysis of ECASS, ATLANTIS, NINDS, and EPITHET trials. Lancet 2010; 375(9727): 1695-703.
[http://dx.doi.org/10.1016/S0140-6736(10)60491-6] [PMID: 20472172]

[6]   Goyal M, Menon BK, van Zwam WH, *et al.* HERMES collaborators. Endovascular thrombectomy after large-vessel ischaemic stroke: a meta-analysis of individual patient data from five randomised trials. Lancet 2016; 387(10029): 1723-31.
[http://dx.doi.org/10.1016/S0140-6736(16)00163-X] [PMID: 26898852]

[7]   Wardlaw JM, Murray V, Berge E, *et al.* Recombinant tissue plasminogen activator for acute ischaemic stroke: an updated systematic review and meta-analysis. Lancet 2012; 379(9834): 2364-72.
[http://dx.doi.org/10.1016/S0140-6736(12)60738-7] [PMID: 22632907]

[8]   Marler JR, Tilley BC, Lu M, *et al.* Early stroke treatment associated with better outcome: the NINDS rt-PA stroke study. Neurology 2000; 55(11): 1649-55.
[http://dx.doi.org/10.1212/WNL.55.11.1649] [PMID: 11113218]

[9]   The National Institute of Neurological Disorders and Stroke rt-PA Stroke Study Group. Tissue plasminogen activator for acute ischaemic stroke. N Engl J Med 1995; 333: 1581.
[http://dx.doi.org/10.1056/NEJM199512143332401] [PMID: 7477192]

[10]  Hacke W, Kaste M, Bluhmki E, *et al.* ECASS Investigators. Thrombolysis with alteplase 3 to 4.5 hours after acute ischemic stroke. N Engl J Med 2008; 359(13): 1317-29.
[http://dx.doi.org/10.1056/NEJMoa0804656] [PMID: 18815396]

[11]  Wahlgren N, Ahmed N, Dávalos A, *et al.* SITS investigators. Thrombolysis with alteplase 34.5 h after acute ischaemic stroke (SITS-ISTR): an observational study. Lancet 2008; 372(9646): 1303-9.
[http://dx.doi.org/10.1016/S0140-6736(08)61339-2] [PMID: 18790527]

[12]  Sandercock P, Wardlaw JM, *et al.* The benefits and harms of intravenous thrombolysis with

recombinant tissue plasminogen activator within 6 h of acute ischaemic stroke (the third international stroke trial [IST-3]): a randomised controlled trial. Lancet 2012; 379: 2352.
[http://dx.doi.org/10.1016/S0140-6736(12)60768-5] [PMID: 22632908]

[13]   Emberson J, Lees KR, Lyden P, *et al.* Stroke Thrombolysis Trialists Collaborative Group. Effect of treatment delay, age, and stroke severity on the effects of intravenous thrombolysis with alteplase for acute ischaemic stroke: a meta-analysis of individual patient data from randomised trials. Lancet 2014; 384(9958): 1929-35.
[http://dx.doi.org/10.1016/S0140-6736(14)60584-5] [PMID: 25106063]

[14]   Parsons M, Spratt N, Bivard A, *et al.* A randomized trial of tenecteplase versus alteplase for acute ischemic stroke. N Engl J Med 2012; 366(12): 1099-107.
[http://dx.doi.org/10.1056/NEJMoa1109842] [PMID: 22435369]

[15]   Anderson CS, Robinson T, Lindley RI. Low-dose *versus* standard-dose intravenous alteplase in acute ischemic stroke. N Engl J Med 2016; 374(24): 2313-23.
[http://dx.doi.org/ 10.1056/NEJMoa1515510]

[16]   Ricci S, Dinia L, Del Sette M, *et al.* Sonothrombolysis for acute ischaemic stroke. Cochrane Database Syst Rev 2012; 6: CD008348.

[17]   Alexandrov AV, Molina CA, Grotta JC, *et al.* Ultrasound-enhanced systemic thrombolysis for acute ischemic stroke. N Engl J Med 2004; 351: 2170-8.
[PMID: 15548777]

[18]   Schellinger PD, Alexandrov AV, Barreto AD, *et al.* CLOTBUSTER Investigators. Combined lysis of thrombus with ultrasound and systemic tissue plasminogen activator for emergent revascularization in acute ischemic stroke (CLOTBUST-ER): design and methodology of a multinational phase 3 trial. Int J Stroke 2015; 10(7): 1141-8.
[http://dx.doi.org/10.1111/ijs.12536] [PMID: 26120902]

[19]   Jauch EC, Saver JL, Adams HP Jr, *et al.* American Heart Association Stroke Council; Council on Cardiovascular Nursing; Council on Peripheral Vascular Disease; Council on Clinical Cardiology. Guidelines for the early management of patients with acute ischemic stroke: a guideline for healthcare professionals from the American Heart Association/American Stroke Association. Stroke 2013; 44(3): 870-947.
[http://dx.doi.org/10.1161/STR.0b013e318284056a] [PMID: 23370205]

[20]   European Stroke Organisation (ESO) Executive Committee; ESO Writing Committee. Guidelines for management of ischaemic stroke and transient ischaemic attack 2008. Cerebrovasc Dis 2008; 25(5): 457-507.
[http://dx.doi.org/10.1159/000131083] [PMID: 18477843]

[21]   Welcome to portal lines ISO-SPREAD guide.  http://www.iso-spread.it/ raccomandazioni ictus acuto, 31 Marzo 2015.

[22]   Miedema I, Luijckx G-J, De Keyser J, Koch M, Uyttenboogaart M. Thrombolytic therapy for ischaemic stroke in patients using warfarin: a systematic review and meta-analysis. J Neurol Neurosurg Psychiatry 2012; 83(5): 537-40.
[http://dx.doi.org/10.1136/jnnp-2011-301794] [PMID: 22378917]

[23]   Jacques De Keyser MD. Intravenous alteplase for stroke beyond the guidelines and in particular

clinical situations stroke 2007; 38: 2612-8.
[PMID: 17656661]

[24]   Smith EE, Abdullah AR, Petkovska I, Rosenthal E, Koroshetz WJ, Schwamm LH. Poor outcomes in patients who do not receive intravenous tissue plasminogen activator because of mild or improving ischemic stroke. Stroke 2005; 36(11): 2497-9.
[http://dx.doi.org/10.1161/01.STR.0000185798.78817.f3] [PMID: 16210552]

[25]   Tong DC. Avoiding thrombolysis in patients with mild stroke: is it SMART? Stroke 2012; 43(3): 625-6.
[http://dx.doi.org/10.1161/STROKEAHA.111.643346] [PMID: 22308248]

[26]   Tassi R, Acampa M, Marotta G, *et al.* Systemic thrombolysis for stroke in pregnancy. Am J Emerg Med 2013; 31(2): 448.e1-3.
[http://dx.doi.org/10.1016/j.ajem.2012.05.040] [PMID: 22867835]

[27]   del Zoppo GJ, Higashida RT, Furlan AJ, Pessin MS, Rowley HA, Gent M. PROACT: a phase II randomized trial of recombinant pro-urokinase by direct arterial delivery in acute middle cerebral artery stroke. PROACT Investigators. Prolyse in Acute Cerebral Thromboembolism. Stroke 1998; 29(1): 4-11.
[http://dx.doi.org/10.1161/01.STR.29.1.4] [PMID: 9445320]

[28]   Furlan A, Higashida R, Wechsler L, *et al.* Intra-arterial prourokinase for acute ischemic stroke. The PROACT II study: a randomized controlled trial. Prolyse in Acute Cerebral Thromboembolism. JAMA 1999; 282(21): 2003-11.
[http://dx.doi.org/10.1001/jama.282.21.2003] [PMID: 10591382]

[29]   Lee M, Hong KS, Saver JL. Efficacy of intra-arterial fibrinolysis for acute ischemic stroke: meta-analysis of randomized controlled trials. Stroke 2010; 41(5): 932-7.
[http://dx.doi.org/10.1161/STROKEAHA.109.574335] [PMID: 20360549]

[30]   Ciccone A, Valvassori L, Nichelatti M, *et al.* SYNTHESIS Expansion Investigators. Endovascular treatment for acute ischemic stroke. N Engl J Med 2013; 368(10): 904-13.
[http://dx.doi.org/10.1056/NEJMoa1213701] [PMID: 23387822]

[31]   Broderick JP, Palesch YY, Demchuk AM, *et al.* Interventional Management of Stroke (IMS) III Investigators. Endovascular therapy after intravenous t-PA *versus* t-PA alone for stroke. N Engl J Med 2013; 368(10): 893-903.
[http://dx.doi.org/10.1056/NEJMoa1214300] [PMID: 23390923]

[32]   Campbell BC, Donnan GA, Lees KR, *et al.* Endovascular stent thrombectomy: the new standard of care for large vessel ischaemic stroke. Lancet Neurol 2015; 14(8): 846-54.
[http://dx.doi.org/10.1016/S1474-4422(15)00140-4] [PMID: 26119323]

[33]   Powers WJ, Derdeyn CP, Biller J, *et al.* AHA/ASA focused update of the 2013 guidelines for the early management of patients with acute ischaemic stroke regarding endovascular treatment: A guideline for healthcare professionals from the American heart association/American stroke association. Stroke 2015; 46: 3020-35.
[http://dx.doi.org/10.1161/STR.0000000000000074]

[34]   Broderick JP, Schroth G. What the SWIFT and TREVO II trials tell us about the role of endovascular therapy for acute stroke. Stroke 2013; 44(6): 1761-4.

[http://dx.doi.org/10.1161/STROKEAHA.113.000740] [PMID: 23686978]

[35]   Meyers PM, Schumacher HC, Higashida RT, *et al.* Indications for the performance of intracranial endovascular neurointerventional procedures: a scientific statement from the American Heart Association Council on Cardiovascular Radiology and Intervention, Stroke Council, Council on Cardiovascular Surgery and Anesthesia, Interdisciplinary Council on Peripheral Vascular Disease, and Interdisciplinary Council on Quality of Care and Outcomes Research. Circulation 2009; 119(16): 2235-49.
[http://dx.doi.org/10.1161/CIRCULATIONAHA.109.192217] [PMID: 19349327]

[36]   Berkhemer OA, Fransen PS, Beumer D, *et al.* MR CLEAN Investigators. A randomized trial of intraarterial treatment for acute ischemic stroke. N Engl J Med 2015; 372(1): 11-20.
[http://dx.doi.org/10.1056/NEJMoa1411587] [PMID: 25517348]

[37]   Campbell BC, Mitchell PJ, Kleinig TJ, *et al.* EXTEND-IA Investigators. Endovascular therapy for ischemic stroke with perfusion-imaging selection. N Engl J Med 2015; 372(11): 1009-18.
[http://dx.doi.org/10.1056/NEJMoa1414792] [PMID: 25671797]

[38]   Saver JL, Goyal M, Bonafe A, *et al.* SWIFT PRIME Investigators. Stent-retriever thrombectomy after intravenous t-PA *vs.* t-PA alone in stroke. N Engl J Med 2015; 372(24): 2285-95.
[http://dx.doi.org/10.1056/NEJMoa1415061] [PMID: 25882376]

[39]   Goyal M, Demchuk AM, Menon BK, *et al.* ESCAPE Trial Investigators. Randomized assessment of rapid endovascular treatment of ischemic stroke. N Engl J Med 2015; 372(11): 1019-30.
[http://dx.doi.org/10.1056/NEJMoa1414905] [PMID: 25671798]

[40]   Jovin TG, Chamorro A, Cobo E, *et al.* REVASCAT Trial Investigators. Thrombectomy within 8 hours after symptom onset in ischemic stroke. N Engl J Med 2015; 372(24): 2296-306.
[http://dx.doi.org/10.1056/NEJMoa1503780] [PMID: 25882510]

[41]   Turk AS, Frei D, Fiorella D, *et al.* ADAPT FAST study: a direct aspiration first pass technique for acute stroke thrombectomy. J Neurointerv Surg 2014; 6(4): 260-4.
[http://dx.doi.org/10.1136/neurintsurg-2014-011125] [PMID: 24569575]

[42]   Kidwell CS, Jahan R, Gornbein J, *et al.* MR RESCUE Investigators. A trial of imaging selection and endovascular treatment for ischemic stroke. N Engl J Med 2013; 368(10): 914-23.
[http://dx.doi.org/10.1056/NEJMoa1212793] [PMID: 23394476]

[43]   Pexmana JHW, Barbera PD, Hilla MD, *et al.* Use of the alberta stroke program early CT score (ASPECTS) for assessing CT scans in patients with acute stroke. AJNR 2001; 22: 1534-42.

[44]   Fransen PS, Berkhemer OA, Lingsma HF, *et al.* Time to reperfusion and treatment effect for acute ischemic stroke: A randomized clinical trial. JAMA Neurol 2016; 73(2): 190-6.
[http://dx.doi.org/10.1001/jamaneurol.2015.3886] [PMID: 26716735]

[45]   Prabhakaran S, Ruff I, Bernstein RA. Acute stroke intervention: a systematic review. JAMA 5 2015; 313: 1451.
[http://dx.doi.org/10.1001/jama.2015.3058]

[46]   Hacke W. Interventional thrombectomy for major strokea step in the right direction. N Engl J Med 2015; 372(1): 76-7.
[http://dx.doi.org/10.1056/NEJMe1413346] [PMID: 25517349]

[47]    Hill MD, Lye T, Moss H, *et al.* Hemi-orolingual angioedema and ACE inhibition after alteplase treatment of stroke. Neurology 2003; 60(9): 1525-7.
[http://dx.doi.org/http:/dx.doi.org/10.1212/01.WNL.0000058840.66596.1A] [PMID: 12743244]

# CHAPTER 12

# Neuroregeneration after Stroke

**Marco Bacigaluppi***, **Gianluca Luigi Russo** and **Gianvito Martino**

*Neuroimmunology Unit, Institute of Experimental Neurology, Division of Neuroscience, San Raffaele Scientific Institute, Via Olgettina 58, 20132 Milan, Italy*

**Abstract:** Promoting tissue plasticity is a very important therapeutic approach to reduce post-stroke disability. The neurological damage occurring after stroke indeed is a consequence of disrupted brain connectivity circuits due to cellular degeneration and impairment of plasticity processes. Axonal degeneration is also invariably seen in remote brain structures that have neuroanatomical links to the ischemic area. Recovery from stroke is thus very much depending on the possibility to develop treatments able to halt the neurodegenerative process and to foster adaptive tissue plasticity. Due to the intricacy of the systems involved, therapies that foster endogenous repair processes in a spatially and time targeted manner are required. We here discuss the physiology of recovery processes occurring after stroke and the main strategies to foster compensatory neuronal networks aiming to reduce stroke-related disability.

**Keywords:** Axonal sprouting, Critical period, Growth factors, Inflammation, Ischemic stroke, Neural stem cell, Plasticity, Transplantation.

## INTRODUCTION

Stroke is a highly disabling neurological disease representing, the third leading cause of death worldwide. Whatever the cause that triggers the occlusion of the brain artery, the inadequate blood supply initiates a series of pathophysiological events that, if not reversed quickly in time, results in irreversible damage of the brain tissue. Victims of stroke experience different clinical manifestations depending on the brain area(s) affected: symptoms might include hemiparalysis,

* **Corresponding author Marco Bacigaluppi:** Neuroimmunology Unit, Institute of Experimental Neurology, Division of Neuroscience, San Raffaele Scientific Institute, Via Olgettina 58, 20132 Milan, Italy; Tel; +390226434958; Fax +390226434855; Email: bacigaluppi.marco@hsr.it

impairment of speech, or loss of vision and many other neurological dysfunctions. Partial functional recovery can occur and depends on the entity of damage and on the spared neuronal networks that can take over the lost brain functions. Unfortunately of all stroke patients about 50% are left with a motor impairment, 30% are not able to walk and about 26% have a severe disability requiring care [1].

Following the acute and the subacute phase of stroke, that are characterized by acute injury mechanisms such as spreading depressions, excitotoxicity, calcium release, formation of free radicals, endoplasmic reticulum dysfunction and mitochondria failure, the chronic phase, lasting for months after ischemic insult, follows [2, 3]. Even though in this phase secondary injury mechanisms contribute to the progression of tissue damage, repair mechanisms begin to emerge. Inflammation, which begins few hours after the onset of ischemia, importantly shapes also this delayed injury phase. Early after stroke microglia and astrocytes are activated as well blood borne cells (*e.g.* neutrophils, lymphocytes and monocytes) are recruited to the brain by locally expressed cytokines, adhesion molecules and chemokines. Even areas remote from the site of injury, degenerate and induce an inflammatory response resulting in secondary damage and atrophy. Consequently, loss of function during stroke is on the one hand due to brain tissue loss in the infarct site and on the other hand due to neuronal dysfunction in the non-ischemic peri-ischemic zone and in more remote areas connected to the infarct core. In the months following stroke some neurological functions spontaneously recover [1, 4]. In fact it is essential to remember that ischemic tissue, and especially the peri-infarct zone, are also sites of active recovery processes. Many evidences support the concept that mechanisms underlying recovery and damage are not separate entities but often diverge in time or space and components involved in damage in the acute phase of stroke can, early after, contribute to recovery processes.

Indeed the transition from injury to repair is guided by mediators of the extracellular matrix, components of the excitatory pathway and from signals derived from activated inflammatory cells; the same players which have a key role in the initial neurodegeneration [5]. An example can be the N- methyl-D-aspartate (NMDA) receptors: in the acute phase their over-activation seems detrimental while, in the chronic phase, the same receptor activation is important to stimulate neuroplasticity and protection against apoptosis. Further examples are matrix metalloproteinases (MMP): although MMPs are able to degrade the neurovascular matrix and to mediate damage of the blood-brain barrier contributing to neuronal death, oedema and haemorrhagic transformation [6] the same MMPs can at a later stage also promote plasticity processes such as remodelling of the neurovascular unit in the boundary of the lesion. Accordingly while inhibitors of MMPs in acute stroke have been shown to reduce tissue infarction, the same inhibitors worsen in sub-acute or chronic phases of stroke the outcome, since they inhibit plasticity processes [7].

These examples show that at the same time of degeneration restorative processes are initiated in brain tissue in response to cerebral ischemia. Recovery after stroke comprehends also central nervous system (CNS) reorganization. The multifaceted mechanisms such as vascular remodelling, neurogenesis and gliogenesis, axonal sprouting, dendritic arborisation modification, spine remodelling and cortical function relocation are often synergistic and tightly orchestrated in time. For succeeding in favourably manipulating neuroregeneration it is essential to study and comprehend in the minimal detail the pathophysiology of stroke. All too often broad pharmacological approaches have failed in triggering effective neuroregeneration since timing, location, duration or dosages were not properly set. In this chapter we review the main biological mechanism underlying regeneration and discuss how these processes can be fostered for eliciting neuroregeneration.

## Reparative Processes after Stroke

### *Inflammation*

Inflammation is a very important actor in the pathophysiology of stroke. Recent evidence suggests that the immune system is involved in all stages of the ischemic cascade, from the very acute vascular occlusion phase, or even before, to the ensuing tissue repair [8]. The past decade has witnessed a revolution in our understanding of CNS inflammation, in particular regarding the involvement of immune cells in CNS maintenance and repair [9]. Although an inflammatory response is known to be essential for healing throughout the body, inflammation in the CNS was up to recent times considered to be merely detrimental. Among innate immune cells, microglia and infiltrating monocyte-derived macrophages are separate populations with distinct ontogeny [10] and different activities following ischemic stroke [11]. Although the role of microglial cells in stroke still remains elusive, initial studies have shown that macrophages might be protective following acute CNS injury, such as ischemic stroke. Indeed reduction of circulating monocytes leads to ischemic lesion volume expansion [12] and to haemorrhagic transformation [13, 14] of stroke. Increasing evidence suggests that a subset of inflammatory cells is fundamental not only for neuroregenerative processes to occur but also for neuroprotection. Inflammatory cells can remove dead cells, help in the development of an anti-inflammatory milieu (*e.g.* TGF-β, IL-4 and IL-10 and IL-13) and release pro-survival factors (*e.g.* growth factors such as VEGF, BDNF, IGF), fostering tissue reconstruction and repair [8].

## Neurogenesis

Adult mammalian brains continue to exhibit focal areas of on-going neurogenesis, namely in the subventricular zone (SVZ) close to the lateral ventricles and in the subgranular zone (SGZ) of the hippocampus. Under physiological conditions these new-born cells replace neurons in the olfactory bulb and in the hippocampus [15]. While the presence of neurogenic niches in the hippocampus and in the SVZ seem to be established also in the adult human brain, the function, role and migratory pathways of these cells have only partly been defined. After cerebral ischemia or hemorrhage, the rate of neurogenesis increases in the SVZ (the most studied area of neurogenesis in stroke) and the newly generated cells follow chemoattractive gradients towards the lesioned tissue, perhaps as part of an endogenous attempt of the brain to repair itself [16]. Although this neurogenic response seems to persist for surprisingly long periods of time, the majority of these new-born cells survive only for a few days [17, 18]. Whether and how these new neurons significantly contribute to functional recovery remains still unclear. Recent studies have suggested that endogenous neural precursor cells (NPCs) of the subventricular zone exert a neuroprotective role in experimental stroke and epilepsy by dampening striatal excitotoxicity though the secretion of cannabinoids [19]. This direct protective effect is observed very early after injury, thus pointing out that the expansion and differentiation of neural precursor cells is not required. Other recent studies have also shown that SVZ derived neural precursor cells migrate towards the ischemic lesion and differentiate mainly into astrocyte stabilizing the glial scar [20]. Interestingly, also exogenous transplantation of neural stem cells has been shown to exert various protective effect acting on modulating detrimental secondary injury mechanisms, such as inflammation and gliosis [21]. These neuroprotective effects of NPCs could also be attributed to their ability to modulate the microenvironment in the vicinity of the ischemic lesion, for example acting on endogenous microvasculature, on peri-ischemic astrocytes and on dendritic plasticity to promote brain recovery [22, 23]. In concert with neurogenesis the recovering brain exhibits complex patterns of vascular remodelling.

## *Angiogenesis*

Brain angiogenesis is a tightly controlled process that is down-regulated beyond the third postnatal week and reactivated in pathological conditions such as hypoxia/ischemia and brain tumour growth. In fact the brain after stroke exhibits complex patterns of vascular remodelling. Angiogenesis and vasculogenesis in peri- infarct regions have been detected in rodent as well as in human stroke [24], and both angiogenic and neurogenic responses are tightly regulated after stroke and contribute to promote recovery [25]. This is not surprising since molecular mechanisms of neurogenesis and angiogenesis have been evolutionary conserved [26]. Indeed promotion of neurogenesis enhances vascular re-growth and conversely, angiogenic stimulation enhances neurogenesis [27]. The importance of neo-angiogenesis for a proper recovery after stroke has been also highlighted by a recent report, showing that *in vivo* inhibition of miR-155 reduced brain tissue damage, and improved the animal functional recovery by supporting brain microvasculature (improved blood flow and microvascular integrity in the peri-infarct area) [28].

## *Astrogliosis*

Astrogliosis, and in particular the proliferation and/or hypertrophy of astrocytes close to damaged areas of the CNS, mainly characterized by enhanced vimentin and glial fibrillary acidic protein (GFAP) expression, strongly influences post-stroke regenerative processes. The astrocytic response is a critical step in the acute phase of stroke as well as in the recovery phase.

On the one hand astrocytes activation in the acute phase of stroke is protective against the expansion of the ischemic lesion, confining inflammation and limiting excitotoxicity and haemorrhagic transformation of the ischemic tissue [29, 30]. Glial cells, especially astrocytes, control brain homeostasis and create a microenvironment for successful brain repair, removing excitatory neurotransmitters and electrolytes from the extracellular space. Reactive astrocytes participate in neuronal remodelling processes by releasing growth factors and furthermore providing lipids for myelination and glial-neuronal interactions [31]. Further studies have shown the beneficial role of GFAP/vimentin reactive astrocytes for axonal remodelling and motor behavioural recovery in mice after stroke [30]. The protective role of activated astrocytes is also supported by studies with GFAP-null mice. GFAP knock-out mice, despite a normal CNS development and function, appear more sensitive to middle cerebral artery occlusion (MCAO), the experimental model of stroke, than wild-type mice, even if infarcted volume is comparable [32].

On the other hand, the formation of glial scar is considered one of the barriers to repair of CNS. Proliferating astrocytes secrete numerous proteins of the extracellular matrix, such as proteoglycans and growth inhibitors factors that create a tenacious growth-blocking membrane, which hampers axonal survival and regeneration [1]. Chondroitinase ABC treatment after experimental focal ischemic stroke in the elderly was shown to promote neuroanatomical and functional recovery [33, 34]. The role of the glial scar and of chondroitin sulfate proteoglycans (CSPGs) as growth inhibitors is however not a simple 'all or none' phenomenon: it is rather a fine and complex titration of proteoglycan concentrations, and their balance with other molecules during their interactions with growth cones, regulating the overall patterning of axonal bundling or branching fate of axons. The particular intricate regulation over time and space of the glial scar composition, as mentioned above for other repair mechanism, results in an extraordinary complexity difficult to be favourably modulated.

## Neuronal Plasticity Processes

The cross-talk between microvessels, neuroblast, inflammatory cells and astrocytes is a tight interplay that creates a (semi-) permissive environment for recovery mechanisms, such as induction of axonal sprouting and neuronal plasticity. Although robust neuroregeneration is desirable to recover function, the dynamic responses of neurons after stroke also requires efficient mechanisms to prevent uncontrolled axonal or dendritic growth that might result in maladaptive sprouting. Indeed, recovery after stroke requires the establishment of specific new functional neuronal networks, while avoiding potential maladaptive connections that might lead to epileptic seizures or allodynia.

### *Axonal Sprouting*

Stroke induces anterograde Wallerian degeneration of pyramidal tract axons, the degree of which depends on the severity of the ischemic insult [35, 36]. Subsequently, axonal fiber tracts reorganize along the infarct rim [37, 38]. Surviving pyramidal tracts, distal to the site of ischemic injury, grow and terminal axonal sprouting is enhanced in the ipsilesional as well as in the contralesional pyramidal tract [4, 39]. Axonal sprouting is the process by which a differentiated neuron initiates a growth program, elaborates a growth cone and extends an axon or an axon collateral to form a new connection. Recovery of function after cortical damage seems to be related to the degree of enhanced axonal growth in the vicinity of the lesion. While small ischemic lesions trigger horizontal axonal sprouting so to enhance connection that are not normally present [40], larger ischemic lesions rather induce long distance axonal sprouting [41]. Post-ischemic endogenous axonal sprouting thus partly compensates for the loss of axons in specific target structures at various levels of the brain (*i.e.*, red nucleus and facial nucleus) and spinal cord [36].

### *Dendritic Remodelling*

Dendrites are key players in the plasticity processes taking place after ischemia. Due to the fact that in the ischemic core neurons are dead, the dendritic remodelling particularly refers to surviving peri-infarct neurons. Brain ischemia induces synaptic rearrangements in neurons adjacent to the lesioned tissue, and these plastic phenomena seem to be responsible for the partial recovery of function that occurs after stroke, and that can be enhanced by rehabilitation [42, 43]. Dendritic growth (and new synapse formation), possibly related to the up-regulation of trophic factors in the ischemic tissue, represents one of the main pathophysiological processes that occurs in neurons adjacent to the infarct zone [44]. While dendritic trees are stable over several weeks in the healthy animal, dendritic tree remodelling is increased in particular in the first weeks after cerebral ischemia [4].

## *Spine Remodelling*

Dynamic changes in spine morphology are important during learning and adaptive plasticity [45]. Spines are indeed highly dynamic structures mediating post- stroke recovery [4]. Alterations include spine retraction, changes in spine length, enhanced spine turnover and reversible dendritic blebbing [46 - 49]. Repeated imaging studies have demonstrated that in the first hours after stroke a loss of dendritic spines takes place, followed soon after by augmented spine turnover (consisting in both the formation and elimination of spines), in particular in the peri-infarct area, that continues for weeks after stroke [46]. Since the degree of tissue reperfusion influences spine density, increased spine densities are associated with high blood perfusion rates in the long- term recovery [50].

## Post-Stroke Adaptive Plasticity Processes

Recovery mechanisms are based on both structural and functional changes of brain circuits that have a close functional relationship to those affected by stroke. Indeed plasticity processes in the adult brain are allowed by a surprisingly amount of diffuse and redundant connectivity, which induces formation of new structural functional circuits through remapping between related cortical regions. The capacity to restructure cortical representational maps is at the maximum level early in development. As an example for this, lesion of the corpus callosum during early childhood is associated with extensive remapping of motor, language and other functions to regions within the remaining hemisphere [51]. Similarly reorganization of cortical representational maps occurs also after stroke in the adult. Indeed cortical-map plasticity is a normal event in adulthood that is highly amplified after ischemia [52].

Thus one way in which the human brain can restore its function after stroke is through the use of a distributed neural network involving brain regions that, in a functional hierarchy, are both upstream and downstream to the affected region. These networks can include healthy brain areas in adjacent regions or even in the intact contralesional hemisphere. In animal models that experience relatively small size strokes altered brain circuits compete for map territory with adjacent healthy tissue [53]. By contrast, after an extensive stroke that destroys wide brain areas deputed to a specific function, tissue that has a similar function might only be found at more distant sites, such as the pre-motor cortex, if primary motor cortex is affected, or even regions in the contralateral hemisphere [54]. Bilateral activation of brain areas for a specific function might therefore indicate an inability of compensatory mechanisms to restore normal neuronal signalling inside the ipsilateral hemisphere. At the structural level mechanisms underlying this recovery of lost neurological functions are defined in terms of dendritic and axonal arborisation and changes in spine density, synapse number and size, receptor density, and in some brain regions also the number of neurons. These elements control neuronal activity, which is temporally and spatially regulated in adaptive plasticity processes. These characteristics together determine the complexity of neuronal network and their activity contribute to the rescue of the lost functions due to stroke [55].

## Re-emergence of a Critical Period after Stroke

In most organisms, neuronal connections underlying specific neuronal functions are still immature at birth. Successively over time they are refined and this process in some species, may last up to several years. Indeed during the early phase of nervous system development, molecular guidance molecules play a fundamental role, whereas neuronal activity becomes the key player during later stages of development. The patterned neuronal activity important for this development is generated either by the developing brain or, once the peripheral sensory organs are functional, is driven by external stimuli. Often, the influence of sensory input on nervous-system organization is robust during a brief, well-defined phase of nervous system development. This phase of increased receptiveness to sensory input has been termed the *"critical period"* for plasticity. Hubel and Wiesel coined this term in 1970, demonstrating that environmental experience, specifically during early infancy, is able to shape and trigger new connection formation and removal, affecting the subsequent properties and function of adult brain. In particular, they demonstrated how visual deprivation during the *critical period* can permanently alter the physiological features of the visual cortex, resulting in a missing ability to develop this specific neurological function [56].

Specifically, both environment-dependent factors, such as the exposure to a certain stimuli at a given time, and neuronal-mediated elements, such as gene expression levels that underlies the critical period itself, are essential for this process to occur. The ability to adapt in response to environmental cues is a fundamental property of the nervous tissue and constitutes the basis for the ability to adapt and learn in an experience-dependent manner throughout life. Animal studies have shown that genes and proteins that underlie neuronal growth, synaptogenesis and reorganization of dendritic spines, are highly expressed during early brain development and subsequently decline with age [57]. The hypothesis of the re-emergence of a *critical period* after stroke relies on the fact that after cerebral ischemia, gene expression, protein and neuronal excitability patterns resemble in part plasticity processes, which physiologically occur in early development. In fact several studies point out that developmental proteins and gene expression normally absent or present at very low levels in the adult brain recur for a short period after an ischemic brain insult [58, 59]. Brain ischemia induces in fact neuronal growth-promoting genes that can be divided in early response genes (*e.g.* SPRR1), early/ sustained response genes (*e.g.* the transcription factor c-Jun and growth cone lipid raft proteins GAP43, CAP23, and MARCKS), middle response genes (*e.g.* cyclin-dependent kinase inhibitor p21/waf1, cell adhesion molecule L1, and embryonic tubulin isoform T$\alpha$1 tubulin), and late response genes (*e.g.* cytoskeletal reorganizing genes SCLIP and SCG10) [59]. Interestingly the dynamic of neuronal growth-promoting genes expressed in the cortex after stroke is unique compared to patterns occurring during neuronal development and also in other CNS lesions [60]. Nonetheless axonal sprouting after stroke requires both the presence of a growth-promoting program within peri-infarct neurons, and a favourable environment. However the surrounding environment is often hampered in stroke patients by coexisting morbidities such as microvascular diseases, advanced age, chronic inflammation and other plasticity-hindering processes, that result in a brain less responsive to neural remodelling [55]. In particular, age has been shown in experimental stroke models to be linked to the up-regulation of myelin and ephrin receptors in sprouting neurons limiting plasticity processes [61]. Thus a *critical period* of augmented neuroplasticity after stroke, similar to what occurs during visual system development, becomes evident for a limited time. A challenge to improve plasticity processes would be to widen the duration of the *critical period* to optimize and increase post-stroke recovery.

## *Brakes of Plasticity after Stroke*

A primary target to enhance plasticity processes is to remove its brakes, that are both structural, such as perineuronal nets of the glial scar and myelin which drastically reduce neurite outgrowth, and functional, consisting of a consolidated excitatory-inhibitory (E-I) balance within established neural networks.

Recently, several molecular brakes involved in the structural process have been identified. In the adult brain, neurons and synapses of the cortical and subcortical regions are surrounded by extracellular matrix (ECM) that stabilize synapses, control ion homeostasis and provide neuroprotection. This ECM, known as the perineuronal nets, consists mostly of chondroitin sulfate proteoglycans (*e.g.* brevican, neurocan, versican, aggrecan and phosphacan) [62], which are produced during central nervous system maturation [63]. The stabilization operated by the ECM is beneficial, because it protects the adult brain against disturbances in functional connectivity. However, to restore functions after CNS injuries such as ischemic stroke, plasticity has to be fostered by circumventing the inhibition of CSPGs on axonal sprouting. In the 1990s, it was shown for the first time that CSPGs might limit the regeneration of the CNS after injury. In adult mammals CSPGs are secreted often soon (within 24 hours) after injury and then persist for months. Interestingly, increased plasticity processes are observed in the CNS of pre-critical period embryos that do not up-regulate CSPGs after injury [64]. Moreover cold-blooded species that are able to successfully regenerate axons have a minimal up-regulation of CSPGs in reactive glia [65]. Specific neurite growth inhibitory factors, many of which are enriched in myelin, are for example Nogo-A, the myelin proteins, oligodendrocyte-myelin glycoprotein (OMgp) and myelin associated glycoprotein (MAG), several semaphorins and ephrins [66]. In particular the well-studied Nogo receptor expressed on neurons binds to various inhibitors of axonal growth expressed by myelin, such as Nogo-A/B, myelin-associated glycoprotein, oligodendrocyte-myelin glycoprotein. Interestingly an alternative receptor for Nogo, paired immunoglobulin-like receptor B (PirB), is expressed at low levels in different parts of the adult CNS, but its expression is increased during neural development or after ischemia [67, 68]. When these receptors are activated they initiate growth cone collapse and growth arrest of neurites [69]. Accordingly genetic deletion of the Nogo receptor, or of its ligand Nogo-A/B, in mice revealed increased spike plasticity after the usual end of the critical period, suggesting their role as a brake for regeneration [70].

A second important target to induce a pre-critical period is to reset the excitatory-inhibitory (E-I) balance [71]. The transition from pre-critical period to critical period is elicited when a severe change of the excitatory-inhibitory balance occurs, reflecting the development of specific inhibitory circuits that usually follow the maturation of excitatory connections [72]. Indeed reduction of inhibitory transmission disrupts ocular dominance plasticity [73], whereas the early enhancement of inhibitory transmission promotes a precocious period plasticity [74]. Furthermore it has been demonstrated that cortical plasticity can be induced by transplantation of inhibitory neurons of a cellular age equivalent to that of endogenous inhibitory neurons during the normal critical period [75]. These findings suggest that the critical period is tuned by the accomplishment of a developmental program intrinsic to inhibitory neurons. Thus, resetting the excitatory-inhibitory balance to mimic critical period onset, or affecting molecular brakes that strengthen structural changes after this period are a possible strategies to foster functional recovery in the adult.

### Alteration of Brain Excitability after Stroke

During the first weeks after cerebral ischemia brain excitability is characterised by two main opposing phases interlinked through γ-Aminobutyric Acid (GABA) and glutamate signalling [76, 77]. In the acute phase of stroke brain excitability levels are elevated due to massive glutamate release from damaged tissue, leading to cell death and neurodegeneration. In this early phase, reducing glutamate or enhancing GABA signalling triggers neuroprotection, at least in animal models of stroke [76]. In the subacute phase however, the E-I balance seems to have different effects. After brain infarction has fully developed the brain tissue begins to reorganize, down-tuning inhibition to favour plasticity processes. Indeed glutamatergic signal activation after 5 days from experimental stroke, possibly through BDNF modulation, induces motor recovery [77]. Moreover genetic and pharmacological reduction of excessive GABAergic tonic inhibition, from day 3 after ischemia on, promotes functional recovery [77]. To better understand the complex mechanisms, which regulate excitatory and inhibitory signals in the different phases of stroke, and how to modulate this balance to promote functional and effective recovery, it is necessary to discuss the molecular elements that regulate these processes.

## *GABA Signalling in Stroke*

Extrasynaptic GABA signalling controls neuronal excitability and drugs blocking this tonic signal promote neuronal excitability, enhance Long Term Potentiation (LTP) formation, and lead to improvements in learning. The inhibitory neurotransmitter GABA is thus important for cortical plasticity. Modulation of GABAergic transmission changes sensory maps during the critical period of cortical development [78] and produces rapid alterations in adult cortical maps that resemble changes occurring after stroke.

Several studies demonstrate that stroke causes an increase in tonic GABA currents for several weeks after injury [77]. Indeed peri-infarct cortex exhibits decreased activation to motor and sensory stimulation early after stroke. In experimental stroke it was shown that neurons in recovering motor cortex are hypoexcitable since a substantial increase in the tonic GABA current affects peri-infarct neurons. This alteration seems to be due to increased tonic GABA currents because of reduced GABA reuptake. In particular a reduced expression of the GABA transporter GAT-3/4 in reactive astrocytes in peri-infarct cortex has been described [77]. Thus the evidence that blocking extrasynaptic $GABA_A Rs$ three days after stroke has an effect on cellular excitability and plasticity, and the indication that these changes in neuronal excitability underlie functional reorganization in peri-infarct cortex, have shown that this system is important in stroke recovery. Thus a fine modulation of GABAergic signalling could promote plasticity and recovery after pathological processes [77].

## *Glutamate Signalling in Stroke*

It has been shown that modifications in the equilibrium between synaptic and extrasynaptic NMDA receptors subunit expression contribute to neuronal dysfunction in acute ischemia. Indeed mice deficient in the NMDA subunit NR2A are more resistant to ischemia [79, 80], while pharmacological blockade of NR2B-NMDA receptors in a model of focal ischemia causes amelioration of neurological outcome and inhibition of detrimental post- ischemic LTP, favouring plasticity processes [81].

As occurs for GABA transporters also the main glutamate transporters, known as excitatory amino acid transporters 2 (EAAT2 or GLT1) and EAAT1 (or GLAST), are down-regulated immediately after ischemia. In particular the expression of GLT1 protein decreases in several experimental models of ischemia, already 6h after transient focal ischemia [82]. Successively at later time point, an up-regulation of GLT1 is present [83], probably indicating an attempt of peri-ischemic tissue to preserve itself from prolonged glutamate-induced damage, augmenting its buffering. Analogous is the regulation of GLAST. Glutamate transporters are down-regulated in the subacute phase of stroke, and then up-regulated later on. Indeed a polymorphism in the EAAT2 promoter has been discovered to be important in stroke. This polymorphism creates a binding site for the repressor transcription factor GC-binding factor 2 (GCF2), highly expressed immediately after stroke, thus leading to a 30% reduction in the basal promoter activity. As a result patients with this polymorphisms in EAAT2 have increased plasma glutamate levels and a trend towards worse neurological outcome after stroke [84]. The role of the toxic effect of glutamate in acute stroke has been amply documented; nonetheless numerous clinical trials aiming to reduce NMDA and AMPA receptor activation have so far failed [105]. As alternative another line of research tries to foster recovery after stroke by exploiting the glutamate signalling to enhance plasticity mechanisms.

A complex balance between excitatory and inhibitory signals emerges, in which modulating GABAergic and Glutamatergic currents seems to be necessary immediately after stroke to limit the damage and the cell death. Soon after however an early increase in glutamatergic signal and a reduction of GABAergic extrasynaptic currents is fundamental to favor plasticity processes, the basis for functional recovery. It is thus necessary to regulate this balance carefully, taking into account that it evolves quickly over time, from being deleterious to promoting recovery.

## Approaches to Modulate Neural Plasticity

Fostering tissue plasticity is one of the major goals of neuroprotective therapies still challenging with incurable neurological disorders such as cerebral ischemia. Various approaches have been suggested to increase the connections of surviving neurons on both the ischemic and contralateral hemisphere [86, 87]. Despite several approaches spanning from pharmacological modulation of the peri-ischemic milieu to electrical stimulation procedures, the results are, so far, mostly elusive when applied into clinical practice. Among developing techniques, cell treatments are emerging as a valid alternative to foster post-stroke plasticity and recovery [88]. In the next paragraphs we will discuss current strategies to try to modulate neural plasticity.

### *Rehabilitation*

Experimental stroke models suggest that increased plasticity processes occur in particular in the first month after brain ischemia. As discussed above, during this initial period, peri-infarct and remote areas undergo changes in excitatory/inhibitory balance and in structural remodelling. Nonetheless the optimal timeframe to improve neurological functions through rehabilitation is still quite unclear. In animal models, very early and intense training seems to lead to increased damage. Recently also a clinical trial on early rehabilitation 'A Very Early Rehabilitation Trial (AVERT)' demonstrated that very early mobilization afters stroke was linked to a less favourable outcome compared to the usual care group [89, 90]. Conversely, late rehabilitation (after one month) seems to be less efficacious in terms of reducing disability. In clinical practice, rehabilitation after disabling stroke involves a 1-2 months of inpatient therapy that although partially effective, often does not match the intensity levels investigated in animal models and includes the training of compensatory strategies that have minimal impact on impairment. It is also important to notice that although early training is more effective, many stroke patients also continue to improve over time after their original injury due to spontaneous recovery processes, home-based rehabilitation or as a result of constraint-induced movement therapy. This points out that the exact timeframe for stroke recovery to occur, as with that of learning is not strictly time-limited. Nonetheless, the plasticity processes that characterize early brain development and the subacute phase after stroke diminish steadily over time.

Wahl *et al.* [91] showed that in experimental stroke a correct timing of sequential interventions could maximise the recovery. Indeed a first reduction of the endogenous growth-inhibitory factor Nogo-A by immunotherapy was able to reduce constraints on lesion-induced structural plasticity [55] and to pave the way for rehabilitative training that was successively necessary to shape the spared and new circuits by selection and stabilization of functional connections and pruning of non-functional ones. This demonstration is an important milestone in exploring growth-inhibitor blockade in combination with rehabilitative training as a treatment strategy for stroke.

## Non-Invasive Transcranial Stimulation

In the last 20 years, due to technological improvements, non- invasive transcranial stimulation has emerged as an appealing and promising approach to be used in different fields of neurology. In particular two major techniques are available; the transcranial magnetic stimulation (TMS) and the transcranial direct current stimulation (tDCS). Beside clinical relevant conventional brain stimulation methods such as deep brain stimulation (DBS) or electroconvulsive therapy, TMS and tDCS have advantages in terms of reduced invasiveness and safety although are not used routinely in clinical practice in stroke. The ability of transcranial stimulation to foster (or dampen) cortical activity of the lesioned (or the unaffected) hemisphere has been used to improve motor- and gait impairment, post-stroke depression, as well as cortical deficits (e.g. aphasia) in stroke patients [86, 92, 93]. Direct current stimulation of the peri-infarct cortex using a protocol that boosts local neuronal excitability improved the use of the affected limb in patients with chronic stroke [85]. Currently, the most promising approach seem to be to trigger durable modifications of neuronal circuits in the ischemic hemisphere or to inhibit the contralesional unaffected hemisphere that might be improperly activated. Different stimulation protocols at different times of application may represent future fields of investigation [94].

### Pharmacological Modulation of Neural Plasticity

Various approaches to enhance recovery after stroke through pharmacological stimulation of neural plasticity have been explored in experimental models of brain ischemia. Studies in animals show that the effects of drugs on neurotransmitters in the CNS can modulate the rate and extent of functional recovery after brain injury. Although its translation to human stroke is quite difficult and not yet possible in clinical practice, important insights in the pathophysiology and possible repair strategies for stroke are given by discussing these examples. Moreover several of the promising compounds are often already in clinical use for other indications so that safety issues might be of less concern.

In the post-ischemic brain, selective serotonin reuptake inhibitors such as fluoxetine seem to act as neuroprotectants both by reducing inflammation but also by promoting hippocampal neurogenesis in experimental stroke and thus ameliorating cognitive defects [95]. In a phase II clinical trial entitled ,Fluoxetine for motor recovery after acute ischemic stroke' (FLAME) it was shown that motor rehabilitation in combination with early fluoxetine treatment ameliorated motor recovery and reduced disability compared to patients exposed to rehabilitative therapy alone [96].

Neurorestorative treatments do not necessarily need to promote the growth of terminal axons distal to the site of injury, but can also trigger homologous fibres originating from the contralesional motor cortex growing out across the midline to reach denervated neurons in target structures of the lesioned pyramidal tract [35, 87].

Vascular endothelial growth factor (VEGF) stimulates neurogenesis and angiogenesis [97] but in stroke a too early administration is detrimental since it promotes blood– brain barrier leakage and haemorrhagic transformation. On the opposite timely administration of VEGF starting 3 days after middle cerebral artery occlusion was observed to trigger neurological stroke recovery by promoting angiogenesis in the ischemic hemisphere, and axonal sprouting in the contralesional hemisphere [87].

Similarly erythropoietin (EPO), a growth factor used for the treatment of anaemia, was observed to be deleterious when applied in the acute phase of stroke in particular when combined with tissue plasminogen activator (tPA). Indeed both drugs acted in synergy on the blood–brain barrier permeability and augmented in this way the occurrence of haemorrhagic transformation [98]. Again, similarly to VEGF, delayed EPO treatment starting 3 days after stroke induction improved functional recovery by promoting neuronal survival and angiogenesis in the peri-ischemic tissue, and contralesional plasticity [35].

Granulocyte colony stimulating factor (G-CSF) has been shown experimentally to improve long-term functional recovery after stroke even when delayed for days [99]. In humans however G-CSF did not show any clinical benefit. Only a trend for reduced infarct growth in the G-CSF group was noticed at the expenses of a strong increase in leukocytes and monocytes that might have offset the potential beneficial effect of G-CSF [100].

Brain derived neurotrophic factor (BDNF) seems to exert a powerful effect on neuronal plasticity, synapse development and dendritic and axonal sprouting. In stroke systemic administration of BDNF promotes recovery [101], while brain infusion of a BDNF antisense oligonucleotide impairs recuperation [102]. Interestingly subjects with a val66met polymorphism in the brain-derived neurotrophic factor (BDNF) gene, have reduced plasticity processes after transcranial magnetic stimulation as compared to subjects without the polymorphism. These results suggest that BDNF is involved in mediating experience-dependent plasticity of human motor cortex [103, 104].

### *Modulation of GABA Signalling to Promote Plasticity*

Potential benefits derived from GABA regulation in post-stroke recovery have been highlighted recently. It has been demonstrated that chronic treatment with an inverse agonist- specific for GABAα5 subunit of GABA$_A$Rs, starting 3 days after experimental cortical stroke (in the subacute phase) reduced the excessive GABA-mediated tonic inhibition, resulting in early and sustained recovery of motor function in mice [77]. In contrast stroke volume was increased when mice were treated with same drug from stroke onset. Genetically lowering the number of α5 or δ-subunit-containing GABA$_A$Rs, responsible for tonic inhibition, also was found to be effective in augmenting stroke recovery. Nonetheless a prolonged treatment with the inverse agonist-specific for GABAα5 subunit produced a deterioration in motor function at late period after stroke, suggesting that increasing cortical excitability or reducing phasic inhibition for too prolonged time negatively impacts on functional recovery [77]. With any stroke treatment the timing of drug delivery is key.

### *Modulation of Glutamate Homeostasis to Promote Plasticity*

Studies on stroke recovery suggest that glutamate and possibly AMPA receptor signalling play a role in the synaptic plasticity that underlies recovery. AMPA stimulation promotes recovery beginning 5 days after stroke, improving limb control [77]. Accordingly blocking AMPA receptor signalling during the same period impedes recovery. AMPA receptor signalling seems thus to have a delayed and causal effect on motor recovery after stroke. Enhancing AMPA receptor activity can mediate improved recovery through its downstream effect of BDNF induction within the peri-infarct cortex.

### *Neural Stem Cell-based Therapies*

The ability of transplanted neural progenitor cells to protect the CNS from diverse injuries through their 'bystander' effect [106] has been demonstrated in experimental neurological diseases such as stroke [21], spinal cord injury [107], epilepsy [108] and experimental multiple sclerosis [109, 110]. Neural progenitor cells are able to sense the environment and to adapt their fate and functionality to the tissue context in which they are transplanted and to exert different therapeutic effects such as cell replacement, neurotrophic support, immunomodulation and angiogenesis, a mode of action that has been called 'therapeutic plasticity' [111 - 114]. In particular the characteristic of stem cells to migrate specifically to the injured tissue site, a property called pathotropism, and the capacity to adapt their function in space and time on the basis of tissue needs is a major advantage compared to pharmacological treatment that are often systemic and not specifically targeted to the tissue needs.

Neural progenitor cell transplantation may indeed promote the formation of new local circuits by releasing neurotrophic growth factors and stem cell regulators at the site of tissue damage [22, 23]. In particular neural progenitor cells surviving in the perilesional milieu were shown to be capable of reducing white matter atrophy, to increase dendritic arborisations of layer V pyramidal neurons in both hemispheres as well as to increase contralateral cortico-cortical, cortico-striatal and cortico-spinal axonal projections. These findings were attributed to the secretion by neural progenitor cells of guidance molecules (*i.e.* slit, thrombospondin 1 and 2) and vascular endothelial growth factor [22, 23], but also other growth factors might be involved. Besides the possible ‚bystander' effect, transplanted NPCs can also exert, in specific cases, a direct repair of injured tissue. After transplantation into the stroke-damaged striatum and cortex, neuroepithelial-like stem (NES) derived from human induced pluripotent stem cells were shown to generate a high proportion of cells with morphological and electrophysiological properties of neurons, thus providing evidence that iPSCs derived NES can be used for neuronal replacement in stroke [115, 116]. Nonetheless, whether integrated transplanted cells effectively contribute to tissue recovery still need to be demonstrated by loss of function experiments. Currently clinical trials with stem cell delivery in stroke patients are on-going, aiming at triggering improvements in the chronic phase after stroke (www.clinicaltrials.gov).

## CONCLUSION

A detailed knowledge of the pathophysiology of post-acute stroke provides an important framework for the development of novel pharmacological strategies to promote recovery. The translation of these approaches from animal models to humans requires a profound understanding of the transition between different phases of stroke, in which a plasticity potential is present but often suppressed. Although the replacing endogenous damaged neurons and brain tissue by transplanting functional cells is still not completely possible after stroke, the prospect that therapeutical strategies can optimize and foster plastic abilities endowed in the CNS using molecules constitutively expressed during development and adulthood is noteworthy.

## TAKE HOME MESSAGE

Recovery from disabling cerebral ischemia can be enhanced by treatments able to halt the neurodegenerative process and to foster adaptive tissue plasticity. Due to the multifaceted pathophysiology of stroke and of the systems involved, therapies that promote repair processes should act in a spatially and timely targeted manner to avoid detrimental effects.

## CONFLICT OF INTEREST

The authors confirm that they have no conflict of interest to declare for this publication.

## ACKNOWLEDGEMENTS

This work has been in part supported by TargetBrain (EU Framework 7 project HEALTH-F2-2012–279017) to GM and by Ministero della Salute Italiana (Progetto Giovani Ricercatori 58/GR-2011-02348160) to MB.

## REFERENCES

[1]     Wieloch T, Nikolich K. Mechanisms of neural plasticity following brain injury. Curr Opin Neurobiol 2006; 16(3): 258-64.
        [http://dx.doi.org/10.1016/j.conb.2006.05.011] [PMID: 16713245]

[2]     Dirnagl U, Iadecola C, Moskowitz MA. Pathobiology of ischaemic stroke: an integrated view. Trends Neurosci 1999; 22(9): 391-7.
        [http://dx.doi.org/10.1016/S0166-2236(99)01401-0] [PMID: 10441299]

[3]     Hossmann KA. Pathophysiology and therapy of experimental stroke. Cell Mol Neurobiol 2006; 26(7-8): 1057-83.
        [http://dx.doi.org/10.1007/s10571-006-9008-1] [PMID: 16710759]

[4]     Sist B, Jesudasan S, Winship IR. Diaschisis, degeneration, and adaptive plasticity after focal ischemic stroke. In: Garcia Rodríguez J, Ed. Acute Ischemic Stroke: InTech. 2012.
        [http://dx.doi.org/10.5772/28577]

[5]     Lo EH. A new penumbra: transitioning from injury into repair after stroke. Nat Med 2008; 14(5): 497-500.

[http://dx.doi.org/10.1038/nm1735] [PMID: 18463660]

[6]　Cunningham LA, Wetzel M, Rosenberg GA. Multiple roles for MMPs and TIMPs in cerebral ischemia. Glia 2005; 50(4): 329-39.
[http://dx.doi.org/10.1002/glia.20169] [PMID: 15846802]

[7]　Zhao BQ, Tejima E, Lo EH. Neurovascular proteases in brain injury, hemorrhage and remodeling after stroke. Stroke 2007; 38(2) (Suppl.): 748-52.
[http://dx.doi.org/10.1161/01.STR.0000253500.32979.d1] [PMID: 17261731]

[8]　Iadecola C, Anrather J. The immunology of stroke: from mechanisms to translation. Nat Med 2011; 17(7): 796-808.
[http://dx.doi.org/10.1038/nm.2399] [PMID: 21738161]

[9]　Moalem G, Leibowitz-Amit R, Yoles E, Mor F, Cohen IR, Schwartz M. Autoimmune T cells protect neurons from secondary degeneration after central nervous system axotomy. Nat Med 1999; 5(1): 49-55.
[http://dx.doi.org/10.1038/4734] [PMID: 9883839]

[10]　Ginhoux F, Greter M, Leboeuf M, Nandi S, See P, Gokhan S, *et al.* Fate mapping analysis reveals that adult microglia derive from primitive macrophages. Science 2010; 330(6005): 841-5.
[http://dx.doi.org/10.1126/science.1194637]

[11]　Li T, Pang S, Yu Y, Wu X, Guo J, Zhang S. Proliferation of parenchymal microglia is the main source of microgliosis after ischaemic stroke. Brain 2013; 136(Pt 12): 3578-88.
[http://dx.doi.org/10.1093/brain/awt287] [PMID: 24154617]

[12]　Chu HX, Broughton BR, Kim HA, Lee S, Drummond GR, Sobey CG. Evidence that Ly6C(hi) monocytes are protective in acute ischemic stroke by promoting M2 macrophage polarization. Stroke 2015; 46(7): 1929-37.
[http://dx.doi.org/10.1161/STROKEAHA.115.009426] [PMID: 25999385]

[13]　Gliem M, Mausberg AK, Lee JI, *et al.* Macrophages prevent hemorrhagic infarct transformation in murine stroke models. Ann Neurol 2012; 71(6): 743-52.
[http://dx.doi.org/10.1002/ana.23529] [PMID: 22718543]

[14]　Kokaia Z, Martino G, Schwartz M, Lindvall O. Cross-talk between neural stem cells and immune cells: the key to better brain repair? Nat Neurosci 2012; 15(8): 1078-87.
[http://dx.doi.org/10.1038/nn.3163] [PMID: 22837038]

[15]　Altman J, Das GD. Autoradiographic and histological evidence of postnatal hippocampal neurogenesis in rats. J Comp Neurol 1965; 124(3): 319-35.
[http://dx.doi.org/10.1002/cne.901240303] [PMID: 5861717]

[16]　Zhang R, Zhang Z, Zhang C, *et al.* Stroke transiently increases subventricular zone cell division from asymmetric to symmetric and increases neuronal differentiation in the adult rat. J Neurosci 2004; 24(25): 5810-5.
[http://dx.doi.org/10.1523/JNEUROSCI.1109-04.2004] [PMID: 15215303]

[17]　Arvidsson A, Collin T, Kirik D, Kokaia Z, Lindvall O. Neuronal replacement from endogenous precursors in the adult brain after stroke. Nat Med 2002; 8(9): 963-70.
[http://dx.doi.org/10.1038/nm747] [PMID: 12161747]

[18] Thored P, Arvidsson A, Cacci E, *et al.* Persistent production of neurons from adult brain stem cells during recovery after stroke. Stem Cells 2006; 24(3): 739-47.
[http://dx.doi.org/10.1634/stemcells.2005-0281] [PMID: 16210404]

[19] Butti E, Bacigaluppi M, Rossi S, *et al.* Subventricular zone neural progenitors protect striatal neurons from glutamatergic excitotoxicity. Brain 2012; 135(Pt 11): 3320-35.
[http://dx.doi.org/10.1093/brain/aws194] [PMID: 23008234]

[20] Benner EJ, Luciano D, Jo R, *et al.* Protective astrogenesis from the SVZ niche after injury is controlled by Notch modulator Thbs4. Nature 2013; 497(7449): 369-73.
[http://dx.doi.org/10.1038/nature12069] [PMID: 23615612]

[21] Bacigaluppi M, Pluchino S, Peruzzotti-Jametti L, *et al.* Delayed post-ischaemic neuroprotection following systemic neural stem cell transplantation involves multiple mechanisms. Brain 2009; 132(Pt 8): 2239-51.
[http://dx.doi.org/10.1093/brain/awp174] [PMID: 19617198]

[22] Andres RH, Horie N, Slikker W, *et al.* Human neural stem cells enhance structural plasticity and axonal transport in the ischaemic brain. Brain : a journal of neurology 2011; 134(Pt 6): 1777-89.
[http://dx.doi.org/10.1093/brain/awr094]

[23] Bacigaluppi M, Russo GL, Peruzzotti-Jametti L, *et al.* Neural stem cell transplantation induces stroke recovery by upregulating glutamate transporter GLT-1 in astrocytes. J Neurosci 2016; 36(41): 10529-44.
[http://dx.doi.org/10.1523/JNEUROSCI.1643-16.2016] [PMID: 27733606]

[24] Krupinski J, Kumar P, Kumar S, Kaluza J. Increased expression of TGF-beta 1 in brain tissue after ischemic stroke in humans. Stroke 1996; 27(5): 852-7.
[http://dx.doi.org/10.1161/01.STR.27.5.852] [PMID: 8623105]

[25] Chopp M, Zhang ZG, Jiang Q. Neurogenesis, angiogenesis, and MRI indices of functional recovery from stroke. Stroke 2007; 38(2) (Suppl.): 827-31.
[http://dx.doi.org/10.1161/01.STR.0000250235.80253.e9] [PMID: 17261747]

[26] Carmeliet P, Tessier-Lavigne M. Common mechanisms of nerve and blood vessel wiring. Nature 2005; 436(7048): 193-200.
[http://dx.doi.org/10.1038/nature03875] [PMID: 16015319]

[27] Ohab JJ, Fleming S, Blesch A, Carmichael ST. A neurovascular niche for neurogenesis after stroke. J Neurosci 2006; 26(50): 13007-16.
[http://dx.doi.org/10.1523/JNEUROSCI.4323-06.2006] [PMID: 17167090]

[28] Caballero-Garrido E, Pena-Philippides JC, Lordkipanidze T, *et al.* *In Vivo* Inhibition of miR-155 Promotes Recovery after Experimental Mouse Stroke. J Neurosci 2015; 35(36): 12446-64.
[http://dx.doi.org/10.1523/JNEUROSCI.1641-15.2015] [PMID: 26354913]

[29] Hayakawa K, Nakano T, Irie K, *et al.* Inhibition of reactive astrocytes with fluorocitrate retards neurovascular remodeling and recovery after focal cerebral ischemia in mice. J Cereb Blood Flow Metab 2010; 30(4): 871-82.
[http://dx.doi.org/10.1038/jcbfm.2009.257] [PMID: 19997116]

[30] Liu Z, Li Y, Cui Y, *et al.* Beneficial effects of gfap/vimentin reactive astrocytes for axonal remodeling

and motor behavioral recovery in mice after stroke. Glia 2014; 62(12): 2022-33.
[http://dx.doi.org/10.1002/glia.22723] [PMID: 25043249]

[31]   Busch SA, Silver J. The role of extracellular matrix in CNS regeneration. Curr Opin Neurobiol 2007; 17(1): 120-7.
[http://dx.doi.org/10.1016/j.conb.2006.09.004] [PMID: 17223033]

[32]   Nawashiro H, Brenner M, Fukui S, Shima K, Hallenbeck JM. High susceptibility to cerebral ischemia in GFAP-null mice. J Cereb Blood Flow Metab 2000; 20(7): 1040-4.
[http://dx.doi.org/10.1097/00004647-200007000-00003] [PMID: 10908037]

[33]   Soleman S, Yip PK, Duricki DA, Moon LD. Delayed treatment with chondroitinase ABC promotes sensorimotor recovery and plasticity after stroke in aged rats. Brain 2012; 135(Pt 4): 1210-23.
[http://dx.doi.org/10.1093/brain/aws027] [PMID: 22396394]

[34]   Gherardini L, Gennaro M, Pizzorusso T. Perilesional treatment with chondroitinase ABC and motor training promote functional recovery after stroke in rats. Cereb Cortex 2015; 25(1): 202-12.
[http://dx.doi.org/10.1093/cercor/bht217] [PMID: 23960208]

[35]   Reitmeir R, Kilic E, Kilic U, *et al.* Post-acute delivery of erythropoietin induces stroke recovery by promoting perilesional tissue remodelling and contralesional pyramidal tract plasticity. Brain 2011; 134(Pt 1): 84-99.
[http://dx.doi.org/10.1093/brain/awq344] [PMID: 21186263]

[36]   Hermann DM, Chopp M. Promoting brain remodelling and plasticity for stroke recovery: therapeutic promise and potential pitfalls of clinical translation. Lancet Neurol 2012; 11(4): 369-80.
[http://dx.doi.org/10.1016/S1474-4422(12)70039-X] [PMID: 22441198]

[37]   Liu XS, Chopp M, Zhang XG, *et al.* Gene profiles and electrophysiology of doublecortin-expressing cells in the subventricular zone after ischemic stroke. J Cereb Blood Flow Metab 2009; 29(2): 297-307.
[http://dx.doi.org/10.1038/jcbfm.2008.119]

[38]   Jiang Q, Zhang ZG, Chopp M. MRI evaluation of white matter recovery after brain injury. Stroke 2010; 41(10) (Suppl.): S112-3.
[http://dx.doi.org/10.1161/STROKEAHA.110.595629] [PMID: 20876482]

[39]   Liu Z, Li Y, Zhang X, Savant-Bhonsale S, Chopp M. Contralesional axonal remodeling of the corticospinal system in adult rats after stroke and bone marrow stromal cell treatment. Stroke 2008; 39(9): 2571-7.
[http://dx.doi.org/10.1161/STROKEAHA.107.511659] [PMID: 18617661]

[40]   Dancause N, Barbay S, Frost SB, *et al.* Extensive cortical rewiring after brain injury. J Neurosci 2005; 25(44): 10167-79.
[http://dx.doi.org/10.1523/JNEUROSCI.3256-05.2005] [PMID: 16267224]

[41]   Buchli AD, Schwab ME. Inhibition of Nogo: a key strategy to increase regeneration, plasticity and functional recovery of the lesioned central nervous system. Ann Med 2005; 37(8): 556-67.
[http://dx.doi.org/10.1080/07853890500407520] [PMID: 16338758]

[42]   Rossini PM, Calautti C, Pauri F, Baron JC. Post-stroke plastic reorganisation in the adult brain. Lancet Neurol 2003; 2(8): 493-502.

[http://dx.doi.org/10.1016/S1474-4422(03)00485-X] [PMID: 12878437]

[43]    Briones TL, Suh E, Jozsa L, Woods J. Behaviorally induced synaptogenesis and dendritic growth in the hippocampal region following transient global cerebral ischemia are accompanied by improvement in spatial learning. Exp Neurol 2006; 198(2): 530-8.
[http://dx.doi.org/10.1016/j.expneurol.2005.12.032] [PMID: 16483572]

[44]    Mattson MP, Meffert MK. Roles for NF-kappaB in nerve cell survival, plasticity, and disease. Cell Death Differ 2006; 13(5): 852-60.
[http://dx.doi.org/10.1038/sj.cdd.4401837] [PMID: 16397579]

[45]    Majewska AK, Newton JR, Sur M. Remodeling of synaptic structure in sensory cortical areas *in vivo*. J Neurosci 2006; 26(11): 3021-9.
[http://dx.doi.org/10.1523/JNEUROSCI.4454-05.2006] [PMID: 16540580]

[46]    Brown CE, Wong C, Murphy TH. Rapid morphologic plasticity of peri-infarct dendritic spines after focal ischemic stroke. Stroke 2008; 39(4): 1286-91.
[http://dx.doi.org/10.1161/STROKEAHA.107.498238] [PMID: 18323506]

[47]    Li P, Murphy TH. Two-photon imaging during prolonged middle cerebral artery occlusion in mice reveals recovery of dendritic structure after reperfusion. J Neurosci 2008; 28(46): 11970-9.
[http://dx.doi.org/10.1523/JNEUROSCI.3724-08.2008] [PMID: 19005062]

[48]    Zhang S, Murphy TH. Imaging the impact of cortical microcirculation on synaptic structure and sensory-evoked hemodynamic responses *in vivo*. PLoS Biol 2007; 5(5): e119.
[http://dx.doi.org/10.1371/journal.pbio.0050119] [PMID: 17456007]

[49]    Tran S, Chen S, Liu RR, Xie Y, Murphy TH. Moderate or deep local hypothermia does not prevent the onset of ischemia-induced dendritic damage. J Cereb Blood Flow Metab 2012; 32(3): 437-42.
[http://dx.doi.org/10.1038/jcbfm.2011.178] [PMID: 22167237]

[50]    Mostany R, Chowdhury TG, Johnston DG, Portonovo SA, Carmichael ST, Portera-Cailliau C. Local hemodynamics dictate long-term dendritic plasticity in peri-infarct cortex. J Neurosci 2010; 30(42): 14116-26.
[http://dx.doi.org/10.1523/JNEUROSCI.3908-10.2010] [PMID: 20962232]

[51]    Benecke R, Meyer BU, Freund HJ. Reorganisation of descending motor pathways in patients after hemispherectomy and severe hemispheric lesions demonstrated by magnetic brain stimulation. Experimental brain research Experimentelle Hirnforschung 1991; 83(2): 419-26.
[http://dx.doi.org/10.1007/BF00231167]

[52]    Cramer SC, Chopp M. Recovery recapitulates ontogeny. Trends Neurosci 2000; 23(6): 265-71.
[http://dx.doi.org/10.1016/S0166-2236(00)01562-9] [PMID: 10838596]

[53]    Nudo RJ, Wise BM. Neural substrates for the effects of rehabilitative training on motor recovery after ischemic infarct. Science 1996; 272(5269): 1791-4.

[54]    Biernaskie J, Szymanska A, Windle V, Corbett D. Bi-hemispheric contribution to functional motor recovery of the affected forelimb following focal ischemic brain injury in rats. Eur J Neurosci 2005; 21(4): 989-99.
[http://dx.doi.org/10.1111/j.1460-9568.2005.03899.x] [PMID: 15787705]

[55]    Murphy TH, Corbett D. Plasticity during stroke recovery: from synapse to behaviour. Nature reviews

2009; 10(12): 861-72.
[http://dx.doi.org/10.1038/nrn2735]

[56]    Hubel DH, Wiesel TN. The period of susceptibility to the physiological effects of unilateral eye closure in kittens. J Physiol 1970; 206(2): 419-36.
[http://dx.doi.org/10.1113/jphysiol.1970.sp009022] [PMID: 5498493]

[57]    Shetty AK, Hattiangady B, Shetty GA. Stem/progenitor cell proliferation factors FGF-2, IGF-1, and VEGF exhibit early decline during the course of aging in the hippocampus: role of astrocytes. Glia 2005; 51(3): 173-86.
[http://dx.doi.org/10.1002/glia.20187] [PMID: 15800930]

[58]    Johansson BB. Brain plasticity and stroke rehabilitation. The Willis lecture. Stroke 2000; 31(1): 223-30.
[http://dx.doi.org/10.1161/01.STR.31.1.223] [PMID: 10625741]

[59]    Carmichael ST, Archibeque I, Luke L, Nolan T, Momiy J, Li S. Growth-associated gene expression after stroke: evidence for a growth-promoting region in peri-infarct cortex. Exp Neurol 2005; 193(2): 291-311.
[http://dx.doi.org/10.1016/j.expneurol.2005.01.004] [PMID: 15869933]

[60]    Carmichael ST. Cellular and molecular mechanisms of neural repair after stroke: making waves. Ann Neurol 2006; 59(5): 735-42.
[http://dx.doi.org/10.1002/ana.20845] [PMID: 16634041]

[61]    Li S, Overman JJ, Katsman D, *et al.* An age-related sprouting transcriptome provides molecular control of axonal sprouting after stroke. Nat Neurosci 2010; 13(12): 1496-504.
[http://dx.doi.org/10.1038/nn.2674] [PMID: 21057507]

[62]    Brückner G, Bringmann A, Köppe G, Härtig W, Brauer K. *In vivo* and *in vitro* labelling of perineuronal nets in rat brain. Brain Res 1996; 720(1-2): 84-92.
[http://dx.doi.org/10.1016/0006-8993(96)00152-7] [PMID: 8782900]

[63]    Silver J, Miller JH. Regeneration beyond the glial scar. Nature reviews 2004; 5(2): 146-56.
[http://dx.doi.org/10.1038/nrn1326]

[64]    McKeon RJ, Schreiber RC, Rudge JS, Silver J. Reduction of neurite outgrowth in a model of glial scarring following CNS injury is correlated with the expression of inhibitory molecules on reactive astrocytes. J Neurosci 1991; 11(11): 3398-411.
[PMID: 1719160]

[65]    Becker CG, Becker T. Repellent guidance of regenerating optic axons by chondroitin sulfate glycosaminoglycans in zebrafish. J Neurosci 2002; 22(3): 842-53.
[PMID: 11826114]

[66]    Schwab ME. Nogo and axon regeneration. Curr Opin Neurobiol 2004; 14(1): 118-24.
[http://dx.doi.org/10.1016/j.conb.2004.01.004] [PMID: 15018947]

[67]    Schwab ME. Functions of Nogo proteins and their receptors in the nervous system. Nature reviews 2010; 11(12): 799-811.
[http://dx.doi.org/10.1038/nrn2936]

[68]    Gou X, Zhang Q, Xu N, *et al.* Spatio-temporal expression of paired immunoglobulin-like receptor-B in

the adult mouse brain after focal cerebral ischaemia. Brain Inj 2013; 27(11): 1311-5.
[http://dx.doi.org/10.3109/02699052.2013.812241] [PMID: 23927735]

[69]  Schwab ME, Strittmatter SM. Nogo limits neural plasticity and recovery from injury. Curr Opin Neurobiol 2014; 27: 53-60.
[http://dx.doi.org/10.1016/j.conb.2014.02.011] [PMID: 24632308]

[70]  McGee AW, Yang Y, Fischer QS, Daw NW, Strittmatter SM. Experience-driven plasticity of visual cortex limited by myelin and Nogo receptor. Science 2005; 309(5744): 2222-6.
[http://dx.doi.org/10.1126/science.1114362]

[71]  Morishita H, Hensch TK. Critical period revisited: impact on vision. Curr Opin Neurobiol 2008; 18(1): 101-7.
[http://dx.doi.org/10.1016/j.conb.2008.05.009] [PMID: 18534841]

[72]  Fagiolini M, Hensch TK. Inhibitory threshold for critical-period activation in primary visual cortex. Nature 2000; 404(6774): 183-6.
[http://dx.doi.org/10.1038/35004582] [PMID: 10724170]

[73]  Hensch TK, Gordon JA, Brandon EP, McKnight GS, Idzerda RL, Stryker MP. Comparison of plasticity *in vivo* and *in vitro* in the developing visual cortex of normal and protein kinase A RIbeta-deficient mice. J Neurosci 1998; 18(6): 2108-17.
[PMID: 9482797]

[74]  Fagiolini M, Fritschy JM, Low K, Mohler H, Rudolph U, Hensch TK. Specific GABAA circuits for visual cortical plasticity. Science 2004; 303(5664): 1681-3.
[http://dx.doi.org/10.1126/science.1091032]

[75]  Southwell DG, Froemke RC, Alvarez-Buylla A, Stryker MP, Gandhi SP. Cortical plasticity induced by inhibitory neuron transplantation. Science 2010; 327(5969): 1145-8.
[http://dx.doi.org/10.1126/science.1183962]

[76]  Carmichael ST. Brain excitability in stroke: the yin and yang of stroke progression. Arch Neurol 2012; 69(2): 161-7.
[http://dx.doi.org/10.1001/archneurol.2011.1175] [PMID: 21987395]

[77]  Clarkson AN, Huang BS, Macisaac SE, Mody I, Carmichael ST. Reducing excessive GABA-mediated tonic inhibition promotes functional recovery after stroke. Nature 2010; 468(7321): 305-9.
[http://dx.doi.org/10.1038/nature09511] [PMID: 21048709]

[78]  Hensch TK. Critical period plasticity in local cortical circuits. Nature reviews 2005; 6(11): 877-8.
[http://dx.doi.org/10.1038/nrn1787]

[79]  Gouix E, Léveillé F, Nicole O, Melon C, Had-Aissouni L, Buisson A. Reverse glial glutamate uptake triggers neuronal cell death through extrasynaptic NMDA receptor activation. Mol Cell Neurosci 2009; 40(4): 463-73.
[http://dx.doi.org/10.1016/j.mcn.2009.01.002] [PMID: 19340933]

[80]  Morikawa E, Mori H, Kiyama Y, Mishina M, Asano T, Kirino T. Attenuation of focal ischemic brain injury in mice deficient in the epsilon1 (NR2A) subunit of NMDA receptor. J Neurosci 1998; 18(23): 9727-32.
[PMID: 9822733]

[81]  Picconi B, Tortiglione A, Barone I, *et al.* NR2B subunit exerts a critical role in postischemic synaptic plasticity. Stroke 2006; 37(7): 1895-901.
[http://dx.doi.org/10.1161/01.STR.0000226981.57777.b0] [PMID: 16741178]

[82]  Torp R, Lekieffre D, Levy LM, *et al.* Reduced postischemic expression of a glial glutamate transporter, GLT1, in the rat hippocampus. Experimental brain research Experimentelle Hirnforschung 1995; 103(1): 51-8.
[PMID: 7615037]

[83]  Yatomi Y, Tanaka R, Shimura H, *et al.* Chronic brain ischemia induces the expression of glial glutamate transporter EAAT2 in subcortical white matter. Neuroscience 2013; 244: 113-21.
[http://dx.doi.org/10.1016/j.neuroscience.2013.04.018] [PMID: 23602887]

[84]  Mallolas J, Hurtado O, Castellanos M, *et al.* A polymorphism in the EAAT2 promoter is associated with higher glutamate concentrations and higher frequency of progressing stroke. J Exp Med 2006; 203(3): 711-7.
[http://dx.doi.org/10.1084/jem.20051979] [PMID: 16520390]

[85]  Hummel FC, Cohen LG. Non-invasive brain stimulation: a new strategy to improve neurorehabilitation after stroke? Lancet Neurol 2006; 5(8): 708-12.
[http://dx.doi.org/10.1016/S1474-4422(06)70525-7] [PMID: 16857577]

[86]  Schlaug G, Renga V, Nair D. Transcranial direct current stimulation in stroke recovery. Arch Neurol 2008; 65(12): 1571-6.
[http://dx.doi.org/10.1001/archneur.65.12.1571] [PMID: 19064743]

[87]  Reitmeir R, Kilic E, Reinboth BS, *et al.* Vascular endothelial growth factor induces contralesional corticobulbar plasticity and functional neurological recovery in the ischemic brain. Acta Neuropathol 2012; 123(2): 273-84.
[http://dx.doi.org/10.1007/s00401-011-0914-z] [PMID: 22109109]

[88]  Martino G, Bacigaluppi M, Peruzzotti-Jametti L. Therapeutic stem cell plasticity orchestrates tissue plasticity. Brain : a journal of neurology 2011; 134(Pt 6): 1585-7.
[http://dx.doi.org/10.1093/brain/awr115]

[89]  Bernhardt J, Langhorne P, Lindley RI, *et al.* Efficacy and safety of very early mobilisation within 24 h of stroke onset (AVERT): a randomised controlled trial. Lancet 2015; 386(9988): 46-55.
[http://dx.doi.org/10.1016/S0140-6736(15)60690-0] [PMID: 25892679]

[90]  Krakauer JW, Carmichael ST, Corbett D, Wittenberg GF. Getting neurorehabilitation right: what can be learned from animal models? Neurorehabil Neural Repair 2012; 26(8): 923-31.
[http://dx.doi.org/10.1177/1545968312440745] [PMID: 22466792]

[91]  Wahl AS, Omlor W, Rubio JC, *et al.* Neuronal repair. Asynchronous therapy restores motor control by rewiring of the rat corticospinal tract after stroke. Science 2014; 344(6189): 1250-5.

[92]  Wessel MJ, Zimerman M, Hummel FC. Non-invasive brain stimulation: an interventional tool for enhancing behavioral training after stroke. Front Hum Neurosci 2015; 9: 265.
[http://dx.doi.org/10.3389/fnhum.2015.00265] [PMID: 26029083]

[93]  Chieffo R, Comi G, Leocani L. Noninvasive neuromodulation in poststroke gait disorders: Rationale, feasibility, and state of the art. Neurorehabil Neural Repair 2016; 30(1): 71-82.

[http://dx.doi.org/10.1177/1545968315586464] [PMID: 25967759]

[94] Peruzzotti-Jametti L, Bacigaluppi M, Sandrone S, Cambiaghi M. Emerging subspecialties in Neurology: transcranial stimulation. Neurology 2013; 80(4): e33-5.
[http://dx.doi.org/10.1212/WNL.0b013e3182833d74] [PMID: 23339212]

[95] Li WL, Cai HH, Wang B, *et al.* Chronic fluoxetine treatment improves ischemia-induced spatial cognitive deficits through increasing hippocampal neurogenesis after stroke. J Neurosci Res 2009; 87(1): 112-22.
[http://dx.doi.org/10.1002/jnr.21829] [PMID: 18711744]

[96] Chollet F, Tardy J, Albucher JF, *et al.* Fluoxetine for motor recovery after acute ischaemic stroke (FLAME): a randomised placebo-controlled trial. Lancet Neurol 2011; 10(2): 123-30.
[http://dx.doi.org/10.1016/S1474-4422(10)70314-8] [PMID: 21216670]

[97] Sun Y, Jin K, Xie L, *et al.* VEGF-induced neuroprotection, neurogenesis, and angiogenesis after focal cerebral ischemia. J Clin Invest 2003; 111(12): 1843-51.
[http://dx.doi.org/10.1172/JCI200317977] [PMID: 12813020]

[98] Ehrenreich H, Weissenborn K, Prange H, *et al.* Recombinant human erythropoietin in the treatment of acute ischemic stroke. Stroke 2009; 40(12): e647-56.
[http://dx.doi.org/10.1161/STROKEAHA.109.564872] [PMID: 19834012]

[99] Schneider A, Wysocki R, Pitzer C, *et al.* An extended window of opportunity for G-CSF treatment in cerebral ischemia. BMC Biol 2006; 4: 36.
[http://dx.doi.org/10.1186/1741-7007-4-36] [PMID: 17049076]

[100] Ringelstein EB, Thijs V, Norrving B, *et al.* Granulocyte colony-stimulating factor in patients with acute ischemic stroke: results of the AX200 for Ischemic Stroke trial. Stroke 2013; 44(10): 2681-7.
[http://dx.doi.org/10.1161/STROKEAHA.113.001531] [PMID: 23963331]

[101] Schäbitz WR, Steigleder T, Cooper-Kuhn CM, *et al.* Intravenous brain-derived neurotrophic factor enhances poststroke sensorimotor recovery and stimulates neurogenesis. Stroke 2007; 38(7): 2165-72.
[http://dx.doi.org/10.1161/STROKEAHA.106.477331] [PMID: 17510456]

[102] Binder DK, Scharfman HE. Brain-derived neurotrophic factor. Growth Factors 2004; 22(3): 123-31.
[http://dx.doi.org/10.1080/08977190410001723308] [PMID: 15518235]

[103] Kleim JA, Chan S, Pringle E, *et al.* BDNF val66met polymorphism is associated with modified experience-dependent plasticity in human motor cortex. Nat Neurosci 2006; 9(6): 735-7.
[http://dx.doi.org/10.1038/nn1699] [PMID: 16680163]

[104] Di Pino G, Pellegrino G, Capone F, *et al.* Val66Met BDNF polymorphism implies a different way to recover from stroke rather than a worse overall recoverability. Neurorehabil Neural Repair 2016; 30(1): 3-8.
[http://dx.doi.org/10.1177/1545968315583721] [PMID: 25896987]

[105] Ginsberg MD. Current status of neuroprotection for cerebral ischemia: synoptic overview. Stroke 2009; 40(3) (Suppl.): S111-4.
[http://dx.doi.org/10.1161/STROKEAHA.108.528877] [PMID: 19064810]

[106] Martino G, Pluchino S. The therapeutic potential of neural stem cells. Nature reviews 2006; 7(5): 395-406.

[http://dx.doi.org/10.1038/nrn1908]

[107]  Cusimano M, Biziato D, Brambilla E, *et al.* Transplanted neural stem/precursor cells instruct phagocytes and reduce secondary tissue damage in the injured spinal cord. Brain 2012; 135(Pt 2): 447-60.
[http://dx.doi.org/10.1093/brain/awr339] [PMID: 22271661]

[108]  Waldau B, Hattiangady B, Kuruba R, Shetty AK. Medial ganglionic eminence-derived neural stem cell grafts ease spontaneous seizures and restore GDNF expression in a rat model of chronic temporal lobe epilepsy. Stem Cells 2010; 28(7): 1153-64.
[PMID: 20506409]

[109]  Laterza C, Merlini A, De Feo D, *et al.* iPSC-derived neural precursors exert a neuroprotective role in immune-mediated demyelination *via* the secretion of LIF. Nat Commun 2013; 4: 2597.
[http://dx.doi.org/10.1038/ncomms3597] [PMID: 24169527]

[110]  Pluchino S, Zanotti L, Rossi B, *et al.* Neurosphere-derived multipotent precursors promote neuroprotection by an immunomodulatory mechanism. Nature 2005; 436(7048): 266-71.
[http://dx.doi.org/10.1038/nature03889] [PMID: 16015332]

[111]  Ourednik J, Ourednik V, Lynch WP, Schachner M, Snyder EY. Neural stem cells display an inherent mechanism for rescuing dysfunctional neurons. Nat Biotechnol 2002; 20(11): 1103-10.
[http://dx.doi.org/10.1038/nbt750] [PMID: 12379867]

[112]  Einstein O, Karussis D, Grigoriadis N, *et al.* Intraventricular transplantation of neural precursor cell spheres attenuates acute experimental allergic encephalomyelitis. Mol Cell Neurosci 2003; 24(4): 1074-82.
[http://dx.doi.org/10.1016/j.mcn.2003.08.009] [PMID: 14697670]

[113]  Pluchino S, Quattrini A, Brambilla E, *et al.* Injection of adult neurospheres induces recovery in a chronic model of multiple sclerosis. Nature 2003; 422(6933): 688-94.
[http://dx.doi.org/10.1038/nature01552] [PMID: 12700753]

[114]  Hayase M, Kitada M, Wakao S, *et al.* Committed neural progenitor cells derived from genetically modified bone marrow stromal cells ameliorate deficits in a rat model of stroke. J Cereb Blood Flow Metab 2009; 29(8): 1409-20.
[http://dx.doi.org/10.1038/jcbfm.2009.62] [PMID: 19436312]

[115]  Tornero D, Wattananit S, Grønning Madsen M, *et al.* Human induced pluripotent stem cell-derived cortical neurons integrate in stroke-injured cortex and improve functional recovery. Brain 2013; 136(Pt 12): 3561-77.
[http://dx.doi.org/10.1093/brain/awt278] [PMID: 24148272]

[116]  Oki K, Tatarishvili J, Wood J, *et al.* Human-induced pluripotent stem cells form functional neurons and improve recovery after grafting in stroke-damaged brain. Stem Cells 2012; 30(6): 1120-33.
[http://dx.doi.org/10.1002/stem.1104] [PMID: 22495829]

# CHAPTER 13

# Post-Stroke Rehabilitation

**Michela Coccia** and **Leandro Provinciali**[*]

*Department of Experimental and Clinical Medicine, Neurological Section, Marche Polytechnic University, Ancona, Italy*

**Abstract:** Stroke is one of the main cause of chronic disability in industrialized countries and, in 2010, it was among the top eighteen diseases that most frequently lead to "years lived with disability". All the quoted conditions decreased between 1990 and 2010, with the exception of the age-standardized rates for stroke. Caring addressed to post-stroke patients involves multiple challenges, due to stroke causes a wide range of impairments, among them motor skills deficits are the most common, even if should be enumerated other areas of impairment such as sensory, visual, swallowing, cognitive and language related. Rehabilitation provides the possibility of reducing the burden of disability and, nowadays, one of the most exciting areas of stroke research is the prospect to increase rehabilitation effectiveness, influence neurological recovery and, subsequently, impact clinical outcomes. In recent years, following the spreading of studies regarding neuroplasticity, innovative rehabilitative approaches have been based on reasonable and intriguing theoretical assumptions. The restorative methods represent significant tools for stroke rehabilitation; nevertheless, they become meaningless if not integrated within the context of a rigorously personalized care plan. A comprehensive rehabilitation plan should begin as soon as the stroke occurs. Management must be directed toward preventing functional deterioration, restoring lost abilities and functions, gaining compensatory strategies, suggesting environmental changes, increasing participation and consequently achieving the highest quality of life after the brain damage. The grade to which a rehabilitation program meets the challenge of improving dignity and independence of stroke survivors is assessable through the adoption of a systematic approach that relates the diseased-state and disability to outcomes of care. The following can be considered as stroke rehabilitation strongholds: (1) to provide a consistent rehabilitation plan throughout the acute, sub-acute, and chronic phases: stroke rehabilitation is a dynamic pathway starting following the

---

[*] **Corresponding author Leandro Provinciali**: Department of Experimental and Clinical Medicine, Marche Polytechnic University, Ancona, Italy; Tel; +39 0715964530; Fax; +39 071887262; Email: l.provinciali@univpm.it

Alberto Radaelli, Giuseppe Mancia, Carlo Ferrarese & Simone Beretta (Eds.)

symptoms onset and accompanying the patient in the care pathway until his going back to community; (2) to set goals based on the prediction of the single cases evolution (short, medium and long-term goals) and design an appropriate pathway: the first step for a well-conceived rehabilitation management is to establish appropriate setting addressed to the patient; (3) to provide a comprehensive, coordinated, interdisciplinary approach: since the strokes clinical manifestations are multidimensional, rehabilitation is best realized through the coordinated and well harmonized actions among the whole members of a specialized team; (4) to build up a tailored rehabilitative treatment.

**Keywords:** Action observation, Comprehensive approach, Individual rehabilitation project, Multidisciplinary, Neuroplasticity, Non Invasive brain stimulation, Prognosis, Robotic device, Setting, Tailored treatment, Task-oriented treatment.

## POST-STROKE REHABILITATION: ACUTE PHASE MANAGEMENT

Systematic Reviews of clinical trials have formerly demonstrated that Stroke Unit, decisively, contributes to reduce mortality, institutionalization and long-term disability compared to general wards [1]. Common characteristics that establish effectiveness of Stroke Unit appear to be:

1. medical and nursing staff deep specialization;
2. multidimensional assessment;
3. early management of risk factors for complications;
4. early mobilization out of bed;
5. caregivers involving;
6. timely design of discharge plan [2].

Most of them belong to acute stroke rehabilitation domain and contribute to the success of Stroke Units indeed (Table **1**).

Early mobilization (out of bed mobilization) is perceived as one of the strategic constituents of acute stroke care responsible for good outcomes. It reduces bedsores, orthostatic hypotyension, deep venous thrombosis and pulmonary embolism, pneumonia. In such a context, a significant issue appears to be the standardization in terms of timing, duration and intensity of treatment: mobilization procedures remain poorly defined and differ both geographically and by the characteristics of the unit where patients are being managed.

**Table 1. Model of rehabilitation care in stroke acute phase.**

| Objectives | Actions | Operators |
|---|---|---|
| Functional Assessment | Evaluation of consciousness, comorbidity, continence, mobility, depression, language, cognitive abilities, global and selective disability. Swallowing Screening Test | Physician (Neurologist, Physiatrist, Nutritionist), Nurse, Physiotherapist, Speech Therapist, Neuropsychologist, Occupational Therapist |
| Prognosis definition | Definition of the real level of global and selective functional recovery achievable on the basis of identified clinical elements | Physiatrist |
| Management of continuity of care and definition of rehabilitation plan | Choice of rehabilitation setting. Information and education for the patient and the caregiver | Physiatrist |
| Prevention of complications | Management of dysphagia, early mobilization, positioning, falls risk management | Nurse, Physiotherapist, Speech Therapist, Occupational Therapist |
| Promotion of independence in primary Activity Daily Living (ADL) | Early mobilization, occupational therapy | Nurse, Physiotherapist, Speech Therapist, Occupational Therapist |

In this background the AVERT [3], published in 2015, is the first randomized controlled clinical trial, conducted on a sample of 2104 patients, that has evaluated the effect of intensive and early mobilization (a few hours after stroke) on medium-term outcome of stroke subjects. The working hypothesis was intended to prove the efficacy of precocious and intensive treatment to improve functional outcome three months after the acute event. The results showed that in the precocious and intensive treatment group, the outcome at three months was worse, in terms of mortality and disability, mainly in patients suffering from severe ischemic stroke and intraparenchymal hemorrhage [3]. The results of the AVERT are still under discussion within the scientific community: far from reducing the emphasis on the importance of early mobilization in stroke patients [4], the stated outcome show that the definition of the timing, frequency and duration of the mobilization "out of bed" in the acute phase is more complex than believed until now.

Baseline assessment should include evaluation of: consciousness level, presence of comorbid diseases, a measure of global disability (Barthel Index -BI [5] and Functional Independence Measure-FIM) [6], motor skills, trunk control, cognitive, language and communication impairment, depression. Measures of Primary and Instrumental Activities of Daily Living and evaluation of social background are supportive in assessment of the possibility of returning home [7].

Swallowing assessment and dysphagia management deserve nonetheless a separate discussion. Dysphagia is really common following strokes, affecting 13%–94% of acute stroke subjects. It is associated with increased risk of aspiration pneumonia, malnutrition and dehydration, increases the risk of mortality in the acute phase, influences independently the global functional prognosis and reduces the quality of life [8]. In the acute phase after a stroke, early identification and management of dysphagia have been associated with reduced risk of complications. Dysphagia screening, performed during the acute phase before administering any type of liquid or solid orally, represent an essential element of stroke care [9]. Baseline evaluation is essential to define a functional prognosis. This is one of the most meaningful rehabilitative skills in the acute phase of stroke and the starting point for the planning of patients' pathway.

## Prognosis

In the context of Framingham Study cohort [10], among ischemic stroke survivors at 6 months, it has been recorded the following: 50% had hemiparesis; 30% were unable to walk without assistance; 46% experienced cognitive deficits; 35% suffered from depressive symptoms; 19% had aphasia; 26% were dependent in Activities of Daily Living (ADL) and last 26% were institutionalized in a nursing home. Early identification of prognostic factors regarding functional recovery enable to draw a rehabilitation project tailored to the patient, as well as to plan the discharge and the continuity of care along with the allocation of the appropriate financial and human resources. Moreover, the rapid development of a prognosis allows defining feasible goals together with achieving the therapeutic compliance concerning patient and caregiver. The timing of functional assessment is crucial in order to express the prognosis of recovery. The right moment to combine biological and functional factors is between the first and second week after the stroke's onset. However, if a persistent lack of trunk control is a predictor of unfavorable global recovery after a week [11], should be considered it will take at least 15-20 days before declaring that a patient, with upper limb plegia, will not recover dexterity [12], and at least one month before giving a prognosis on language impairment [13]. A range of biological and environmental factors influences functional recovery and recovery profiles are characterized by a high inter-individual variability. To date, according to the International Classification of Functions International Classification of Functioning, Disability and Health [14], it is possible to rank the different prognostic factors of post-stroke disability in the following cases, "individual" and "extra-individual", "pre-existing" and "emerging" (Table **2**).

Table 2. Prognostic factors of post-stroke disability.

|  | Individual | Extra-Individual |
|---|---|---|
| **Pre-Existing** | • Age<br>• Sex<br>• Previous functional status<br>• Previous stroke events<br>• Comorbid diseases | • Socio-economic environment<br>• Independence of house mate<br>• Organization of the health care |
| **Emerging** | • Severity of clinical presentation:<br>  - Loss of strength<br>  - Urinary and bowel continence<br>  - Muscular tone<br>  - Neglect<br>  - Aphasia<br>  - Cognitive impairment<br>  - Dysphagia<br>• Severity of functional impairment<br>  - Trunk control<br>  - Autonomy in ADL<br>• Depression and cognitive disorders | • Organization of health care in acute phase post stroke:<br>  - Setting<br>  - Timeliness of rehabilitation treatment<br>  - Continuity of care<br>  - Emotional / affective reaction of caregiver |

Within the prognostic factors, the individual ones, which are expression of cognitive-behavioral features and patients' personal skills, are pivotal in the right choice of the rehabilitation treatment, hence influence its efficacy. The familiar, socio-cultural and political environment along with the rehabilitation care system are involved in the adaptation to the individual disability and in promoting social participation.

## *Recovery of Independence in ADL and Social Participation*

A timely and specific prediction of stroke patient's functional prognosis is crucial in simplifying both homecoming and social participation. The main indicators of functional prognosis are severity of stroke, dysphagia, trunk control, neglect, aphasia [15]. Functional Ambulation Category (FAC) [16], global disability, mood depression, age and other non-motor features, like dementia and autonomic dysfunctions are associated with participation restriction in the chronic phase after a stroke [17]. The severity of clinical expression, which includes neurological impairment, loss of consciousness, urinary incontinence, dysphagia and plegia, is the most significant predictive factors for complications in the acute phase and functional recovery [18]. The performance in ADL correlates strongly with motricity [19] as well as motor recovery is mainly affected by the initial level of paresis [20]. There is strong evidence of the predictive value of functional indexes such as trunk control on independence in the home and community [11, 21]. Cognitive deficits such as neglect are considered negative prognostic factors: patients with Unilateral Spatial Neglect (USN) show lower admission and discharge BI scores [22] and longer rehabilitation periods [23], less independence at home following the discharge and high risk of functional worsening at 1 year follow up [24]. Aphasia patients with comprehension deficit have a meaningfully more severe basal neurological and functional status upon admission and a higher percentage of disability and urinary incontinence upon discharge, as well as a risk of low therapeutic response being nearly 4 times higher than other patients [25]. Gialanella *et al.* [26] demonstrate that, among cognitive deficits, USN influences mainly motor recovery, being a predictor of motor FIM, while aphasia is a predictor of cognitive FIM scores. The role that gender plays on functional prognosis is controversial. In the last years, it is reported that women have significantly worse functional outcomes than men [27]. Factors that contribute to poorer functional outcomes in women include pre-stroke condition, marital status, nursing home residence, history of stroke and stroke severity, most of which are not amended at stroke onset. Being widow, along with social isolation, represents another factor associated with a poorer outcome [28]. The correlation between increasing age and disability is not well established yet. In recent times, it has been evaluated that subjects >85 years have a risk of low recovery in ADL that is about ten times greater than younger's [29]. Nevertheless, in other cases, high age is not considered itself as a limit to functional recovery if not associated with other parameters.

## *Gait*

The recovery of walking ability is considered one of the weightiest goals after a stroke. Currently in the acute phase, approximately 50% of the patients cannot walk and 12% needs assistance to gait [30]. Rehabilitation Units constitute a significant setting for regaining the walking ability, engraving with a substantial percentage: 60% *versus* 39% in an Acute Unit. These results visibly emphasize the importance of the rehabilitation effort [31]. Age and sex, stroke severity, pathogenesis, trunk control, health care/timing of rehabilitation caregiving, and cognitive deficit, all of them are prognostic factors related to the recovery of gait. Trunk control is undoubtedly an early prognostic factor for the recovery of postural control and independent walking [32]. Trunk Control Tests [33] evaluated 14 days after the stroke with a score < than 50 can predict non-independent walkers (FAC< 4) [16, 34]. In acute stroke patients, leg motor impairment and disability evaluation predict the recovery: in the early phase, active ankle dorsiflexion and the Mingazzini maneuver are related to the prognosis of lower limb function, standing and walking [35]. Moreover, the probability of regaining patient's walking ability is higher when the Modified Barthel Index (MBI) score is 50 or more and lower limb strength recovers within the first week. On the other hand, in the first week, MBI < 20 associated with poor limb strength, significantly reduce the chance of walking improvement [36]. It has been even established that Rehabilitation Units represent a positive prognostic factor for both functional and walking recovery. Patients in Rehabilitation Units have 21% more chance to regain independent walking [31]. Paolucci *et al.* describe stroke patients' walking abilities after discharging from a Rehabilitation Unit as following: 5% are independent even in stair climbing; 9% walk outside and 14% walk inside, 27% walk with a support, while 45% have to use a wheelchair [37]. There is certain variability between the sexes; in particular, male patients have a higher probability to reach good autonomy in stair climbing, whereas female patients have a higher probability of walking with a cane [38]. Cognitive skills are prognostic factors of motor recovery [40] due to their own involvement in postural control and in patient's compliance in rehabilitation treatment [39].

Additionally, the probability of walking recovery could depend on the etiopathogenesis of the stroke. Paolucci *et al.* proved that hemorrhagic stroke patients show a higher mobility recovery in 22% rather than 11.6% of ischemic patients [41]. A study conducted by Baer *et al.* [42] revealed that distinct sub-classifications of strokes have dissimilar impact of gait recovery: particularly subjects sustaining total anterior circulation infarct (TACI) have overall the worst prognosis. About 63% of TACI patients did not regain independent walking ability.

### Upper Limb

The ability of stroke survivors to independently undertake ADL depends on the recovery of the upper limb [43]. About 70% of the stroke patients suffers an involvement of upper extremity (UE) [44]. The recovery is scarce: 18%, 25% and 31% improved limb dexterity respectively at 3, 6 and 12 months after stroke. The factors related to the recovery of upper limb function are: age, UE Motricity Index Scores at the time of rehabilitation admission, UE function, UE muscle tone, global disability, cognitive abilities, visuo-spatial impairment at onset [45, 46] and characteristics of motor-evoked or somatosensory potentials [47]. Active range of motion [48] muscle strength, and 2-point discrimination [49] evaluated within the first 4 weeks after a stroke, predict six-month improvement. Furthermore, despite the improvement in the ability to move the UE, the use in ADL of the affected UE, is restricted in the chronic phase. UE dexterity, proprioception, and grip strength, measured at discharge from Rehabilitation Units, predict daily use of the affected UE at 12 months [50].

The study conducted by Smania *et al.* [51] prove that active finger extension is a strong early predictor of short, medium and long-term post-stroke recovery. It suggests that preservation of this movement may be related to the amount of corticospinal neurons spared. Patients with a basal active finger extension score of more than 3 (MRC) have a high probability of reaching the top Motricity Index arm subtest.

USN and anosognosia affect prognosis of UE motor skills [52, 53]. Lastly, patients with apraxia, despite recovery of the UE strength, have difficulty in managing ADL [54], especially patients with ideational apraxia.

## Continuity of Care Management

Post-stroke rehabilitation may take place throughout:

- intensive rehabilitation in inpatient Rehabilitation Unit;
- home rehabilitation;
- rehabilitation in an outpatient facility;
- rehabilitation in a nursing home;
- rehabilitation in long-term care.

Clinical stability/instability, functional disability, physical endurance and ability to learn are key conditions for choosing a setting after the acute phase of stroke. Subjects with severe cognitive deficits are unable to learn new strategies and are not candidates for intensive rehabilitation programs. Patients with a poor prognosis or unable to tolerate intense treatment are suitable to follow lower level program such as extensive rehabilitation in nursing homes. Patients with severe comorbidity need long-term care facilities, and the transition to intensive rehabilitation may always be proposed after clinical stabilization [7].

## POST-STROKE REHABILITATION: SUB-ACUTE PHASE MANAGEMENT

A mainstay in sub-acute phase is the modality of planning the rehabilitation project.

The conventional rehabilitation approach is a well-defined process that includes:

- assessment;
- definition of prognosis;
- description of the long, medium, short-term goals;
- explanations of assessment measures;
- intervention;
- progress evaluation in comparison to the fixed goals.

Only this approach can ensure the efficiency and the efficacy of the whole rehabilitation process.

Stroke rehabilitation uses multiple operating modalities, nevertheless none of them is superior to another in achieving the best outcome [55]: rehabilitation treatment should be tailored to the patients.

There are many factors to be taken into account in the implementation of a rehabilitation project: the possibility to realize a gait training appears related to the acquisition of adequate trunk and postural control and a sufficient aerobic capacity, alternatively drugs can interfere in the functional recovery, and moreover caregivers' training is crucial in the creation of a rehabilitation program.

Recent researches regarding brain plasticity have provided some key elements in the application of rehabilitation treatments. Specifically, neural plasticity after brain lesion is mainly influenced by repetitive, intensive, task-oriented, and multisensory interventions [55, 56].

This concept is currently the mainstream of stroke rehabilitation and every single rehabilitative approach must be based on such a knowledge. The intensity of practice is a key factor in meaningful training following a stroke and it is generally associated with a better outcome [57] even if the modalities of clinical applications are controversial yet [58]. Task-oriented training is a specific process of motor learning that focuses on skill acquisition in the contest of a particular functional activity [56, 59].

Based on this assumption in the last few years there has been ever-growing evidence on Enriched Environment (EE) effectiveness. EE is a setting which offers great opportunity for performing motor and cognitive activities, receiving multi-sensory stimuli and gaining motivation. Thus, it provides the possibility to create meaningful, intensive, repetitive and task-oriented training that promote functional recovery. Janssen *et al.* [60] accomplished a systematic review to evaluate the efficacy of EE on outcome and mortality in animal models of ischemic stroke and as aftermath EE results in an improvement of sensorimotor function. In a non-randomized trial, the same Author [61] directly observed the impact of EE in motor, cognitive, social activity in stroke patients admitted in a

Rehabilitation Unit. The preliminary results suggest that the model of EE in a Rehabilitation Unit is effective in increasing activity in stroke patients and even in reducing time spent passively and inactively.

## Main Sub-acute Phase Issues

### Post-stroke Cognitive Impairment

Cognitive impairment is a common consequence following a stroke. Prevalence data shows that 10% of patients already has dementia at the time of the stroke, 10% develops dementia subsequently the first stroke and 30% develops dementia after stroke relapse.

The 3-month post-stroke rates of dementia vary from 6% to more than 30%. Percentages increase when considering cognitive disorders not dementia: 20-90% of stroke patients exhibit Mild Cognitive Impairment at 3 months after a stroke [62]. The underlying mechanisms of Post-Stroke Cognitive Impairment (PSCI) are not known in detail. The neuroanatomical lesions caused by strokes on strategic areas such as the hippocampus, the white matter lesions, the neurodegenerative changes previous and/or subsequent a stroke, alone or in combination, contribute to the pathogenesis of PSCI. From a clinical point of view, PSCI is characterized by prevalent damage in executive functions, which comprise planning, maintaining switching attention and making decisions using one's judgment. These abilities are necessary for IADL and for functioning independently. PSCI is one of the silent unmet needs in more than 50% of stroke survivors and causes greater functional impairment, increases mortality and influences quality of life determining a patient and a caregiver's distress. In mild stroke and in young patients PSCI is the main factor that affects returning to work or to a familial role [63]. Despite this strong burden, effective interventions on increasing the autonomy and quality of life in PSCI are not defined yet.

For the time being, no drug or rehabilitative treatment has shown strong clinical evidence of influencing cognitive functions [64]. The only way is a correct diagnosis and behavioral management through prompt and careful caregiver's information and education.

## *Depression*

Mood depression is a frequent and clinically significant occurrence in patients who have suffered single or repeated cerebrovascular lesions.

Post-stroke depression (PSD) has a cumulative incidence of up to 52% within 5 years of a stroke, with a pooled prevalence of 29% that remained stable in the first 10 years after a stroke across different study settings. Most patients who have suffered depression after stroke become depressed shortly after the acute event. A significant proportion of them recover from depression in subsequent assessments and the rise of new cases stabilize the overall prevalence of depression [65]. Due to different methods in the clinical approach to the PSD, such as timing of assessment, different study settings, dissimilar approaches used to diagnose depression, the available data provide prevalence rates of depressive disorders ranging from 25-79% [66]. Besides, a relevant number of studies do not include aphasics and dementia patients because of the obvious complexity in evaluating depressive symptoms. The social impact of depression following cerebrovascular disease is due to its prevalence as well as the negative influence on the patient's quality of life. PSD increases death risks, is a caregiver's burden, makes the cognitive impairment worse and can determine a negative impact on functional recovery. Social costs may be presumed but are not defined: it has been observed that depressed stroke patients are more often institutionalized, are assiduous users of the health services, and the presence of PSD is associated with a less efficient rehabilitative practice, leading to an increased stay in the hospital.

The effects of antidepressant drugs on post-stroke depression have been extensively explored and studies documented positive results [67]. The potential effect of these drugs on brain plasticity, motor recovery, cognitive activation and ultimately on the functional recovery and the improvement of quality of life is a decisive challenge. The characterization of the features of post-stroke depression, the potential identification of subtypes, combined with a definition of the molecular mechanisms of depressive disorder in stroke, are crucial in future research in order to identify molecules or associations of molecules targeted to the disorder treatment.

## Spasticity

Spasticity following stroke, interferes with the quality of movement and contributes to functional limitations in mobility, personal cares, comfort and many ADL. In the chronic phase, the emergence and worsening of spasticity can lead the patient to a neurologist, reporting a deterioration of dexterity or gait. Stroke patients with upper or lower limb spasticity have a greater waste of energy, have difficult in positioning and using orthosis and splint, have a higher risk of developing joint stiffness, pressure sores and pain. Recognition of spasticity as a cause of the deterioration of the function is essential for a correct diagnosis and planning of treatment. It is agreed that the treatment of spasticity is led by the definition of functional objectives shared with the patient and the caregiver. The principal aims of spasticity treatment are to increase patient function and to reduce the burden of care. Often patients show complex spastic motor patterns, so clinicians should examine patients carefully both at rest and during activities. The understanding of the motor patterns drives the clinician in choosing the most appropriate treatment aimed at improving function. A comprehensive assessment includes physical examination, standard and dynamic electromyography, quantitative gait analysis [68]. The decision concerning whether, when, and how to manage spasticity is influenced by many factors such as its severity, distribution and duration, patients' global disabilities and comorbidities and lastly a reachable end state. Treatment options of spasticity should be considered in connection with its distribution: antispastic drugs administered orally in multifocal spasticity and the treatment using botulinum toxin for the management of focal spasticity. It is relevant to consider the pharmacological treatment of spasticity as part of a broader rehabilitation program, which takes even into due consideration the following: casting, stretching, muscle strengthening and occupational therapy.

## Pain

Post-stroke Pain (PSP) refers to a broad range of clinical conditions responsible of pain after stroke, not only restricted to central post-stroke pain, which affects from 10% to 50% of patients [69]. PSP is often an under-recognized and under-treated phenomenon: some general practitioners believe that pain is a natural and inevitable condition for stroke survivors; furthermore, patients have often difficulty to explain their symptoms. There are also disagreements about the use of drugs for pain treatment in stroke patients due to the alarm of side effects and medication interactions. Risk factors for the development of PSP are age at stroke onset, female sex, depression, peripheral vascular disease, spasticity, severe UE motor impairment, sensory deficits, and stroke localization [70]. Patients with PSP suffer greater cognitive and functional disorders, depression and worst quality of life. In any stroke phases, every procedure necessary to investigate the presence of painful symptoms and assess the specific characteristics and intensity is recommended in order to implement specific pharmacological or rehabilitative measures in a multidisciplinary approach.

PSP can be categorized in Central Post-Stroke Pain (CPSP), pain associated to spasticity, shoulder pain, Complex Regional Pain Syndrome (CRPS), tension type headache, lumbar and dorsal pain [69]. Most of the patients complains more than one condition.

The pathogenesis of PSP is complex, multifactorial and several elements influence the clinical features: central neuropathic and peripheral nociceptive mechanisms, autonomic system involvement, inflammatory disorders, joint and muscle complications, psychological aspects [71]. The relative influences of these aspects may change between subjects and over time [72]. Shoulder pain is one of the most frequent manifestation of PSP and commonly affect 25-50% of stroke patients: its etiology can depend on the following: reduced UE strength, glenohumeral subluxation, adhesive capsulitis, rotator cuff strain, spasticity and CRPS.

Dorsal and lumbar pain may result from reduced muscle strength and spasticity. CRPS is a disorder characterized by sensory deficits (dysesthesia, allodynia, hyperesthesia), autonomic disorders (vasodilatation or vasoconstriction, edema, variations in temperature, abnormal sweating), functional impairment. A correct diagnosis allows setting a therapeutic approach that, given the complexity of the conditions, is often multidimensional.

The treatment of a painful shoulder in hemiplegic patients' needs a multidisciplinary management with pharmacological and non-pharmacological procedures such as appropriate positioning (both in bedridden patients and during transfers), mobilization of the limb, treatment of spasticity and physical therapies. Among the useful pharmacological methods to reduce shoulder pain syndromes is counted intra-articular injections of steroids.

In cases of persistent CPSP a treatment with antiepileptic drugs is recommended (Lamotrigine, Gabapentin, Pregabalin) or tricyclic antidepressants (Amitriptyline) personalizing the dosage [4].

The appearance of post-stroke CRPS is always a problem for the clinician because the management is complex and currently there are no effective treatments. An interdisciplinary approach involving pharmacological treatment, mobilization, motor training, desensitization techniques, occupational therapy is a keystone of care concerning such kind of patients [73].

## POST-STROKE REHABILITATION: CHRONIC PHASE MANAGEMENT

The end of a formal rehabilitation program is usually signaled by a functional plateau, after which little or no recovery occurs. Could be not so easy to identify the latter, nevertheless if no improvement occurs over 4 weeks' treatment in significant outcome measure, further substantial restorative improvement is roughly unlikely, although patients may still learn other compensatory strategies. Ending up a proper rehabilitation program does not mean to conclude patient's health care. In order to reduce hospital readmission, to avoid unsuitable repetitions of rehabilitation training sessions and to enable patients' social reintegration, an adequate management of the chronic phase is essential. Therefore, the main goals of a stroke's chronic phase are:

• to restrain functional decline;
• to maintain cardiorespiratory fitness;
• to optimize social participation;
• to ensure longitudinal follow-up aimed at identifying complications.

In such a specific phase, occupational therapy can improve performance and reduce the risk of functional deterioration. Occupational therapy is a rehabilitative intervention aimed to increasing autonomy in ADL. The main used processes are: improving relevant activity, environmental changes, training compensatory strategies.

Among the whole setting of the pointed out compensatory strategy, the most frequently chosen by the caregiver regard self-care activities focused training, leisure activities guidance as well as recommendation regarding mobility equipment or assistive devices. Moreover, the "occupational therapist" both educates and shares information with family members and designated primary caregiver for the purpose of providing him right and proper assistance. Carefully selected meaningful activities taken from real life, performed in an EE, used as a strategy for intervention, provide multidimensional learning opportunities. The efficacy of occupational therapy in improving functional task performance is well-documented [74].

Interventions with an aerobic activity can improve cardiorespiratory fitness after a stroke; cardiorespiratory training involving walking improves speed, tolerance, and independence [75].

In most cases, unspecific repetitions of rehabilitation trainings are not effective.

Chronic stroke survivors often exhibit a conspicuous restriction of their participation years after the event, in spite of a recovered independence in the basic ADL [17]. Participation restriction was associated with global disability, mood depression, age, and dementia.

Remarkably, over 50% of the variance of participation measures could not be clearly explained, it could depend on a maladaptive adjustment. A Cochrane review in 2002 [76] reported care pathways in stroke units resulted in significant lower patient satisfaction and worse quality of life: this apparent paradox may signify the importance of using evidence or guideline to assist clinicians in individualizing a tailored approach as opposed to a "one size fits all" approach [77]. Although not investigated in a formal manner yet, the evidence that social support improves outcomes is strongly sustained by clinical practices.

A better understanding of the clinical and vocational patients' features is desirable as it may influence participation in daily activities and social roles and thus improves rehabilitation outcomes. The General Practitioner (GP) is always considered a critical member of the team; GP's role becomes paramount in this phase so when, especially, he has to help patients and caregivers in understanding the real difficulties they are going to face.

At this time, the clear and correct identification of the following complications is crucial: pain, spasticity, dementia, and depression. Specific regard must be even given to caregivers, who often bear even more of a burden than the patient does. This is particularly true when cognitive and behavioral problems showed up or when dementia is unmasked. The latter may be offset by the involvement of the caregiver in goal setting, as well as educational programs and counseling.

## WHAT'S NEW IN STROKE REHABILITATION

Recently, advancements in technologies employing non-invasive techniques in studying human brain, have improved the knowledge about the neural plasticity and its relationship to stroke recovery. Many original stroke rehabilitative approaches have been developed based on basic science and clinical studies concerning brain remodeling. The Systematic Reviews and meta-analysis have however revealed that these rehabilitation interventions show large inter-individual difference in efficacy because the processes underlying motor recovery are dissimilar across patients. These mechanisms involve multifaceted processes comprising spontaneous recovery, neuroplasticity, learning-dependent processes, compensatory activities indeed [56]. Therefore, to clarify how to use innovative knowledge about brain plasticity, to adapt technological aids to the principles of neuroplasticity and to build up treatments increasingly tailored to the patient, can be considered the new challenges of stroke rehabilitation.

### Constraint Induced Movement Therapy (CIMT)

In patients with cerebrovascular disease, the prevailing use of the unaffected limb implicates the phenomenon of so-called "learned non-use" of the paretic limb. This condition reduces the possibility of paretic limb improvements. In particular, stroke often results in a significant impairment in both sensitive and motor functions.

In the case of injury to the areas delegated to the upper limb motor control, the use of the paretic arm will require more effort than the unaffected limb. In this situation, the patient tends to maximize the usage of the unaffected limb. The limited use of paretic limb causes a reduction in sensory input. The lack of sensory information also leads to a reduction in the activity level of the related sensorial and motor central circuits. This loss of functionality will make less efficient those areas which, spared by the lesion, may be able to support the recovery. In summary, the "learned-non-use" generates additional functional loss, not only directly dependent on the primary lesion.

CIMT is a therapeutic strategy in which the use of the unaffected limb is constrained, obliging the patient to use the affect limb. The distinctive characteristics of this rehabilitative treatment include intense, repetitive, task-oriented training of the paretic limb and immobilization of the unaffected arm. This approach is considered significant for promoting neural plasticity [78]. A novel Cochrane Review decreases the emphasis on the effectiveness of CIMT in both improvement of motor deficit and long-term disability [79]. Further studies with detailed and standardized protocols regarding optimal timing and intensity of training are desirable to evaluate CIMT efficacy.

## Body Weight-Supported Treadmill Training (BWSTT)

BWSTT is a rehabilitation approach in which patients, who have suffered a stroke, walk on a treadmill that supports their body weight. The added value of this type of treatment is the opportunity to offer a repetitive and intensive training, and to put the focus on the gait pattern. Using BWSTT therapist can dedicate to recover trunk control, improve knee alignment, increase stride length and walking speed, set the step symmetry avoiding compensatory walking behaviors, such as hip hiking and circumduction.

A Systematic Cochrane Review has established that only stroke patients who are able to walk seem to advantage from this type of treatment: in detail, walking speed and endurance are the improved parameters.

Enhancement in walking endurance for stroke patients may have persisting positive effects in a long term [80].

The proposed studies do not allow to translate this treatment in clinical practice effectively because there are no specific details of the method of application of this technique, in particular, the duration, frequency and intensity of training, as well as the use of handrails [80].

## Robotic Devices

During the last decades, robotic devices have been studied to improve rehabilitation techniques in stroke patients.

Robotic devices offer several theoretical advantages in stroke rehabilitation. In detail, they can make objective and quantifiable the measurements of subject performance and provide a way that has proven effective for promoting motor learning: an accurate sensory feedback together with tools to increase the intensity, the number of repetition of task, and to tailor the characteristics of activity. Robots used in stroke rehabilitation can precisely monitor assistance, resistance, speed, direction, rate of movement and coordination [81]. The devices currently available can be classified as robots for the upper limbs and robots intended for the lower limbs. Another classification can divide robots in exoskeleton categories (*e.g.* Lokomat) and end-effector based (*e.g.* G-EO-System, MIT Manus).

An updated Cochrane review [82] have recently documented the efficacy of electromechanical-assisted gait training in combination with physiotherapy in achieving independent walking in stroke patients than conventional training alone.

In detail, severely affected stroke patients who are not able to walk in the first three months after the event seem to advantage most from this approach. Specifically, Morone *et al.* [83] found that severe patients with subacute stroke are the ideal candidates for a rehabilitative approach in which the gait treatment is accompanied by robotic training. Otherwise, in less severe patients, therapy supported by robotic training adds no advantages compared to conventional therapy.

Another recent Cochrane Review [84] declares that dexterity training dedicated to upper limb supported by electromechanical and robotic device improves upper limb strength, hand function and ADL. Further research is needed to delineate operating protocols. Nonetheless, it necessary to keep in mind that the efficacy of these approaches still depends deeply on the ability of the rehabilitation team to select the type of robotic device and to tailor the treatment protocol to each patient's needs and personal characteristics.

## Virtual Reality (VR)

In the last few years VR technologies have used with increasingly sophisticated methods in stroke rehabilitation. VR offers some of the key elements of brain plasticity: the sensory stimulation and the redundance of the stimuli which can be tailored to the patient's features. Furthermore, this approach can easily make accessible, repetitive, intensive, and task-specific every training and can be pooled with other approaches [85].

VR applications can vary from non-immersive to fully immersive depending on the degree to which the patients are isolated from the real environment when relating with the VR [56]. Despite its great potential, VR has not good evidence of efficacy due to the low quality of the studies carried out: most of them are underpowered and lacking controls. Moreover, these studies do not evaluate the maintenance of long-term results, and lastly it is very problematic to define the successful features of a VR program. In view of this, evidence of the efficacy of VR treatment in stroke rehabilitation is limited.

An updated Cochrane Review conclusion evidences that the use of VR and interactive videogames may be advantageous in improving upper limb function and ADL function when carried out together with conventional therapy. There was not sufficient evidence about the possibility of increasing gait speed or global motor function [86].

## Action Observation (AO)

Rehabilitation based on AO arises from the mirror neurons paradigm. The mirror neurons system has generated great interest over the past two decades: the main reason of attention is the possibility to unify the concepts of "action production" and "action observation". The brain network known as "mirror neurons system" has been early identified in primates in which the inferior parietal lobule, inferior frontal gyrus, and the adjacent ventral premotor cortex are activated by the simple action of observing someone performing a meaningful motor task [87]. The mirror neurons system has been even described in human brain. According to human model, the mirror neuron paradigm is implicated in action understanding, imitation and motor learning. Within this background AO might activate the motor system similarly to execution, by creating a representation of action that can be employed for motor learning [87].

This concept can be translated in stroke rehabilitation: AO may be applicable to recover motor impairment through motor learning. Garrison *et al.* [88] in a study with functional Magnetic Resonance Imaging, has found that, in injured cortical areas after stroke, AO triggers specific motor programs and this activation is related to the motor competence involved in performing the same actions. AO was studied to improve upper limb motor functions [89] too, with a significant effect in patients undergoing experimental treatment. In the study of Ertelt *et al.*, functional Magnetic Resonance Imaging, carried out before and after therapy, exhibited a substantial intensification in activity in the bilateral ventral premotor cortex, bilateral superior temporal gyrus, supplementary motor area and contralateral supramarginal gyrus, which are the motor areas involved in the action observation and action execution in "human mirror neurons system".

Other studies have reported that AO therapy increase upper-limb motor function in patients who have suffered a stroke [90, 91]. Preliminary results have also been gathered in speech recovery [92].

After an initial enthusiasm, evidences of effective use of AO paradigm in clinical practice is still scarce, and future research is required to determine specific characteristics which make it suitable into standard clinical practice.

**Non-Invasive Brain Stimulation (NIBS)**

Repetitive Transcranial Magnetic Stimulation (rTMS) and transcranial Direct Current Stimulation (tDCS) are NIBS techniques that can modulate human cortex excitability. The paradigm of NIBS is founded on the interhemispheric competition model, which suggests that impairments in stroke patients are both consequent to a reduced output from the injured hemisphere and increased interhemispheric inhibition from the unaffected hemisphere to the damaged hemisphere [93]. Therefore, NIBS achieves improvement both increasing the excitability of the injured hemisphere and decreasing the excitability of the unaffected hemisphere. NIBS creates a more fecund environment for neural plasticity through the modulation of motor cortex excitability and for this reason it is considered a precious tool to promote recovery of motor, cognitive and linguistic abilities, mainly in combination with conventional rehabilitative interventions. Both rTMS and tDCS are demonstrated to determine long-term effects on cortical excitability that may lead to long-lasting behavioral modifications [94]. Undoubtedly, NIBS techniques have contributed to physiological and pathophysiological knowledge of motor, cognitive and affective control in human. However, despite the increasing number of investigations designed to specify the therapeutic use of NIBS after a stroke, nowadays, only very low quality evidence exists on the effectiveness of tDCS (anodal/cathodal/dual) for improving ADL and functional activities after stroke [95] and current evidences do not support the routine use of rTMS for the treatment of stroke [96]. At present time, it is crucial to better define the individual response to NIBS methodic. Several potential predictive markers have been already identified, in detail the functional effect of NIBS is determined by the "neural context" of the stimulated brain networks at the time just before and during the administration of NIBS. This context can depend by ipsilateral and/or contralateral injured cortex activity, metabolic markers, neurotransmitter environment, extent of injury and residual perilesional activity [94]. Future researches need to expand these theories in order to increase the NIBS adaptability, applicability and possibility of customization.

## CONCLUSION

Post-stroke rehabilitation is a process that, through a comprehensive and multidisciplinary approach, aims to improve functions, reduce disability, limit the occurrence of complications, control symptoms and improve the patient's quality of life within his family and social background.

Post-stroke rehabilitation always works on two tracks: the knowledge of the neurobiological mechanisms underlying functional recovery to propose treatments founded on rational bases and the intervention within the social and environmental aspects associated with disability. In the last few decades, post-stroke rehabilitation assumes a leading role in stroke care thanks to training of increasingly competent and specialized personnel, change of the concept "disease-based care" in "individual-based care", global care throughout the whole pathway, focusing not only on the acute phase treatment and increasing brain plasticity studies that allowed to develop suitable methods of treatment. Nowadays the challenge is to enhance the relationship between basic sciences and clinical rehabilitation to provide the necessary tools aimed to properly drive the interaction between subject brain activity and behavior, in order to reduce the pathological aspects and encourage the training which facilitate the functional recovery.

## TAKE HOME MESSAGE

Despite the significant steps forward in the field of primary prevention and management of the acute phase, stroke remains the main cause of chronic disability in industrialized countries. Post-stroke rehabilitation is a complex multidimensional process that accompanies the patient from the acute phase to the return to the community, monitors and manages the medium-long term complications. The secret for succeeding in rehabilitation treatment does not lie in a "special therapy": the key words are, undoubtedly, precociousness, customization and goal-directed management. Such approach requires interdisciplinary team specialized in stroke care able to know how to create an effective and efficient rehabilitative pathway.

## CONFLICT OF INTEREST

The authors confirm that they have no conflict of interest to declare for this publication.

## ACKNOWLEDGEMENTS

Declared none.

# REFERENCES

[1]     Stroke Unit Trialists' Collaboration. Organized Inpatient (Stroke Unit) Care After Stroke (Cochrane Review) The Cochrane Library, Issue 1. Oxford: Update Software 2000.

[2]     Langhorne P, Pollock A. Stroke Unit Trialists Collaboration. What are the components of effective stroke unit care? Age Ageing 2002; 31(5): 365-71.
        [http://dx.doi.org/10.1093/ageing/31.5.365] [PMID: 12242199]

[3]     Bernhardt J, Langhorne P, Lindley RI, *et al.* AVERT Trial Collaboration group. Efficacy and safety of very early mobilisation within 24 h of stroke onset (AVERT): a randomised controlled trial. Lancet 2015; 386(9988): 46-55.
        [http://dx.doi.org/10.1016/S0140-6736(15)60690-0] [PMID: 25892679]

[4]     SPREAD-Stroke Prevention and Educational Awareness Diffusion. Ictus cerebrale: linee guida italiane di prevenzione e trattamento VII ed., 2012. http://www.isospread.it

[5]     Mahoney FI, Barthel D. Functional evaluation: the Barthel Index. M. State Med J 1965; 14: 56-61.

[6]     Guide for the Uniform Data System for Medical Rehabilitation (Adult FIM). Version 4.0. Buffalo: State University of New York at Buffalo 1993.

[7]     Gresham GE, Alexander D, Bishop DS, *et al.* American Heart Association Prevention Conference. IV. Prevention and Rehabilitation of Stroke. Rehabilitation. Stroke 1997; 28(7): 1522-6.
        [http://dx.doi.org/10.1161/01.STR.28.7.1522] [PMID: 9227710]

[8]     Martino R, Foley N, Bhogal S, Diamant N, Speechley M, Teasell R. Dysphagia after stroke: incidence, diagnosis, and pulmonary complications. Stroke 2005; 36(12): 2756-63.
        [http://dx.doi.org/10.1161/01.STR.0000190056.76543.eb] [PMID: 16269630]

[9]     Hinchey JA, Shephard T, Furie K, Smith D, Wang D, Tonn S. Formal dysphagia screening protocols prevent pneumonia. Stroke 2005; 36(9): 1972-6.
        [http://dx.doi.org/10.1161/01.STR.0000177529.86868.8d] [PMID: 16109909]

[10]    Kelly-Hayes M, Beiser A, Kase CS, Scaramucci A, DAgostino RB, Wolf PA. The influence of gender and age on disability following ischemic stroke: the Framingham study. J Stroke Cerebrovasc Dis 2003; 12(3): 119-26.
        [http://dx.doi.org/10.1016/S1052-3057(03)00042-9] [PMID: 17903915]

[11]    Franchignoni FP, Tesio L, Ricupero C, Martino MT. Trunk control test as an early predictor of stroke rehabilitation outcome. Stroke 1997; 28(7): 1382-5.
        [http://dx.doi.org/10.1161/01.STR.28.7.1382] [PMID: 9227687]

[12]    Shelton FD, Volpe BT, Reding M. Motor impairment as a predictor of functional recovery and guide to rehabilitation treatment after stroke. Neurorehabil Neural Repair 2001; 15(3): 229-37.
        [http://dx.doi.org/10.1177/154596830101500311] [PMID: 11944745]

[13]    Pedersen PM, Jørgensen HS, Nakayama H, Raaschou HO, Olsen TS. Aphasia in acute stroke: incidence, determinants, and recovery. Ann Neurol 1995; 38(4): 659-66.
        [http://dx.doi.org/10.1002/ana.410380416] [PMID: 7574464]

[14]    World Health Organization. International Classification of Functioning, Disability and Health (ICF), Geneva: World health. Organization 2008.

[15]   Morone G, Paolucci S, Iosa M. In what daily activities do patients achieve independence after stroke? J Stroke Cerebrovasc Dis 2015; 24(8): 1931-7.
[http://dx.doi.org/10.1016/j.jstrokecerebrovasdis.2015.05.006] [PMID: 26051663]

[16]   Holden MK, Gill KM, Magliozzi MR, Nathan J, Piehl-Baker L. Clinical gait assessment in the neurologically impaired. Reliability and meaningfulness. Phys Ther 1984; 64(1): 35-40.
[PMID: 6691052]

[17]   Andrenelli E, Ippoliti E, Coccia M, *et al.* Features and predictors of activity limitations and participation restriction 2 years after intensive rehabilitation following first-ever stroke. Eur J Phys Rehabil Med 2015; 51(5): 575-85.
[PMID: 25616152]

[18]   Kalra L, Yu G, Wilson K, Roots P. Medical complications during stroke rehabilitation. Stroke 1995; 26(6): 990-4.
[http://dx.doi.org/10.1161/01.STR.26.6.990] [PMID: 7762051]

[19]   Kong KH, Lee J. Temporal recovery of activities of daily living in the first year after ischemic stroke: a prospective study of patients admitted to a rehabilitation unit. NeuroRehabilitation 2014; 35(2): 221-6.
[PMID: 24990018]

[20]   Hendricks HT, van Limbeek J, Geurts AC, Zwarts MJ. Motor recovery after stroke: a systematic review of the literature. Arch Phys Med Rehabil 2002; 83(11): 1629-37. [Review].
[http://dx.doi.org/10.1053/apmr.2002.35473] [PMID: 12422337]

[21]   Hsieh CL, Sheu CF, Hsueh IP, Wang CH. Trunk control as an early predictor of comprehensive activities of daily living function in stroke patients. Stroke 2002; 33(11): 2626-30.
[http://dx.doi.org/10.1161/01.STR.0000033930.05931.93] [PMID: 12411652]

[22]   Kalra L, Perez I, Gupta S, Wittink M. The influence of visual neglect on stroke rehabilitation. Stroke 1997; 28(7): 1386-91.
[http://dx.doi.org/10.1161/01.STR.28.7.1386] [PMID: 9227688]

[23]   Katz N, Hartman-Maeir A, Ring H, Soroker N. Functional disability and rehabilitation outcome in right hemisphere damaged patients with and without unilateral spatial neglect. Arch Phys Med Rehabil 1999; 80(4): 379-84.
[http://dx.doi.org/10.1016/S0003-9993(99)90273-3] [PMID: 10206598]

[24]   Paolucci S, Grasso MG, Antonucci G, *et al.* One-year follow-Up in stroke patients discharged from rehabilitation hospital. Cerebrovasc Dis 2000; 10(1): 25-32.
[http://dx.doi.org/10.1159/000016021] [PMID: 10629343]

[25]   Paolucci S, Matano A, Bragoni M, *et al.* Rehabilitation of left brain-damaged ischemic stroke patients: the role of comprehension language deficits. A matched comparison. Cerebrovasc Dis 2005; 20(5): 400-6.
[http://dx.doi.org/10.1159/000088671] [PMID: 16205059]

[26]   Gialanella B, Ferlucci C. Functional outcome after stroke in patients with aphasia and neglect: assessment by the motor and cognitive functional independence measure instrument. Cerebrovasc Dis 2010; 30(5): 440-7.

[http://dx.doi.org/10.1159/000317080] [PMID: 20720414]

[27]    Di Carlo A, Lamassa M, Baldereschi M, *et al.* Sex differences in the clinical presentation, resource use, and 3-month outcome of acute stroke in Europe: data from a multicenter multinational hospital-based registry. Stroke 2003; 34(5): 1114-9.
    [http://dx.doi.org/10.1161/01.STR.0000068410.07397.D7] [PMID: 12690218]

[28]    Lisabeth LD, Reeves MJ, Baek J, *et al.* Factors influencing sex differences in poststroke functional outcome. Stroke 2015; 46(3): 860-3.
    [http://dx.doi.org/10.1161/STROKEAHA.114.007985] [PMID: 25633999]

[29]    Paolucci S, Antonucci G, Troisi E, *et al.* Aging and stroke rehabilitation. a case-comparison study. Cerebrovasc Dis 2003; 15(1-2): 98-105.
    [http://dx.doi.org/10.1159/000067137] [PMID: 12499718]

[30]    Jørgensen HS, Nakayama H, Raaschou HO, Olsen TS. Recovery of walking function in stroke patients: the Copenhagen Stroke Study. Arch Phys Med Rehabil 1995; 76(1): 27-32.
    [http://dx.doi.org/10.1016/S0003-9993(95)80038-7] [PMID: 7811170]

[31]    Preston E, Ada L, Dean CM, Stanton R, Waddington G. What is the probability of patients who are nonambulatory after stroke regaining independent walking? A systematic review. Int J Stroke 2011; 6(6): 531-40.
    [http://dx.doi.org/10.1111/j.1747-4949.2011.00668.x] [PMID: 22111798]

[32]    Verheyden G, Vereeck L, Truijen S, *et al.* Trunk performance after stroke and the relationship with balance, gait and functional ability. Clin Rehabil 2006; 20(5): 451-8.
    [http://dx.doi.org/10.1191/0269215505cr955oa] [PMID: 16774097]

[33]    Collin C, Wade D. Assessing motor impairment after stroke: a pilot reliability study. J Neurol Neurosurg Psychiatry 1990; 53(7): 576-9.
    [http://dx.doi.org/10.1136/jnnp.53.7.576] [PMID: 2391521]

[34]    Duarte E, Marco E, Muniesa JM, Belmonte R, Aguilar JJ, Escalada F. Early detection of non-ambulatory survivors six months after stroke. NeuroRehabilitation 2010; 26(4): 317-23.
    [PMID: 20555154]

[35]    Smania N, Gambarin M, Paolucci S, Girardi P, Bortolami M. FIaschi A, Santilli V, Picelli A. Active ankle dorsiflexion and the Mingazzini manoeuvre: two clinical bedside tests related to prognosis of postural transferring, standing and walking ability in patients with stroke. Eur J Phys Med 2011; 47: 435-40.

[36]    Wandel A, Jørgensen HS, Nakayama H, Raaschou HO, Olsen TS. Prediction of walking function in stroke patients with initial lower extremity paralysis: the Copenhagen Stroke Study. Arch Phys Med Rehabil 2000; 81(6): 736-8.
    [http://dx.doi.org/10.1016/S0003-9993(00)90102-3] [PMID: 10857515]

[37]    Paolucci S, Bragoni M, Coiro P, *et al.* Quantification of the probability of reaching mobility independence at discharge from a rehabilitation hospital in nonwalking early ischemic stroke patients: a multivariate study. Cerebrovasc Dis 2008; 26(1): 16-22.
    [http://dx.doi.org/10.1159/000135648] [PMID: 18511867]

[38]    Paolucci S, Bragoni M, Coiro P, *et al.* Is sex a prognostic factor in stroke rehabilitation? A matched

comparison. Stroke 2006; 37(12): 2989-94.
[http://dx.doi.org/10.1161/01.STR.0000248456.41647.3d] [PMID: 17082475]

[39]   Brown LA, Sleik RJ, Winder TR. Attentional demands for static postural control after stroke. Arch Phys Med Rehabil 2002; 83(12): 1732-5.
[http://dx.doi.org/10.1053/apmr.2002.36400] [PMID: 12474178]

[40]   Nijboer T, van de Port I, Schepers V, Post M, Visser-Meily A. Predicting functional outcome after stroke: the influence of neglect on basic activities in daily living. Front Hum Neurosci 2013; 7: 182.
[http://dx.doi.org/10.3389/fnhum.2013.00182] [PMID: 23675336]

[41]   Paolucci S, Antonucci G, Grasso MG, *et al.* Functional outcome of ischemic and hemorrhagic stroke patients after inpatient rehabilitation: a matched comparison. Stroke 2003; 34(12): 2861-5.
[http://dx.doi.org/10.1161/01.STR.0000102902.39759.D3] [PMID: 14615613]

[42]   Baer G, Smith M. The recovery of walking ability and subclassification of stroke. Physiother Res Int 2001; 6(3): 135-44.
[http://dx.doi.org/10.1002/pri.222] [PMID: 11725595]

[43]   Veerbeek JM, Kwakkel G, van Wegen EE, Ket JC, Heymans MW. Early prediction of outcome of activities of daily living after stroke: a systematic review. Stroke 2011; 42(5): 1482-8.
[http://dx.doi.org/10.1161/STROKEAHA.110.604090] [PMID: 21474812]

[44]   Nakayama H, Jørgensen HS, Raaschou HO, Olsen TS. Recovery of upper extremity function in stroke patients: the Copenhagen Stroke Study. Arch Phys Med Rehabil 1994; 75(4): 394-8.
[http://dx.doi.org/10.1016/0003-9993(94)90161-9] [PMID: 8172497]

[45]   Kong KH, Lee J. Temporal recovery and predictors of upper limb dexterity in the first year of stroke: a prospective study of patients admitted to a rehabilitation centre. NeuroRehabilitation 2013; 32(2): 345-50.
[PMID: 23535798]

[46]   Sone T, Nakaya N, Iokawa K, *et al.* Prediction of upper limb recovery in the acute phase of cerebrovascular disease: evaluation of functional hand using the manual function test. J Stroke Cerebrovasc Dis 2015; 24(4): 815-22.
[http://dx.doi.org/10.1016/j.jstrokecerebrovasdis.2014.11.018] [PMID: 25687939]

[47]   Coupar F, Pollock A, Rowe P, Weir C, Langhorne P. Predictors of upper limb recovery after stroke: a systematic review and meta-analysis. Clin Rehabil 2012; 26(4): 291-313.
[http://dx.doi.org/10.1177/0269215511420305] [PMID: 22023891]

[48]   Beebe JA, Lang CE. Active range of motion predicts upper extremity function 3 months after stroke. Stroke 2009; 40(5): 1772-9.
[http://dx.doi.org/10.1161/STROKEAHA.108.536763] [PMID: 19265051]

[49]   Au-Yeung SS, Hui-Chan CW. Predicting recovery of dextrous hand function in acute stroke. Disabil Rehabil 2009; 31(5): 394-401.
[http://dx.doi.org/10.1080/09638280802061878] [PMID: 18608431]

[50]   Rand D, Eng JJ. Predicting daily use of the affected upper extremity 1 year after stroke. J Stroke Cerebrovasc Dis 2015; 24(2): 274-83.
[http://dx.doi.org/10.1016/j.jstrokecerebrovasdis.2014.07.039] [PMID: 25533758]

[51]    Smania N, Paolucci S, Tinazzi M, *et al.* Active finger extension: a simple movement predicting recovery of arm function in patients with acute stroke. Stroke 2007; 38(3): 1088-90.
[http://dx.doi.org/10.1161/01.STR.0000258077.88064.a3] [PMID: 17255546]

[52]    Nijboer TC, Kollen BJ, Kwakkel G. The impact of recovery of visuo-spatial neglect on motor recovery of the upper paretic limb after stroke. PLoS One 2014; 9(6): e100584.
[http://dx.doi.org/10.1371/journal.pone.0100584] [PMID: 24950224]

[53]    Gialanella B, Monguzzi V, Santoro R, Rocchi S. Functional recovery after hemiplegia in patients with neglect: the rehabilitative role of anosognosia. Stroke 2005; 36(12): 2687-90.
[http://dx.doi.org/10.1161/01.STR.0000189627.27562.c0] [PMID: 16269649]

[54]    Foundas AL. Apraxia: neural mechanisms and functional recovery. Handb Clin Neurol 2013; 110: 335-45.
[http://dx.doi.org/10.1016/B978-0-444-52901-5.00028-9] [PMID: 23312653]

[55]    Veerbeek JM, van Wegen E, van Peppen R, *et al.* What is the evidence for physical therapy poststroke? A systematic review and meta-analysis. PLoS One 2014; 9(2): e87987.
[http://dx.doi.org/10.1371/journal.pone.0087987] [PMID: 24505342]

[56]    Takeuchi N, Izumi S. Rehabilitation with poststroke motor recovery: a review with a focus on neural plasticity. Stroke Res Treat 2013; 2013: 128641.
[http://dx.doi.org/10.1155/2013/128641] [PMID: 23738231]

[57]    Langhorne P, Bernhardt J, Kwakkel G. Stroke rehabilitation. Lancet 2011; 377(9778): 1693-702.
[http://dx.doi.org/10.1016/S0140-6736(11)60325-5] [PMID: 21571152]

[58]    English C, Veerbeek J. Is more physiotherapy better after stroke? Int J Stroke 2015; 10(4): 465-6.
[http://dx.doi.org/10.1111/ijs.12474] [PMID: 25973702]

[59]    Pollock A, Baer G, Campbell P, *et al.* Physical rehabilitation approaches for the recovery of function and mobility following stroke. Cochrane Database Syst Rev 2014; 4(4): CD001920.
[PMID: 24756870]

[60]    Janssen H, Bernhardt J, Collier JM, *et al.* An enriched environment improves sensorimotor function post-ischemic stroke. Neurorehabil Neural Repair 2010; 24(9): 802-13.
[http://dx.doi.org/10.1177/1545968310372092] [PMID: 20834046]

[61]    Janssen H, Ada L, Bernhardt J, *et al.* An enriched environment increases activity in stroke patients undergoing rehabilitation in a mixed rehabilitation unit: a pilot non-randomized controlled trial. Disabil Rehabil 2014; 36(3): 255-62.
[http://dx.doi.org/10.3109/09638288.2013.788218] [PMID: 23627534]

[62]    Brainin M, Tuomilehto J, Heiss WD, *et al.* Post-stroke cognitive decline: an update and perspectives for clinical research. Eur J Neurol 2015; 22(2): 229-238, e13-e16.
[http://dx.doi.org/10.1111/ene.12626] [PMID: 25492161]

[63]    Blackburn DJ, Bafadhel L, Randall M, Harkness KA. Cognitive screening in the acute stroke setting. Age Ageing 2013; 42(1): 113-6.
[http://dx.doi.org/10.1093/ageing/afs116] [PMID: 22923608]

[64]    Gillespie DC, Bowen A, Chung CS, Cockburn J, Knapp P, Pollock A. Rehabilitation for post-stroke cognitive impairment: an overview of recommendations arising from systematic reviews of current

evidence. Clin Rehabil 2015; 29(2): 120-8.
[http://dx.doi.org/10.1177/0269215514538982] [PMID: 24942480]

[65]    Ayerbe L, Ayis S, Wolfe CD, Rudd AG. Natural history, predictors and outcomes of depression after stroke: systematic review and meta-analysis. Br J Psychiatry 2013; 202(1): 14-21.
[http://dx.doi.org/10.1192/bjp.bp.111.107664] [PMID: 23284148]

[66]    Provinciali L, Coccia M. Post-stroke and vascular depression: a critical review. Neurol Sci 2002; 22(6): 417-28.
[http://dx.doi.org/10.1007/s100720200000] [PMID: 11976972]

[67]    Paolucci S. Role, indications, and controversies of antidepressant therapy in chronic stroke patients. Eur J Phys Rehabil Med 2013; 49(2): 233-41.
[PMID: 23558703]

[68]    Gormley ME Jr, OBrien CF, Yablon SA. A clinical overview of treatment decisions in the management of spasticity. Muscle Nerve Suppl 1997; 6: S14-20.
[http://dx.doi.org/10.1002/(SICI)1097-4598(1997)6+<14::AID-MUS3>3.0.CO;2-M]    [PMID: 9826980]

[69]    Harrison RA, Field TS. Post stroke pain: identification, assessment, and therapy. Cerebrovasc Dis 2015; 39(3-4): 190-201.
[http://dx.doi.org/10.1159/000375397] [PMID: 25766121]

[70]    Sommerfeld DK, Welmer AK. Pain following stroke, initially and at 3 and 18 months after stroke, and its association with other disabilities. Eur J Neurol 2012; 19(10): 1325-30.
[http://dx.doi.org/10.1111/j.1468-1331.2012.03747.x] [PMID: 22568638]

[71]    Kumar B, Kalita J, Kumar G, Misra UK. Central poststroke pain: a review of pathophysiology and treatment. Anesth Analg 2009; 108(5): 1645-57.
[http://dx.doi.org/10.1213/ane.0b013e31819d644c] [PMID: 19372350]

[72]    Bruehl S. Complex regional pain syndrome. BMJ 2015; 351: h2730.
[http://dx.doi.org/10.1136/bmj.h2730] [PMID: 26224572]

[73]    Pertoldi S, Di Benedetto P. Shoulder-hand syndrome after stroke. A complex regional pain syndrome. Eura Medicophys 2005; 41(4): 283-92.
[PMID: 16474282]

[74]    Legg L, Drummond A, Leonardi-Bee J, *et al.* Occupational therapy for patients with problems in personal activities of daily living after stroke: systematic review of randomised trials. BMJ 2007; 335(7626): 922.
[http://dx.doi.org/10.1136/bmj.39343.466863.55] [PMID: 17901469]

[75]    Saunders DH, Greig CA, Mead GE. Physical activity and exercise after stroke: review of multiple meaningful benefits. Stroke 2014; 45(12): 3742-7.
[http://dx.doi.org/10.1161/STROKEAHA.114.004311] [PMID: 25370588]

[76]    Kwan J, Sandercock P. In-hospital care pathways for stroke. Cochrane Database Syst Rev 2002; (2): CD002924.
[PMID: 12076460]

[77]    Teasell R. Stroke recovery and rehabilitation. Stroke 2003; 34(2): 365-6.

[http://dx.doi.org/10.1161/01.STR.0000054630.33395.E2] [PMID: 12574538]

[78]    Wolf SL, Winstein CJ, Miller JP, *et al.* Retention of upper limb function in stroke survivors who have received constraint-induced movement therapy: the EXCITE randomised trial. Lancet Neurol 2008; 7(1): 33-40.
[http://dx.doi.org/10.1016/S1474-4422(07)70294-6] [PMID: 18077218]

[79]    Corbetta D, Sirtori V, Castellini G, Moja L, Gatti R. Constraint-induced movement therapy for upper extremities in people with stroke. Cochrane Database Syst Rev 2015; 10(10): CD004433.
[PMID: 26446577]

[80]    Pohl M, Elsner B. Treadmill training and body weight support for walking after stroke. Cochrane Database Syst Rev 2014; 1: CD002840.

[81]    Miller EL, Murray L, Richards L, *et al.* American heart association ouncil on cardiovascular nursing and the stroke council. Stroke 2010; 41(10): 2402-48.
[http://dx.doi.org/10.1161/STR.0b013e3181e7512b] [PMID: 20813995]

[82]    Mehrholz J, Elsner B, Werner C, Kugler J, Pohl M. Electromechanical-assisted training for walking after stroke. Cochrane Database Syst Rev 2013; 7(7): CD006185.
[PMID: 23888479]

[83]    Morone G, Iosa M, Bragoni M, *et al.* Who may have durable benefit from robotic gait training?: a 2-year follow-up randomized controlled trial in patients with subacute stroke. Stroke 2012; 43(4): 1140-2.
[http://dx.doi.org/10.1161/STROKEAHA.111.638148] [PMID: 22180255]

[84]    Mehrholz J. Pohl, Platz T, Kugler J, Elsner B. Electromechanical and robot-assisted arm training for improving activities of daily living, arm function, and arm muscle strength after stroke. Cochrane Database Syst Rev 2012; 3(6): CD006876.

[85]    Broeren J, Claesson L, Goude D, Rydmark M, Sunnerhagen KS. Virtual rehabilitation in an activity centre for community-dwelling persons with stroke. The possibilities of 3-dimensional computer games. Cerebrovasc Dis 2008; 26(3): 289-96.
[http://dx.doi.org/10.1159/000149576] [PMID: 18667809]

[86]    George S, Thomas S, Deutsch JE, Crotty M. Virtual reality for stroke rehabilitation. Cochrane Database Syst Rev 2015; 2: CD008349.

[87]    Gallese V, Fadiga L, Fogassi L, Rizzolatti G. Action recognition in the premotor cortex. Brain 1996; 119(Pt 2): 593-609.
[http://dx.doi.org/10.1093/brain/119.2.593] [PMID: 8800951]

[88]    Garrison KA, Aziz-Zadeh L, Wong SW, Liew SL, Winstein CJ. Modulating the motor system by action observation after stroke. Stroke 2013; 44(8): 2247-53.
[http://dx.doi.org/10.1161/STROKEAHA.113.001105] [PMID: 23743974]

[89]    Ertelt D, Small S, Solodkin A, *et al.* Action observation has a positive impact on rehabilitation of motor deficits after stroke. Neuroimage 2007; 36 (Suppl. 2): T164-73.
[http://dx.doi.org/10.1016/j.neuroimage.2007.03.043] [PMID: 17499164]

[90]    Franceschini M, Ceravolo MG, Agosti M, *et al.* Clinical relevance of action observation in upper-limb stroke rehabilitation: a possible role in recovery of functional dexterity. A randomized clinical trial.

Neurorehabil Neural Repair 2012; 26(5): 456-62.
[http://dx.doi.org/10.1177/1545968311427406] [PMID: 22235059]

[91] Kim K. Action observation for upper limb function after stroke: evidence-based review of randomized controlled trials. J Phys Ther Sci 2015; 27(10): 3315-7.
[http://dx.doi.org/10.1589/jpts.27.3315] [PMID: 26644700]

[92] Marangolo P, Bonifazi S, Tomaiuolo F, *et al.* Improving language without words: first evidence from aphasia. Neuropsychologia 2010; 48(13): 3824-33.
[http://dx.doi.org/10.1016/j.neuropsychologia.2010.09.025] [PMID: 20887740]

[93] Avenanti A, Coccia M, Ladavas E, Provinciali L, Ceravolo MG. Low-frequency rTMS promotes use-dependent motor plasticity in chronic stroke: a randomized trial. Neurology 2012; 78(4): 256-64.
[http://dx.doi.org/10.1212/WNL.0b013e3182436558] [PMID: 22238412]

[94] Raffin E, Siebner HR. Transcranial brain stimulation to promote functional recovery after stroke. Curr Opin Neurol 2014; 27(1): 54-60.
[http://dx.doi.org/10.1097/WCO.0000000000000059] [PMID: 24296641]

[95] Elsner B, Kugler J, Pohl M, Mehrholz J. Transcranial direct current stimulation (tDCS) for improving function and activities of daily living in patients after stroke. Cochrane Database Syst Rev 2013; 11: CD009645.

[96] Hao Z, Wang D, Zeng Y, Liu M. Repetitive transcranial magnetic stimulation for improving function after stroke. Cochrane Database Syst Rev 2013; 5: CD008862.
[http://dx.doi.org/10.1590/1516-3180.20131316T2]

# SUBJECT INDEX

## A

Acetazolamide 121, 123
Actilyse 250, 253
Activation of epigenetic mechanisms 241, 242
Activity daily living (ADL) 302, 303, 304, 305, 307, 312, 315, 319
Acute ischemic stroke 112, 113, 114, 115, 120, 122, 124, 131, 135, 153, 162, 179, 187, 233, 245, 253, 259, 264, 286
Acute phase of stroke 251, 252, 261, 271, 275, 287, 303, 308
Acute therapy 250
AIS treatment 148
Allergic reactions 100, 115, 121
Alteplase 120, 250, 252, 253, 256, 257, 264
Andexanet 103, 104
Andexanet alfa 102, 103
Angiogenesis 198, 239, 274, 286, 287, 288
Angiotensin receptor blockers (ARBs) 10, 12, 19, 20
Anterior cerebral arteries (ACA) 113, 262
Anterior circulation 259, 260, 264
Anticoagulant drugs 85, 89, 227, 228
Anticoagulant therapy 89, 227, 255
Anticoagulant treatment 103, 104
Anticoagulation reversal 85
Antigen-presenting cells (APCs) 68, 238
Anti-platelet 132, 133, 148, 153
Aphasia 200, 285, 303, 304, 305
Apixaban 94, 95, 97, 101, 103
Apoptosis 64, 151, 154, 204, 272
Arrhythmia 199, 216, 222, 223, 227
Arterial occlusion 112, 113, 115, 116, 133, 135, 153, 251, 262
Arteries, occluded 250, 251, 263, 264
Astrocytes 33, 59, 60, 61, 63, 67, 68, 271, 274, 275, 276
Atrial appendage, left 216, 217, 219
Atrial fibrillation 4, 85, 92, 102, 135, 203, 216, 217, 218, 219, 221, 223, 225, 227, 228
Autonomic function 44
Autonomic nervous system 26, 27, 28, 30, 31, 36, 37, 38, 39, 40, 44, 45

Axonal sprouting 270, 272, 276, 279, 280, 287

## B

Baroreflex function 26, 42
Baroreflex impairment 35, 38, 42
Baroreflex sensitivity 34, 35, 38
Bleeding complications 86, 96, 98
Bleeding risk 85, 86, 98
Blood perfusion units (BPUs) 143
Blood pressure variability (BPV) 26, 34, 35, 36, 40, 41
Body weight-supported treadmill training (BWSTT) 317
Bone marrow-derived cells (BMDCs) 59, 60
BP control 5, 9, 20
BP reduction 3, 10, 11, 20, 38
BP variability 38, 39
Brain, stroke-damaged 150
Brain-computer interface (BCI) 151
Brain damage, secondary ischemic 65
Brain-derived neurotrophic factor (BDNF) 242, 273, 287
Brain edema 133, 134
Brain haemorrhages, symptomatic 258, 260
Brain injury 57, 58, 69, 234, 286
    stroke-induced 57, 69
Brain ischemia 64, 234, 276, 279, 284, 286
Brain-MRI 16
Brain parenchyma 250, 251, 260, 263
Brain perfusion 31, 32, 33
Brain plasticity 309, 311, 316, 319
Brain regions 27, 278
Brain repair 132, 151, 233, 275
Brain tissue 117, 134, 235, 240, 270, 272, 282, 289

## C

Calculation of thromboembolic risk 218, 219
Cardiac resynchronisation therapy (CRT) 216, 224
Caregivers 301, 302, 303, 304, 309, 312, 316
Cells, dendritic 59, 68, 238

Alberto Radaelli, Giuseppe Mancia, Carlo Ferrarese & Simone Beretta (Eds.)

www.ingramcontent.com/pod-product-compliance
Lightning Source LLC
Chambersburg PA
CBHW041724210326
41598CB00008B/775

* 9 7 8 1 6 8 1 0 8 4 2 2 0 *